Autonomy a
Mental Diso᠆ᵈᵉᵣ

International Perspectives in Philosophy and Psychiatry

Series editors: Bill (K.W.M.) Fulford, Katherine Morris, John Z. Sadler, and Giovanni Stanghellini

Volumes in the series:

Autonomy and Mental Disorder

Edited by

Lubomira Radoilska

OXFORD
UNIVERSITY PRESS

OXFORD

UNIVERSITY PRESS

Great Clarendon Street, Oxford OX2 6DP

Oxford University Press is a department of the University of Oxford.
It furthers the University's objective of excellence in research, scholarship,
and education by publishing worldwide in

Oxford New York

Auckland Cape Town Dar es Salaam Hong Kong Karachi Kuala Lumpur Madrid
Melbourne Mexico City Nairobi New Delhi Shanghai Taipei Toronto

With offices in

Argentina Austria Brazil Chile Czech Republic France Greece Guatemala Hungary
Italy Japan Poland Portugal Singapore South Korea Switzerland Thailand Turkey
Ukraine Vietnam

Oxford is a registered trade mark of Oxford University Press
in the UK and in certain other countries

Published in the United States
by Oxford University Press Inc., New York

British Library Cataloguing in Publication Data
Data available

Library of Congress Cataloging in Publication Data
Library of Congress Control Number: 2012931993

Typeset by Cenveo, Bangalore, India
Printed in Great Britain
on acid-free paper by
CPI Group (UK) Ltd, Croydon, CR0 4YY

ISBN 978-0-19-959542-6

10 9 8 7 6 5 4 3 2 1

Contents

Part IV: **Emerging alternatives**

List of contributors

Tineke Abma
Department of Medical
Humanities
University of Amsterdam,
The Netherlands

Natalie Banner
Centre for the Humanities
and Health
King's College London, UK

Derek Bolton
Institute of Psychiatry
King's College London, UK

Lisa Bortolotti
Philosophy Department
University of Birmingham, UK

Matthew Broome
Warwick Medical School
University of Warwick;
Coventry and Warwickshire
Partnership Trust;
Institute of Psychiatry
King's College London, UK

Rochelle Cox
ARC Centre of Excellence in
Cognition and its Disorders
Macquarie University
Sydney, NSW, Australia

Elizabeth Fistein
Department of Psychiatry
University of Cambridge, UK

KWM (Bill) Fulford
Faculty of Philosophy and
St Cross College
University of Oxford;
University of Warwick
Medical School
Coventry, UK

Grant Gillett
Otago Bioethics Centre
University of Otago
Medical School
Dunedin, New Zealand

Jane Heal
Faculty of Philosophy
University of Cambridge, UK

Jules Holroyd
Department of Philosophy
Nottingham University, UK

Hallvard Lillehammer
Faculty of Philosophy
University of Cambridge, UK

Matteo Mameli
Department of Philosophy
King's College London, UK

Alfred R. Mele
Department of Philosophy
Florida State University
Tallahassee, FL, USA

Jennifer Radden
Department of Philosophy
University of Massachusetts
Boston, MA, USA

Lubomira Radoilska
Faculty of Philosophy
University of Cambridge, UK

Guy A. M. Widdershoven
Department of Medical
Humanities
University of Amsterdam
Amsterdam, The Netherlands

Introduction: personal autonomy, decisional capacity, and mental disorder

Lubomira Radoilska

Three premises of the autonomy debate

Autonomy is a fundamental yet contested concept in both philosophy and our broader intellectual culture. To a great extent, this is due to the widely accepted idea that, by giving precedence to reason over tradition, to individuals over communities, autonomy epitomizes Enlightenment as an overall project and, more precisely, its core philosophical and political doctrine, liberalism.[1] This genealogy marks the first point of convergence in the current autonomy debate, an illustration of which is the close association between respect for autonomy, on the one hand, and privacy, on the other. For, in both cases, the ambition is to delimit a sphere of individual action which falls beyond the scope of legitimate state authority.[2]

This leads us to a second point of convergence in the current debate, according to which personal autonomy is an individual's right to self-determination, the purpose of which is to protect the exercise of this individual's capacity for self-determination.[3] To simplify, autonomy is

---

[1] Schneewind (1998) offers a comprehensive analysis of the rise of autonomy as a distinctly modern moral concept. On the close links between autonomy and political liberalism, see Christman and Anderson (2005). A succinct and emblematic outline of the project of Enlightenment is to be found in Kant (1784). See also Horkheimer and Adorno (1973) for a classical critique of this project and its underlying presuppositions.

[2] The relationships between autonomy and authority are helpfully explored in Wolff (1990) and Shapiro (2002). On the significance of a recognized sphere of privacy, where consent between legally competent adults suffices in order to make certain behaviour permissible, see Hart (1963).

[3] The dialectic between a capacity and a right aspect in the idea of autonomy is well articulated in Feinberg (1986, chapter 18). It also underpins Ronald Dworkin's 'integrity view

an agency concept aiming to define what a person can (legitimately) do. With respect to this second point of convergence, alternative accounts of autonomy could be seen as competing views on the nature of the capacity for self-determination that is worth protecting,[4] whereas critiques of autonomy target the right to self-determination which according to them involves a problematic conceptualization of freedom in terms of non-interference. In essence, the charge is that, by focusing on *self*-determination, autonomy sets out a misleading ideal of free agency as taking place to the exclusion of others. In doing so, it warrants only a thin 'morality of independence' to the detriment of richer alternatives, such as that of 'mutual responsibility' (Gaylin and Jennings 2003, p. 4).

A third point of convergence has to do with the assumption that personal autonomy and (severe) mental disorder are mutually exclusive. This is to say that participants in the autonomy debate, who otherwise disagree on both the nature of the capacity for self-determination and the appropriate scope for a right to self-determination, often concur on the idea that mental disorder affects this capacity and, consequently, undercuts the corresponding right. For instance, Marina Oshana articulates this idea as one of the considered intuitions against which rival theories of autonomy are to be assessed. The underlying reasoning is as follows:

> It is enough to note that as the possession of these qualities [comprising the capacity for autonomy] is a matter of degree and can be cultivated more or less successfully in persons. A sense of the relevant threshold can be gained by a glance at cases in which *it is clear* that the threshold is not met. The very small child,

---

of autonomy', according to which the right to autonomy is meant to protect 'the ability to act out of genuine preference or character or conviction or a sense of self' (1993, p. 225).

[4] For instance, some of these accounts conceive the capacity at issue in purely psychological terms that, following Christman (2003), can be helpfully divided into two groups, authenticity and competency conditions, the first reflecting the conative and the second the cognitive components of this capacity. In contrast, other accounts point to additional features, which may be psychological or internal as the above, like the capacity to value (Jaworska 1999) but could be also social-relational or external, like being in a position of recognised and secure authority over one's life with respect to powerful others (Oshana 2006).

the individual afflicted with Alzheimer's disease, and the insane person lack the rudimentary ability to self-governing. (Oshana 2006, p. 7)[5]

To reflect the central role in framing discussions of autonomy, I shall refer to the three points of convergence I identified as 'premises of the autonomy debate'. The first is that autonomy is a fundamentally liberal concept. The second is that autonomy as an agency concept, best understood in terms of a capacity-cum-right to self-determination. The third is that autonomy is incompatible with (severe) mental disorder.

A major ambition of the present collection of essays is to critically examine the third premise and, in so doing, to shed new light onto the preceding two. More precisely, the underlying thought is that, by looking in some detail at cases of mental disorder where autonomy seems to be clearly absent, we are in a better position to articulate the implicit intuitions that underpin our thinking about autonomy and, following this trail, to uncover further conceptual and historical roots that may unsettle some standard assumptions but at the same time offer a clearer perspective onto persistent points of disagreement. A related objective, which this overall strategy aims to achieve, is to help address two kinds of emerging scepticism about autonomy questioning, on the one hand, its theoretical appeal and coherence, and, on the other, its relevance to specific areas of normative thought, including medical and, more specifically, psychiatric ethics.[6]

The notion of decisional capacity is central to the present inquiry, for it is meant to work out the conditions under which the third premise of the autonomy debate obtains, that is, when mental disorder should be considered severe enough as to be incompatible with a capacity for self-determination. Thus, to avoid circularity, it is crucial to get clearer about the relationship between these two capacities. The issue is even more pressing if we consider that 'decisional capacity' is sometimes

---

[5] Both the text inserted in square brackets and the italics are mine.

[6] I consider Nomy Arpaly's suggestion that we should either replace 'autonomy' with narrower, qualified autonomy-concepts, e.g. autonomy as authenticity, autonomy as interpersonal authority etc., or abandon 'autonomy' altogether, for it has become an overworked and misleading term (2003, chapter 4) as an example of the first kind of scepticism, and Gaylin and Jennings (2003) as an example of the second kind of scepticism.

used as equivalent of 'autonomy' rather than an independent criterion specifying the interactions between autonomy and mental disorder. Moreover, a closer look at the notion of mental disorder itself suggests that this notion builds on the idea of an impediment, if not breakdown of agency, and, in this sense, may depend upon an implicit conception or conceptions of autonomy. To bring into relief the points made so far and set the scene for the following analysis, the next section will look into the right to refuse treatment and its possible limitations. As we shall see, the topic offers a good meeting ground for the concepts at the heart of the present inquiry—personal autonomy, mental disorder, and decisional capacity—and enables us to explore the close yet challenging links between the three premises of the autonomy debate, with which it began.

Value-neutrality and the capacity threshold

Value-neutrality is a central way of conceptualizing autonomy and, possibly, decisional capacity. This is because it offers a plausible interpretation of the conjunction of the first two premises implying that autonomy is an independent but limited in scope source of justification. Drawing on the previous section, autonomy refers to a protected sphere of actions, which we may call purely, or substantively self-regarding and which are permissible solely by virtue of being this person's own, without the need for further justification.[7] In other words, to say that a choice, relative to this sphere of actions, is autonomous is to shield it from legitimate interference, even though this choice may be met with serious objections on moral or prudential grounds. For instance, it could be that this choice harms or disadvantages in some way the person who makes it. Yet, as long as this is a genuine choice as opposed to being the outcome of coercion, manipulation, or deception and it has no significant negative impact on others than the person who makes this choice, respect for autonomy apparently demands that it remains unopposed. This is the rationale for the so-called Harm principle as a distinctive liberal commitment stating

---

[7] On the notion of substantively self-regarding choices, see Feinberg (1986, chapter 17) and Scoccia (2008).

that a person's freedom may be legitimately constrained only to prevent harm to others, but not harm to self, as long as this is willingly and knowingly incurred (Feinberg 1984). As John Stuart Mill, whose work led to formulating the Harm principle observes in his treatise *On Liberty*:

> If a person possesses any tolerable amount of common sense and experience, his own mode of laying out his existence is the best, not because it is the best in itself, but because it is his own mode. (Mill 1859, p. 114)

In light of these observations, it becomes clear that, by recognizing autonomy as an independent source of justification, we are able to efficiently oppose another conception of moral and political obligation, according to which it may sometimes be permissible to interfere with a person's autonomous choice not because it has an identifiable adverse effect on others, but for his or her own good. This conception is known as paternalism. Although it has been recently argued that respect for autonomy and paternalism may not be incompatible after all, it remains the case that, in so far as autonomy is conceived as an independent, though limited in scope source of justification, it does not square with paternalist interventions.[8]

Having said that, there is room for reasonable disagreement about the exact scope of choices where autonomy could provide protection from interference, irrespective of further normative considerations. This point leads to distinguishing, as indicated earlier, substantively self-regarding choices from self-regarding choices which are to a significant degree also other-regarding. As a result, some autonomous self-regarding choices may be open to legitimate interference on grounds that they effectively harm unwilling third parties, not only the person who makes the choice at issue (Radoilska 2009). Examples include various health and safety measures, such as the prohibition of smoking in public spaces. This is why instances of treatment refusal are

---

[8] Examples of this conciliatory approach to autonomy and paternalism include Scoccia (2008) and Taylor (2004). It builds upon an alternative understanding of autonomy motivated by the rejection of either of the first two premises of the current debate, or an alternative interpretation of their conjunction, which departs from value-neutrality. I shall return to this point in the penultimate section.

particularly to the point. For it is hard to think of a clearer case where a person's choice should be protected from interference merely by virtue of being his or her own than decisions concerning this person's bodily integrity. A further reason to focus on treatment refusals is that it is often fairly clear that this kind of decision will make the person worse off to the point of causing his or her preventable death. In this respect, they also offer plausible ground for paternalist interventions. To bring out this point, let us consider the following excerpt from a recent court ruling:

> A mentally competent patient has an absolute right to refuse to consent to medical treatment for any reason, rational or irrational, or for no reason at all, even where that decision may lead to his or her own death. (*Re MB* 1997)

This piece of legal reasoning is not only consistent with value-neutrality but effectively parallels the previous quote from *On Liberty* in that it articulates mental competence, also referred to as decisional capacity, as a precondition to this absolute right to treatment refusal. To be more specific, the parallel is with 'any tolerable amount of common sense and experience' conceived as threshold for the application of the 'Harm principle' viz. respect for personal autonomy. This is the third premise of the autonomy debate identified in the previous section.

At first sight, the move from the conjunction of the first two premises understood in terms of value-neutrality to the third premise may seem unproblematic. The reason is as follows. If autonomy is a kind of self-determination, then autonomous choices should be in some sense up to the person who makes them as opposed to merely happening to them (Frankfurt 1971). This idea is crucial to appreciating the underlying argument in *Re MB*. For the conclusion is to confirm that a patient was correctly deemed to lack decisional capacity with respect to giving or refusing consent to a particular treatment—the injection of anaesthetics—because of her extreme phobia of needles. The court decision draws on a distinction between inability to make a specific decision because of a phobia, e.g. a person cannot make a choice about receiving an injection, on the one hand, and, on the other, an irrational decision to refuse an injection because, for instance, he or she is afraid of needles and yet recognizes that needles are not scary. The point of the distinction is to show that only the former, that is, inability to make a decision but not the latter, that is, an irrational decision to the same effect offers a sufficient ground for overturning a patient's explicit treatment refusal.

However, the distinction is not self-evident and, unless we are able to present a further argument to support it, it would seem rather arbitrary. For in both cases, we are faced with apparently similar treatment refusals, that is, made for no good reason and, what is more, in the presence of compelling reasons that speak against it. Following this line of reasoning, if autonomy is an independent source of justification that could shield an irrational treatment refusal, it would seem that it should also be able to shield an incompetent one. Yet, as indicated earlier, if we consider the point of a right to self-determination—to protect a distinctive category of actions merely by virtue of being one's own, irrespective of further considerations, the idea of a threshold satisfied by irrational but not incompetent choices becomes persuasive. This leaves us with a conundrum. The third premise of the autonomy debate appears to be both required by value-neutrality as the conjunction of the first two premises and at the same time at odds with it.

To resolve this conundrum, we should be able to reliably distinguish between irrational treatment refusals that are protected by an absolute right and incompetent treatments refusals that can be overridden on paternalist grounds, i.e. in the patient's best interests. In fact, the court judgment in *Re MB* candidly points to this difficulty in the following observation:

> Although it might be thought that irrationality sits uneasily with competence to decide, panic, indecisiveness and irrationality in themselves do not as such amount to incompetence, but they may be symptoms or evidence of incompetence. (*Re MB* 1997)

A related challenge is to work out a criterion that is not implicitly value-laden, that is, dependent upon further considerations than autonomy itself. Unless this is achieved, some substantively self-regarding choices, such as irrational treatment refusals would turn out to be worthy of respect not merely by virtue of being a person's own, but in so far as they also accord with additional values. Similarly, the so-called incompetent treatment refusals would be overridden on other grounds than autonomy. But then, a rift between the first two premises or value-neutrality, on the one hand, and the third premise or a threshold condition for autonomy excluding (severe) mental disorder, on the other, will not be avoided. In this case, we may begin to lose sight of what the notion of autonomy, for which we just specified a reliable (value-laden) threshold, even amounts to.

The Mental Capacity Act, which came into power in England and Wales in 2005, as well as related legislation in other countries (Charland 2008), aims to address this challenge by laying down apparently value-neutral criteria for decisional capacity, the threshold condition at issue. Thus, Part 1, section 3 of the Act states that an adult is deemed unable to make a decision for him or herself if he or she cannot at the time of decision-making:

(a) understand the information relevant to the decision,
(b) retain that information,
(c) use or weigh that information as part of the process of making the decision, or
(d) communicate his/her decision (whether by talking, using sign language or any other means).

The underlying ambition is to focus on cognitive failures, such as various kinds of misperception of reality and mishandling of evidence, but to exclude any substantive or value-laden criteria. For the sake of clarity I shall refer to the latter kind as 'reasonableness requirements', to distinguish them from the previous minimal or formal criteria consistent with a value-neutral understanding of decisional capacity. How successful has been the Act in keeping out reasonableness requirements?

Looking at the conditions (a) and (c), it is plausible to argue that they both present an implicit reasonableness requirement, especially in light of an explanatory point at the end of section 3. This point reads as follows:

(4) The information relevant to a decision includes information about the reasonably foreseeable consequences of –
    (a) deciding one way or another, or
    (b) failing to make the decision. (Mental Capacity Act 2005)

This clarification sits uneasily with one of the principles, set out at the start of the Act, namely: 'A person is not to be treated as unable to make a decision merely because he makes an unwise decision' (Mental Capacity Act 2005, 1.1.4). The reason is that if—in order to pass the capacity threshold—a person is expected to 'use or weigh' relevant information, including the 'reasonably foreseeable consequences' specified earlier in the process of making his or her decision, it becomes difficult to see how this could fail to impose the requirement of making a somewhat wise or at least not particularly unwise decision.

At first sight, this implication may not appear particularly worrying. Yet, accepting it would mean not resolving the difficulty with which we began, that is, how to distinguish between irrational but competent decisions that ought to be protected from interference for the sake of personal autonomy, and incompetent ones that ought to be overruled on paternalist grounds. Instead, some if not all irrational decisions would be assimilated to the category of incompetent decisions and become open to paternalist interventions.

To appreciate this point, suffice to look at the way irrationality consistent with decisional capacity is defined by the ruling in *Re MB* (1997):

> Irrationality is here used to connote a decision which is so outrageous in its defiance of logic or of accepted moral standards that no sensible person who had applied his mind to the question to be decided could have arrived at it.

An intuitive reaction is to conclude that this kind of decisions is not worth protecting from interference in the name of autonomy. However, it is precisely in cases like this, where no further moral or prudential considerations speak in favour of an autonomous decision, that the significance of autonomy as an independent source for justification can be assessed. For if we are not prepared to recognize irrational decisions in the sense described as possibly autonomous, we implicitly deny autonomy any greater role than that of a derivative justification. And if so, nothing of consequence would hang on the question whether a choice is autonomous or not, since the right to self-determination merely stands for a cluster of further substantive rights, like the right to bodily integrity, the right to freedom of religion, etc.[9] By reflecting on

---

[9] See, in particular, Scoccia (2008) advocating such a reductionist account of autonomy.

the scope of these specific rights, we should be able to determine which instances of treatment refusal are to be honoured and which overridden. From this perspective, the question of whether an irrational treatment refusal could be a person's own in the required sense for autonomy becomes rather tangential. As a result, the point of a distinction between irrational and incompetent decisions is no longer apparent.

It may be tempting to avoid the implication that autonomy is a secondary normative concept by confining scepticism about irrational choices as worth protecting out of respect for autonomy to instances of mental disorder. This solution seems to be in tune with the provisions of the Mental Capacity Act (2005, 1.2.1.), according to which a person lacks capacity with respect to a specific decision, if he or she is unable to make such a decision 'because of an impairment of, or a disturbance in the functioning of, the mind or brain'. Following this line of reasoning, we could say that, on its own, neither the irrationality of a decision, nor the presence of mental disorder amount to lack of decisional capacity, however, when put together, the two of them add up to it.

Unfortunately, a closer look at this suggestion reveals it as no more than a reformulation of the initial conundrum the conception of decisional capacity was meant to resolve. To recap, the task at hand is to find a criterion that enables us to reliably distinguish, within the category of substantively self-regarding choices of which treatment refusal is a central example, a subcategory of choices that are a person's own in the required sense and are therefore worth protecting merely on grounds of autonomy, irrespective of further normative considerations. Mental disorder comes to attention in this context in so far as it may affect some of a person's motivations to the extent that, with respect to these, he or she is best understood as a 'passive bystander' rather than a self-determining agent (Frankfurt 1971). Clearly, motivations thus affected are not a person's own in the required sense, what is less clear is how to work out a criterion or criteria which could consistently exclude these motivations from the subcategory of substantively self-regarding choices we are interested in. As argued earlier, irrationality cannot play the role of such a criterion on pain of compromising the underlying commitment to autonomy as an independent source of justification.

So, if irrational decisions associated with mental disorder are deemed to fall beyond the capacity threshold for autonomy, this cannot be by virtue of their irrationality. The fact that it does make a difference with respect to the issue whether decisions associated with mental disorder are open to paternalist interference or not, should not mislead us. All it shows is that, on this view, no decision associated with mental disorder meets the capacity threshold for autonomy, whether it happens to point toward a rational, or an irrational course of action. This is third premise of the autonomy debate reassessed, but still at odds with the conjunction of the first two by which it is, at the same time, required.

Mental disorder and reasonableness

A possible way out of the persisting conundrum is to reconsider decisional capacity as a threshold for paternalist interventions which only has a partial bearing on the distinction between decisions that should to be protected from interference out of respect for autonomy and decisions that should not. Following this lead, the test for capacity is best understood as involving three separate steps. The object of the first or preliminary step is to answer the question whether a mental disorder that could affect a specific decision is present. To give an example, a diagnosis of depression is prima facie relevant in the context of a life-sustaining treatment refusal, since the wish to end one's life is a core depression symptom. The second or central step is to determine whether the decision at issue is in fact affected by the mental disorder present or not. In terms of the earlier example, this second step should make it possible to uphold life-sustaining treatment refusals that, although made in the presence of depression, are not influenced by it. By distinguishing between the first two steps of the capacity test, we are able to make sense of the current legislation, according to which the presence of mental disorder is not a bar to the presumption of capacity.

In contrast, the third and final step relates to decisions that in all probability are affected by mental disorder. The point is to make sure that even these decisions do not become open to paternalist interventions by default. Thus, the third step reflects a corollary of the value-neutrality thesis, according to which autonomy is an independent—but not ultimate—source of justification. So, there might be further moral or prudential reasons that speak in favour of the decisions at issue. In such instances, paternalist interventions still remain out of order although on different grounds than respect for autonomy as conceptualized earlier.[10]

An immediate advantage of this revision is that it helps make room for some reasonableness requirements which, as observed earlier, seem to be both indispensable for setting out the capacity threshold and difficult to square with the value-neutrality thesis. However, to resolve the conundrum rather than postpone it, the question of reasonableness should only arise at the later stages of the capacity test, ideally at the final and under no circumstances at the preliminary one. To appreciate the significance of the task at hand, let us consider a contrast, which is as intuitive as it is difficult to pin down. This contrast is between life-saving treatment refusals made on religious grounds and refusals with equally fatal consequences, but associated with mental disorder. It may be plausible to want to see only the former but not the latter protected by an absolute right, but does the notion of a capacity threshold support this asymmetry?

A recent report in the *Hastings Center Report* suggests that it may not. By reflecting on the interactions between religious beliefs and decisional capacity in instances of blood transfusion refusals by Jehovah's Witnesses, Adrienne Martin, author of this report concludes:

> Respect for autonomy might require that we respect a treatment decision even when the person 'unreasonably' retains that [religious] belief in spite of compelling counter-evidence – even when the belief renders her incapacitated. (Martin 2007, p. 37)

The idea of unreasonableness here indicates that the treatment refusals at issue are unlikely to pass the capacity threshold if criteria like 3.1(a) and 3.1(c) of the Mental Capacity Act (2005) or equivalents are employed. Such criteria, I called earlier 'reasonableness requirements' aim to ascertain a person's (ability to) use relevant information as part

---

[10] A number of these grounds are covered in section 1.4. 'Best interests' of the Mental Capacity Act (2005). I shall return to this point in the final section of this Introduction.

of making the decision under scrutiny. This is not to say that Jehovah's Witnesses are unable to relate relevant treatment refusals back to their core religious convictions,[11] but that, unless these convictions are accepted as self-standing premises not to be further probed, the whole reasoning falls apart or, rather, below the capacity threshold. However, isolating religious convictions from assessment in this way seems to defeat the point of a capacity threshold. For if a person's ultimate convictions are to be taken at face value, many decisions based on delusions, a central symptom of severe mental disorder would also pass the test. This is because, in both instances, resistance to counter-evidence and problematic weighing of pros and cons can be explained away assuming certain first premises. No incoherence need be involved.[12] We are now faced with a dilemma: the capacity test is either arbitrary in its application to relevantly similar cases or unfit for purpose, since it fails to isolate even paradigm cases of severe mental disorder.

To avoid this dilemma, it is tempting to dissociate, as Martin (2007) does, the concepts of decisional capacity and personal autonomy. On this ground, it is possible to argue that, whilst life-saving treatment refusals based on religious considerations may fail the capacity test— given that the underlying decision-making sometimes clearly frustrates the reasonableness requirements of the test—these refusals should all

---

[11] Consider, for instance, the following clarification offered by a Jehovah's Witness in the context of a radio debate on the topic of blood transfusion refusals: 'Our belief is based firmly on what the Bible has to say, just as the Bible, as everybody knows, forbids things like adultery and stealing and lying, it also tells us to abstain from blood. In a number of places it mentions this command and most especially in Acts chapter 15, in verse 28 and 29 the apostles of Jesus Christ wrote: "For it has seen good to the Holy Spirit and to us to lay upon you no greater burden than these necessary things, that you abstain from what has been sacrificed to idols and from blood and from what is strangled and from unchastity." So on the basis of that we feel the need to obey that command, as well as all the others in the Bible to abstain from things which God says are wrong. The reason that we would refuse blood is because we feel that it would endanger our standing with the Almighty, that it could have an effect on our everlasting future and we're convinced of course that this life is not all that there is, we're convinced that there is a life beyond this and we want to preserve our good relationships with the Almighty so that the judgement he would render would be in our favour' (Parry 2005).

[12] See Jackson (1997) and Jackson and Fulford (1997) exploring the links between religious experience and delusion, and the possibility of non-pathological delusions.

the same be shielded from interference out of respect for personal autonomy.

However, this move does not resolve the issue of arbitrariness, for nothing tells us why we should not extend the same protection over treatment refusals associated with mental disorder that fail the reasonableness requirements in a relevantly similar way to that of treatment refusals based on religious considerations. And if we pursue this line of thought to its logical conclusion, we are bound to uphold some life-saving treatment refusals that in all probability are affected by mental disorder.

In the abstract, this conclusion could take two forms: either the claim that both categories of treatment refusals pass the capacity test or, alternatively, that neither does, yet both should be respected for the sake of autonomy. However, by accepting the latter form, we would immediately run into the second horn of the dilemma we were trying to avoid, i.e. the capacity test is unfit for purpose. So it is only the former that stands a chance to transcend the dilemma and it requires that, when considering treatment refusals associated with mental disorder, we ignore the kind of unreasonableness they share with treatment refusals made on religious grounds.

A recent decision to uphold a life-saving treatment refusal made by a person with mental health issues, in the aftermath of her tenth suicide attempt (the Wooltorton case) illustrates this logic. Drawing on McLean (2009), the case could be described as follows. Kerrie Wooltorton, a 26-year-old woman, had ingested antifreeze on nine previous occasions but had accepted life-saving treatment afterwards. She was deemed to have an untreatable emotionally unstable personality disorder and, possibly, to be depressed. In 2007, days before her death, Wooltorton had drafted an advance statement indicating that she did not wish to be treated should the same circumstances arise in the future, even if she called for an ambulance. Rather than being treated, she wanted to die in a situation where she was not alone and where comfort care was provided. A document containing a rejection of treatment was presented by Wooltorton on admission to hospital, after ingesting antifreeze for a tenth time. This document was accepted as valid. In addition, she made a contemporaneous refusal of treatment and was considered to satisfy the criteria for decisional capacity. The medical professionals involved did not give life-saving treatment. A subsequent coroner's ruling upheld their decision as lawful.[13]

The upshot is that we end up with the same difficulty, with which we began: how to draw a principled and reliable distinction between irrational though competent and incompetent treatment refusals. The several potential resolutions that I considered earlier helped confirm the pivotal role of such a distinction, but at the same time failed to provide the required conceptual means for the task.

To help bring out this point, let us briefly return to the latest suggestion, which was to reinterpret the capacity threshold as related directly to paternalist interventions and loosen its links to personal autonomy. The ambition was to explain the need for some reasonableness requirements when ascertaining decisional capacity without giving up the value-neutrality thesis according to which autonomy is an independent source of justification. Yet, the initially plausible strategy of setting out three separate stages of the capacity test so that the reasonableness requirements are not applied to distinguishing between autonomous and non-autonomous choices but only between competent and incompetent choices was ultimately unsuccessful. More specifically, this strategy led to either ad hoc readjustments where some treatment refusals (e.g. made in the presence of mental disorder) are required to pass a reasonableness test from which others (e.g. made on religious grounds) are exempt, or self-defeating applications of the capacity test, like in the Wooltorton case where treatment refusals that are in all probability due to mental disorder are upheld to avoid ad hocery. In neither case does the permissibility of a treatment refusal rest on respect for personal autonomy as an independent source of justification.

Three promising lines of inquiry

Drawing on the preceding analysis, we are not only able to appreciate the nature and significance of the underlying tension between the three premises of the autonomy debate, and more specifically, between

---

[13] For a further discussion of this case and its implications for clarifying the links between personal autonomy and decisional capacity, see Radoilska (in press).

the value-neutrality thesis jointly supported by the first two premises and the third premise as articulated in the notion of a capacity threshold. In addition, three promising lines of inquiry toward resolving the tension at issue emerge from the discussion.

Firstly, we may abandon the value-neutrality thesis about autonomy. An immediate advantage of this approach is to legitimize the use of reasonableness requirements. In particular, by pointing out specific values and principles, the accord or discord with which makes a choice either autonomous or non-autonomous, it becomes possible to spell out the kinds of unreasonableness that distinguish an incompetent from a (merely) irrational decision. To be successful, accounts following this value-laden line of inquiry should be able to rebut two main charges. The first is of arbitrariness. It builds on the first premise of the autonomy debate, according to which a major task of autonomy is to delimit a recognized sphere of individual action—privacy—outside the scope of legitimate state authority. This task appears to be undermined by reliance on further values or norms, for substantively self-regarding choices which happen not to accord with these values or norms would be exposed to intrusion, irrespective of their private character. The second charge is to miss the point of autonomy as an agency concept, the second premise of the autonomy debate. This charge is particularly pressing for value-laden accounts that either remain silent on the nature of value or take it to be a kind of desire.[14]

---

[14] More specifically, valuing could be interpreted as desiring to desire (Lewis 1989). There is an intuitive link between this interpretation and the value-neutrality thesis about autonomy. This link is apparent in the so-called hierarchical accounts and in particular Frankfurt (1971) arguing that second-order endorsement of first-order attitudes, e.g. the desire to desire what one actually desires, is the distinctive feature of personal autonomy. See Smith (1992) for a discussion on the connections between understanding valuing as a kind of desire and a Humean psychology according to which all motivation to act is fully accounted for by a belief–desire model where beliefs are taken to be ultimately inert. The distinction between authenticity and competency conditions for autonomy proposed by Christman (2003) reflects this Humean model, see footnote 4. So, by considering values as strong or long-term preferences, value-laden accounts of autonomy and/or decisional capacity endorse both a conception of value and a philosophical psychology which arguably undermine their objective (e.g. Culver and Gert 2004; Charland 2008).

Secondly, we may distinguish, drawing on Williams (1981), between two kinds of reasonableness—internal and external—and argue that the tension between value-neutrality and a capacity threshold only arises when the latter kind is mistakenly brought into the picture along with the former. This is because when assessing whether a decision is internally reasonable, we assume the evaluative perspective of the person who makes the decision. In contrast, when assessing a decision's external reasonableness, we ask ourselves whether there are reasons that speak in favour of it, irrespective of whether the person who makes the decision is able to appreciate these reasons or not.

To get a handle on the proposed distinction, let us briefly return to the issue of life-saving treatment refusals. The difficulty we faced there was how to reliably differentiate refusals that are merely irrational from refusals that are also incompetent. By distinguishing between two separate categories of reasonableness, it becomes possible to isolate irrationality, that is, failures of external reasonableness as irrelevant to establishing the capacity threshold. If only failures of internal reasonableness are inconsistent with decisional capacity, we seem to have found a logical space for the intuitive yet elusive class of irrational but competent life-saving treatment refusals. An example could be a refusal made by a person who considers life to be no longer worth living since changed circumstances made the pursuit of his or her life project impossible. In so far as the latter assessment is correct, the refusal is internally reasonable and therefore passes the capacity threshold. In this context, the question of whether the life project at issue is worthy of such a commitment should not even arise, for this question illegitimately probes the external reasonableness of the treatment refusal.[15]

This approach is clearly attractive, for it promises to satisfy all three premises of the autonomy debate which, although difficult to reconcile, are extremely plausible each in its own right. However, to be successful, accounts pursuing this line of inquiry should be able to maintain a clear distinction between internal and external reasonableness requirements. The underlying difficulty becomes apparent as soon as we take into

---

[15] See Feinberg (1986, pp. 351–362) considering a relevantly similar case in some detail.

consideration the role of interpersonal comparison in (re)constructing the first-person evaluative perspective that frames considerations of internal reasonableness.[16]

Thirdly, we may choose to explore the claims which underpin the premises of the autonomy debate without expecting them to converge into a coherent conceptualization. More specifically, by assuming a de facto pluralism about the concept(s) of autonomy, we are able to disentangle the variety of intuitions that seem to stand or fall together once we interpret autonomy through the lens of agency (the second premise). Yet, some of these intuitions build on different conceptual grounds. If expressed in terms of agency, their original underpinnings become obfuscated. The upshot is that the credentials of autonomy as an agency concept get undeservedly weakened, since it is evoked as a rationale for a separate group of intuitions. Equally, the intuitions at issue appear as groundless, since they are grafted onto unsuitable roots.

To bring this point to the fore, suffice to look at the three subjects of autonomy attribution as singled out in the *Oxford English Dictionary* (1989) entry on autonomy: institutions and especially states, persons, and organisms. Whilst there is a clear analogy across subjects, the autonomy of each being conceived as independence by virtue of living in accord with one's own laws, the limitations of the analogy are equally clear. This is to say that—by making the kind of autonomy appropriate for one of the subjects above a model for understanding the autonomy of one or both of the remaining two—we would be not merely pushing the analogy too far, but effectively denying the reality of our chosen object of inquiry. For, we would no longer conceive it as governed by its own laws but as following the laws of something or somebody else.

----

[16] Cf. Davidson (2004, p. 67): 'In the process of attributing propositional attitudes like beliefs, desires, and preferences to others, interpersonal comparisons are necessarily made. The values that get compared are those of the person who attributes preferences or desires to someone else, and of the person to whom the attributions are made. I do not mean that in attributing a value to another the attributer consciously or unconsciously makes a comparison, but that in the process of attribution the attributer necessarily uses his own values in a way that provides a basis for comparison; a comparison is implied in the attribution'.

The salient yet possibly misleading analogy between subjects of autonomy attribution complicates the matter most of all with respect to persons who not only partake in the kind of autonomy specific to them, that is, personal autonomy. As members of states and further self-governing bodies, they play an inherent part in another kind of autonomy, which is political in the broad sense and, as such, attaches primarily to groups and institutions and, only by implication to individuals. As living beings, persons also exhibit a third kind of autonomy, which distinguishes organic entities from artefacts. To have a name for it, let us call it organic autonomy.

In light of these remarks, it becomes apparent that claims which superficially share the following logical form: 'We should/should not treat a person in a particular way out of respect for his/her autonomy', may in fact refer to the political or organic meaning of the term as applied to persons rather than specifically to personal autonomy. This is significant because neither political nor organic autonomy requires a notion of full-blown agency, which however is at the heart of personal autonomy. More precisely, political autonomy builds on an alternative notion, that of full-blown membership within a self-governing community. Seen through this lens, autonomy becomes a status rather than an agency concept.[17] In contrast, organic autonomy draws on a notion of naturalness, according to which living beings are ends in themselves. Unlike the Kantian use of the term, which covers only rational beings whose will is able to give itself its own law, apart from any object willed

---

[17] To get clearer on the proposed distinction, we may consider, for instance, Kittay (2005) whose central claim expands on the idea that moral personhood is best defined by the participation in meaningful human relationships instead of the exercise of intricate cognitive capacities allowing one to understand, plan, revise, and, crucially, provide reasons for one's choices and actions. Thus understood, moral personhood is a status, not an agency concept. See also Nussbaum (2009) arguing that no citizen should be excluded from the performance of public functions with deep expressive and symbolic meaning, such as jury service. The ensuing proposal is that people who are unable to do so in person because of, inter alia, severe or profound intellectual disabilities should perform this kind of functions by the proxy of a guardian. Thus understood, citizenship is also a status, not an agency concept. Returning to the autonomy debate, the distinction at issue seems particularly to the point for clarifying the interest and limitations of the so-called relational autonomy, which seems to combine aspects of both a status and an agency concept, e.g. Oshana (2006).

(*Groundwork*, 4: 428), the conceptualization of living beings as ends in themselves points to a norm of doing well or flourishing that each of them possesses by virtue of substantiating a specific—its own— life form.[18] To treat such a natural end in itself as a mere means to the achievement of an external end is to violate its inherent norm of doing well, that is, its organic autonomy.[19] Following this line of thought, it becomes clear that the impermissibility of harm does not have to be grounded in the infringement of rational agency, e.g. going against someone's self-regarding decisions. This point has direct bearing on both gaining clearer understanding of the Harm principle as key expression of respect for autonomy and locating correctly the difficulty raised by self-harm. For instance, if the impermissibility of harm, as opposed to its (tolerable) wrongness is fully accounted for in terms of infringement of rational agency, self-harm would be obviously permissible since it does not involve such an infringement.[20] Yet, as indicated by the preceding discussion of life-saving treatment refusals, such a view could hardly do justice to the complexities of the issue.

So a de facto pluralistic approach to appeals of autonomy could offer the advantage to constructively revisit apparent disagreements on the nature and scope of personal autonomy viz. autonomous agency, as well as explore its possible interactions with the two further notions of autonomy—political and organic—as applicable to persons.

---

[18] The genealogy of the concept of organic autonomy as sketched here can be traced back to Aristotle's definition of nature in *Physics* 2.1. For a recent development, see the notion of natural goodness in Foot (2001, chapter 2).

[19] Some critiques of enhancement vie medical means as opposed to therapy draw on this intuition. See in particular Habermas (2003), whose argument against certain enhancements points to the fact that they obliterate a crucial distinction, that between the 'grown' and the 'made' or, in the terms of the present discussion, a living form and an artefact, brought to existence to serve pre-existing ends.

[20] Cf. Dworkin (1994, p. 156): 'individuals have the right to dispose of their bodily organs and other bodily parts if they so choose. By recognising such a right we respect the bodily autonomy of individuals, that is, their capacity to make choices about how their body is to be treated by others'. Dworkin's conception of bodily autonomy not merely differs from that of organic autonomy but is, in a way, a negation of it. More precisely, it translates into the claim that (a certain version of) personal autonomy always trumps the organic autonomy of a person.

With respect to this approach, an obvious drawback to beware of is that, by positing a variety of potentially incompatible autonomy concepts, it may inadvertently slip into a premature scepticism which forecloses rather than advances our systematic understanding of autonomy.

Overview of the chapters

The twelve contributions which compose the present volume explore in detail particular aspects of the three lines of inquiry identified earlier. More precisely, Chapters 1–3, forming the first section 'Mapping the conceptual landscape', are focused on key methodological and substantive presuppositions related to personal autonomy, on the one hand, and, mental disorder, on the other. By employing explicit accounts of mental disorder as reference points, Chapters 4–6 of the following section 'Autonomy in light of mental disorder' critically examine individual premises of the autonomy debate. Chapters 7–9 of the penultimate section 'Rethinking capacity and respect for autonomy' consider the possible involvement of evaluative commitments both in establishing a capacity threshold and in broadening the scope of respect for autonomy to cover instances where this threshold is unmet. Chapters 10–12 of the final section 'Emerging alternatives' put forth specific accounts of autonomy with reference to mental disorder. In the following, I shall briefly comment on each contribution in turn.

   In 'Mental disorder and the value(s) of autonomy' (Chapter 1), Jane Heal identifies and critically examines a form of thought which is implicit in discussions about what we, as a society, owe to people with mental disorder. This form of thought builds upon intuitions which link respect for a person with respect for this person's autonomy. In light of these intuitions, the issue of how to treat a person with mental disorder may seem to revolve around the question whether or not this person has the capacity for autonomy. However, Heal argues, inquiries that share this logical form are methodologically inappropriate and potentially unhelpful in answering either of the questions they put together: what we owe to people with mental disorder and what is involved in autonomy as a capacity. The reason for this is twofold.

Firstly, the apparent consensus about autonomy as a capacity for self-determination that ought to be protected from interference by a corresponding right to self-determination is too shallow to ground a coherent course of action in terms of respect for autonomy. Even if we work with the assumption that autonomy is part of the Enlightenment project, we face an important dilemma since we have to choose between a Kantian or rationality oriented and a Millian or well-being oriented take on the nature and significance of autonomy. Secondly, even if were to reach a substantive consensus on the concept of autonomy, it would arguably require an intricate array of mental capacities, outside the reach of at least some people with mental disorder. Getting clearer on what autonomy is will not help us find out what it means to treat these people respectfully.

In 'Autonomy and neuroscience' (Chapter 2), Alfred Mele addresses a sceptical challenge about free will raised by some scientists. This challenge has immediate bearing on the prospects of a coherent notion of personal autonomy. For, if free will is shown to be an illusion as these scientists, following Benjamin Libet, contend, no free actions could ever be performed, yet autonomy as self-determination requires the ability to perform some free actions. How cogent is this kind of scepticism? By reviewing experiments in neuroscience and social psychology cited in its support, Mele concludes that the sceptical thesis about free will rests on a mistake. More precisely, it rests on an unwarranted inference about the alleged insignificance of conscious intentions from the fact that, in certain settings, these intentions seem to be preceded by unconscious preparatory brain activity. Yet, to quote Mele's helpful illustration, 'when the lighting of a fuse precedes the burning of the fuse, which in turn precedes a firecracker's exploding, we do not infer that the burning of the fuse plays no causal role in producing the explosion' (p. 31). Drawing on this analysis, it becomes apparent that the sceptical challenge about free will is in fact motivated by an implicit substance dualism, according to which, in order to be free, our will has to be supernatural. This is because, to be free on this view, a mental action, such as making a decision cannot involve brain events or other physical processes. However, as Mele points out, philosophical arguments in support of free will rarely hang on such an implausible claim. What is more, there are good reasons to believe that ordinary views about free will are equally independent from substance dualism. Hence, a refutation of the latter does not support scepticism about free will. This conclusion is very much to the point, for some critiques of personal autonomy as an agency concept effectively target substance dualism, which they take to be its metaphysical underpinnings.

In 'Three challenges from delusion for theories of autonomy' (Chapter 3), K.W.M. Fulford and I consider a series of issues faced by accounts of autonomy as an agency concept. The central claim is that, to avoid circularity in defining autonomy, these accounts need to explicitly address the putative failures of autonomous agency that are suggested by the logical topography of delusions as paradigm symptoms of mental disorder and, in particular, the possibility of non-pathological or autonomy-preserving delusions. By reflecting on the inescapable yet elusive association between delusions and different kinds of breakdowns of intentional agency that emerges from the variety of case vignettes discussed, we reach two related conclusions. Firstly, there are two separate conceptions of objectivity at work in existing accounts of delusions, only one of which—objectivity as non-arbitrariness—is promising, whereas the other—objectivity as mind-independence—is potentially misleading. Secondly, there is an implicit notion of agential success that underlies our thinking about breakdowns of intentional agency in mental disorder viz. failures of autonomous agency. However, none of the three initially plausible interpretations of agential success that we considered—conventionalist, particularist, and universalist—could satisfy the legitimate ideal of non-arbitrariness without renouncing the equally intuitive claim that autonomous agency has to do with some credible form of achievement.

As its title suggests, Chapter 4 'Does mental disorder involve loss of personal autonomy?' by Derek Bolton and Natalie Banner is focused on the assumption that mental disorder is incompatible with personal autonomy or the third premise of the autonomy debate I identified earlier. More specifically, Bolton and Banner argue that this assumption is best understood if we adopt an experiential account of mental disorder in terms of unmanageable distress. In light of this account, mental disorder leads to different kinds of internal breakdowns of what Bolton and Banner call 'pragmatic autonomy' (p. 81), i.e. the freedom to do what one is usually able to do. These breakdowns are particularly distressing not only because of the inability to cope with one's tasks as planned but also because of the resulting disruption of one's self-understanding. This picture may seem familiar from accounts of autonomy which highlight the significance of authenticity and, respectively, consider self-alienation as incompatible with personal autonomy. However, this is a way of thinking about autonomy that Bolton and Banner effectively critique as potentially unhelpful and 'metaphysical', for it seems to stipulate a kind of dualism between a person's real or authentic self and the unauthentic selves, affected by mental disorder. To avoid this unattractive metaphysics of authenticity, Bolton and Banner suggest that we rethink personal autonomy by means of a closer analogy with political autonomy, following recent social-relational accounts.

In 'Rationality and self-knowledge in delusion and confabulation: implications for autonomy as self-governance' (Chapter 5), Lisa Bortolotti, Rochelle Cox, Matthew Broome, and Matteo Mameli reflect upon the nature of autonomy as an agency concept or the second premise of the autonomy debate, with which we began. In particular, by exploring the links between irrationality, pathology, and impaired autonomy in delusions and confabulations, Bortolotti and co-authors are able to shed further light on the implicit success criterion identified in Chapter 3. The central question they consider is as follows. Assuming that the failures of epistemic rationality, including self-knowledge involved in the two symptoms of mental disorder mentioned previously do compromise autonomy, which aspects of it are particularly affected and which possibly left intact? Drawing on a distinction between autonomy as capacity for self-governance, on the one hand, and autonomy as successful self-governance, on the other, Bortolotti and co-authors argue that delusions and confabulations are not necessarily corruptive of the former kind of autonomy and may even enhance it on occasions; however, they are rarely compatible with the latter kind of autonomy. As Bortolotti et al. put it, 'the capacity for self-governance depends on the capacity to develop a self-narrative which encompasses the capacity to endorse attitudes and actions on the basis of reasons. Success in self-governance depends on the coherence of self-narratives and on their correspondence to real life events.' (p. 100). Following this line of thought, it is persuasive to acknowledge that, by allowing a person to strengthen the inner coherence of her self-narrative, some delusions and confabulations, though both irrational and pathological, could be supportive of her capacity for self-governance. Yet, this support is paradoxical to the extent that more coherence comes at the price of less correspondence to reality and so the seeds of unsuccessful self-governance are already sown. In other words, delusions and confabulations could help a person make better sense of herself as a planning agent but this would probably affect her getting things right, the other prerequisite of successful planning.

In 'Privacy and patient autonomy in mental healthcare' (Chapter 6), Jennifer Radden argues for a more comprehensive understanding of respect for the autonomy of psychiatric patients, beyond respect for informed consent. More specifically, the discussion is focused on the 'privacy stakes' for these patients, a term by which Radden refers to the likelihood that their confidentiality will be breached and the degree of harm that they would suffer from it. By reflecting on a series of relevant factors, including: the nature of mental disorder and therapeutic exchange, a normative framework which imposes conflicting professional obligations on mental healthcare professionals, and the persistent societal stigma associated with mental disorder, Radden concludes that there is a combination of high risk of disclosure and highly negative consequences which place people treated for severe mental disorder 'in a situation of extreme and continuing vulnerability' (p. 124) This upshot has immediate bearing on the issue of personal autonomy. For, by denying a secure right to privacy to psychiatric patients, e.g. on grounds of public safety, the current state of affairs effectively and unfairly compromises their autonomy prospects on recovery.

This line of argument sheds light into a major, yet often neglected side of the dialectic between the capacity for and the right to self-determination, which determines autonomy as a liberal concept at the heart of the Enlightenment project, or the first premise of the autonomy debate outlined at the start of this Introduction. To be more specific, by equating respect for patient autonomy with respect for informed consent, discussions in bioethics frequently focus on one side only of the dialectics at issue, namely, the inference from a capacity to self-determination (in the guise of a capacity to give or refuse consent to medical treatment) to a right to self-determination (in the guise of a right to give or refuse consent to medical treatment). This focus inadvertently overshadows the other side of the autonomy dialectic, according to which a secure right to self-determination viz. a protected sphere of privacy is a condition of possibility for the capacity for self-determination just as much as it is dependent upon it. The discussion on privacy stakes in mental healthcare offered by Radden brings to the fore the underlying interdependence between these two sides of personal autonomy.

In 'Clarifying capacity: value and reasons (Chapter 7)', Jules Holroyd examines the conditions for decisional capacity set out by the Mental Capacity Act (2005) and argues that some of these, namely understanding and weighing relevant information are value-laden. On the one hand, the former condition requires the so-called insight into illness, yet the concepts of health and illness have an implicit evaluative component, such as judging a person to be in a good or a bad state. On the other hand, the latter condition seems to require that a person not only values specific things but also values them to a specific degree relative to others. To illustrate this point, Holroyd looks into capacity assessment in cases of anorexia nervosa, where treatment refusals could be interpreted as undervaluing one's life and well-being relative to thinness because of a distorted or 'pathological' pattern of evaluation. In conclusion, Holroyd points to the need for further discussion in order to resolve some remaining dilemmas about the role of evaluative commitments in current thinking about decisional capacity. As Holroyd observes: 'intuitions seem to pull in different directions: it appears intuitively plausible that over-valuing food avoidance or under-valuing continued existence thwarts the ability to weigh information relevant to treatment decisions. On the other hand it is less intuitively compelling to think that under-valuing the risk of death or disability due to a commitment to religious doctrine undermines decisional capacity' (p. 161).

The subsequent Chapter 8 'The Mental Capacity Act and conceptions of the good' by Elizabeth Fistein also reflects on the role of evaluative commitments as stipulated by this piece of legislation, however, it focuses on the aspects relevant to decision-making on behalf of people deemed to lack decisional capacity. In particular, Fistein offers a comparative analysis of the ways in which the central notion of best interests is interpreted in theory, law, and clinical practice. According to Fistein, there are three kinds of theories of the good that could underpin this notion: hedonistic, preference satisfaction, and objective list or ideal theories. Although current legislation, Fistein argues, is moving away from an objective list to a preference satisfaction account of what is in the best interests of a person lacking capacity, there is evidence to suggest that clinical practice still relies heavily on an objective list theory that prioritizes the values of health and safety over a person's known preferences. The case study at the centre of the discussion, which is based on a transcript of clinicians and family members discussing the care of a person, deemed to have lost capacity due to dementia, offers direct insight into the inescapable role played by interpersonal value comparisons in making decisions on behalf of another. Yet, drawing on Fistein's contribution, it is plausible to conclude that this role is not fully recognized by current policy and practice.

In 'Autonomy, value, and the first person' (Chapter 9), Hallvard Lillehammer distinguishes between two separate kinds of autonomy, agent and choice autonomy. The former requires a capacity for substantively self-governing agency as stipulated in the following four necessary conditions: higher-order reflection and endorsement of practical options; planning and executing actions that accord with practical options endorsed; responsiveness of these to minimally intelligible standards of rational argument; and a conception of oneself as a single person living a certain kind of life. On the other hand, the latter or choice autonomy is negative freedom with respect to a certain range of options. Unlike agent autonomy, it does not build upon a set of higher-order capacities for rational thought and action. Instead, it is grounded in us having a first-person perspective on life events, a feature at least partly captured by the notion of voluntariness. The distinction between choice and agent autonomy is significant, for it helps identify and forestall a potential confusion about the nature and scope of respect for autonomy, especially with regard to people with severe mental disorders who, ex hypothesi, do not meet all conditions for agent autonomy. The confusion at issue stems from the tempting yet mistaken assumption that choice autonomy is exclusively grounded in agent autonomy. Drawing on this assumption, respect for choice autonomy in the absence of agent autonomy is then either misconceived as respect for a derivative or incomplete form of agent autonomy, or unduly eclipsed by considerations of best interests. The upshot is that human beings are effectively taken to be worthy of respect only to the extent that they are rational agents rather than by virtue of their humanity as expressed in having a first-person perspective on their lives. Yet, as Lillehammer points out: 'A human being whose mental capacities does not fully meet all the criteria of genuine self-governance need not be thought of as a second-rate person any more than a traffic warden need be thought of as a second-rate policeman or an EU citizen claiming residential rights in the UK need be thought of as a second rate Brit.' (p. 204). Along with the line of argument developed in Chapter 1 by Heal, Lillehammer's contribution supports the conclusion that there are good reasons to doubt the centrality of autonomy as an agency concept for specifying what we, as a society, owe to people with severe mental disorders. At the same time, by introducing choice autonomy as a separate category, this contribution points to a plausible alternative for conceptualizing respect for autonomy as a value which, though independent of full-blown agency, still functions as a constraint on the promotion of further desirable outcomes.

Drawing on Aristotle's conception of phronesis or practical rationality and, more precisely, its developments in the 20th-century hermeneutic tradition, 'Autonomy, dialogue, and practical rationality' (Chapter 10) by Guy Widdershoven and Tineke Abma offers an account of autonomy, which is centred on moral development as dialogical and practical learning. The main claim is that a focus on freedom from interference is generally unhelpful for conceptualizing autonomy and even more so in the context of mental healthcare. Reflecting on a series of interviews with a person who, having committed a sex offence, was sentenced to treatment in forensic psychiatry, Widdershoven and Abma argue that, by urging patients to reflect on their values through dialogue and joint deliberation, clinicians could help them develop a better practical insight into their situations and, in so doing, promote rather than compromise patient autonomy. Unlike the standard cognitive-oriented approach to autonomy as informed consent, which boils down to providing patients with information whilst leaving their preferences unchallenged, the proposed dialogue-based approach requires that the perspectives of both patients and clinicians are open to challenge and possible transformation as a result of the therapeutic exchange.

In 'How do I learn to be me again? Autonomy, life skills, and identity' (Chapter 11), Grant Gillett sets out an account of autonomy as capacity of being-in-the-world-with-others. Drawing on classical works in philosophy and, in particular, Kant's *Critique of Pure Reason* and *Anthropology* which conceptualize insanity as lack of common sense, Gillett argues that mental health recovery hangs on the ability to think of one's life as meaningful, that is, the ability to share in and have an effect upon the meaning given to the world by others. To develop this ability, a person ought to be actively supported in the exercise of relevant discursive skills so that he or she becomes a moral agent and not merely a 'moral patient' (p. 248) made to inhabit an unintelligible and frightening intersubjective world. Following this line of reasoning, it becomes apparent that autonomy as ability to exercise control over one's life-world is inseparable from practical rationality as rationality applicable to the ends and not only means of action.

In the concluding Chapter 12 'Autonomy and Ulysses arrangements', I sketch the structure of a general concept of personal autonomy and then reply to possible objections with reference to Ulysses arrangements in psychiatry. The broad lines of this schema are as follows. Unlike the related freedom of action and intentional agency, autonomy is, firstly, incompatible with passive self-determination and, secondly, dependent upon a temporal asymmetry privileging prior over later commitments. More specifically, it takes the form of active self-determination with respect to one's actions, on the one hand, and, on the other, one's motives. There are two ways to exercise active self-determination: trouble-free xxxviii | INTRODUCTION: PERSONAL AUTONOMY, DECISIONAL CAPACITY, AND MENTAL DISORDER

autonomy and express pre-commitment. The effortlessness that distinguishes the former from the latter makes it difficult to perceive their shared form, which is pre-commitment. In contrast, this comes to light when active self-determination takes place against identifiable threats affecting either a person's authorship (internal obstacles) or ownership (external obstacles) over her actions and motives. The two paradigm kinds of express pre-commitment—trailblazing and character-building—articulate the underlying form, the first with respect to actions, the second with respect to motives.

This analysis points to an implicit hierarchy between three alternative conceptions of autonomy that coexist at present—value-neutral, value-laden, and relational. In particular, a value-neutral approach which conceives autonomy as an independent source of normativity turns out to be central. This is because it covers well the complex relationship of both authorship and ownership over one's actions and motives, at the heart of active self-determination. In contrast, considerations about responsiveness to reasons as opposed to mere incentives, which underpin value-laden conceptions, gain salience only when the presence of significant internal obstacles makes an assumption of non-autonomy plausible. Similarly, concerns about social-relational status, central to relational conceptions, legitimately come to the fore only when the external obstacles present are so overwhelming as to clearly back an assumption of non-autonomy.

By making explicit the structure of the concept of autonomy, we are in a position to see that the paradox, to which Ulysses arrangements seem to give rise in the context of mental disorder, is in fact due to a flawed conceptualization that takes effortlessness to be the form of autonomy, not active self-determination. Once this misconception is dispelled, it becomes clear that obstacles to autonomy associated with mental disorder are not different in kind from the obstacles addressed by paradigm instances of express pre-commitment. This is good reason to doubt an assumption of non-autonomy attaching to mental disorder per se.

Acknowledgements

I would like to thank the participants of the following research seminars and conferences at the University of Cambridge: 'Autonomy and

Mental Health', the Ethics Group, and the Cambridge Forum for Legal and Political Philosophy for many stimulating discussions related to the topics of this volume. I am particularly grateful to Hallvard Lillehammer, Jane Heal, Ulrich Müller, Matthew Kramer, Jennifer Radden, and K.W.M. (Bill) Fulford.

I would also like to acknowledge the Wellcome Trust's support for this project (Ref.: 081498/Z/06/Z; 090536MA).

References

Aristotle. (1984). *Physics* (Trans. R.P. Hardie and R.K. Gaye). In J. Barnes (ed.) *The Complete Works of Aristotle*. Princeton, NJ: Princeton University Press.

Arpaly, N. (2003). *Unprincipled Virtue: An Inquiry into Moral Agency*. Oxford: Oxford University Press.

Charland, L. (2008). Decision-making capacity. In E.N. Zalta (ed.) *The Stanford Encyclopedia of Philosophy* (Winter 2008 Edition) [Online] http://plato.stanford.edu/entries/decision-capacity/

Christman, J. (2003). Autonomy in moral and political philosophy. In E.N. Zalta (ed.) *The Stanford Encyclopedia of Philosophy* (Winter 2008 Edition) [Online] http://plato.stanford.edu/entries/autonomy-moral/

Christman, J. and Anderson, J. (eds.) (2005). *Autonomy and the Challenges to Liberalism: New essays*. Cambridge: Cambridge University Press.

Culvert, C.M. and Gert, B. (2004). Competence. In J. Radden (ed.) *The Philosophy of Psychiatry: A Companion*. Oxford: Oxford University Press, pp. 25–270.

Davidson, D. (2004). The interpersonal comparison of values. In *Problems of Rationality*. Oxford: Oxford University Press, pp. 59–74.

Dworkin, G. (1994). Markets and morals: the case for organ sales. In G. Dworkin (ed.) *Morality, Harm, and the Law*. Boulder, CO: Westview Press, pp. 155–61.

Dworkin, R. (1993). *Life's Dominion: an Argument about Abortion and Euthanasia*. London: Harper Collins.

Feinberg, J. (1984). *The Moral Limits of the Criminal Law: Vol. 1 Harm to Others*. New York: Oxford University Press.

Feinberg, J. (1986). *The Moral Limits of the Criminal Law: Vol. 3 Harm to Self*. New York: Oxford University Press.

Foot, P. (2001). *Natural Goodness*. Oxford: Clarendon Press.

Frankfurt, H. (1971). Freedom of the will and the concept of a person. *Journal of Philosophy* 68: 5–20.

Gaylin, W. and Jennings, B. (2003). *The Perversion of Autonomy: Coercion and Constraints in a Liberal Society*. Washington DC: Georgetown University Press.

Habermas, J. (2003). *The Future of Human Nature*. Cambridge: Polity Press.

Hart, H.L.A. (1963). *Law, Liberty, and Morality*. Oxford: Oxford University Press.

Horkheimer, M. and Adorno, T. (1973). *Dialectic of Enlightenment*. London: Allen Lane.

Jackson, M.C. (1997). Benign schizotypy? The case of spiritual experience. In G.S. Claridge (ed.) *Schizotypy: Relations to Illness and Health*. Oxford: Oxford University Press, pp. 227–50.

Jackson, M. and Fulford, K.W.M. (1997). Spiritual experience and psychopathology. *Philosophy, Psychiatry, & Psychology* 4(1): 4–66.

Jaworska, A. (1999). Respecting the margins of agency: Alzheimer's patients and the capacity to value. *Philosophy and Public Affairs* 28: 105–38.

Kant, I. (1784). An answer to the question: What is enlightenment? In *Practical Philosophy* (ed. and trans. M.J. Gregor) [1996]. Cambridge: Cambridge University Press.

Kant, I. (1785). *Groundwork of the Metaphysics of Morals*. In Kant, I. *Practical Philosophy*. (ed. and trans. Gregor, M.J.) [1996]. Cambridge: Cambridge University Press.

Kittay, E. (2005). At the margins of moral personhood. *Ethics* 116: 100–31.

Lewis, D. (1989). Dispositional theories of value. *Proceedings of the Aristotelian Society* 63(suppl.): 113–38.

Martin, A.M. (2007). Tales publicly allowed: competence, capacity, and religious belief. *Hastings Center Report* 37(1): 33–40.

McLean, S. (2009). Live and let die. *British Medical Journal* 339: b4112.

Mental Capacity Act (2005). Office of Public Sector Information [Online] http://www.opsi.gov.uk/acts/acts2005/ukpga_20050009_en_1

Mill, J.S. (1859). *On Liberty*. Indianapolis, IN: Bobbs Merrill [1959].

Nussbaum, M.C. (2009). The capabilities of people with cognitive disabilities. *Metaphilosophy* 40: 331–51.

Oshana, M. (2006). *Personal Autonomy in Society*. Aldershot: Ashgate.

Parry, V. (2005). Inside the ethics committee: Treating a Jehovah's Witness. BBC Radio 4, 11 May 2005. http://www.bbc.co.uk/radio4/science/ethicscommittee_20050511.shtml

Radoilska, L. (2009). Liberalism and public health ethics. *Public Health Ethics* 2(2): 135–45.

Radoilska, L. (in press). Autonomy and depression. In K.W.M. Fulford, M. Davies, G. Graham, J. Sadler, G. Stanghellini and T. Thornton (eds.) *Oxford Handbook of Philosophy and Psychiatry*. Oxford: Oxford University Press.

Re MB [1997] 2 FLR 426. http://www.bailii.org/ew/cases/EWCA/Civ/1997/3093.html

Schneewind, J.B. (1998). *The invention of autonomy: a history of modern moral philosophy*. Cambridge: Cambridge University Press.

Scoccia, D. (2008). In defense of hard paternalism. *Law and Philosophy* 27: 351–81.

Shapiro, S. (2002). Authority. In J. Coleman and S. Shapiro (eds.) *The Oxford Handbook of Jurisprudence and Philosophy of Law*. Oxford: Oxford University Press, pp. 382–439.

Smith, M. (1992). Valuing: desiring or believing? In D. Charles and K. Lennon (eds.) *Reduction, Explanation, and Realism*. Oxford: Clarendon, pp. 323–59.

Taylor, J.S. (2004). Autonomy and informed consent. *Journal of Value Inquiry* 38: 393–91.

Williams, B. (1981). Internal and external reasons. In: *Moral Luck*. Cambridge: Cambridge University Press, pp. 101–13.

Wolff, R.P. (1990). The conflict between authority and autonomy. In J. Raz (ed.) *Authority*. New York: New York University Press, pp. 20–31.

Part I

Mapping the conceptual landscape

Chapter 1

Mental disorder and the value(s) of 'autonomy'

Jane Heal

1.1 Introduction

'Autonomy' is a word which indicates an area where important things are felt to be at issue but where much is also complex and disputed. As to its broad shape the notion has both a descriptive and a normative face. It is taken that 'autonomous' specifies descriptively a way a person or decision may be and which (many) people and decisions actually are, at least to some extent. But use of the notion also brings with it (at least for many users) acknowledgement of a normative requirement to respect autonomy and an acknowledgement of the value of promoting more autonomy. There is, however, much debate as to how both the descriptive and the normative elements of the notion are to be articulated.

One area where the complexities and disputes manifest themselves is in considering how things should go for the mentally disordered. The need for decisions may arise, for the person him- or herself and for carers, clinicians, and others, concerning what treatment to have, where to live, how to dress, what activities to take up, etc. In making these decisions it is accepted that we should seek, as far as possible, to realize in the lives of the mentally disordered those value(s) we gesture at with talk of autonomy. But in practice we find that, in many cases, we do not know what this requires of us.

Often in a situation of this shape, i.e. one where one has getting G as a goal, but is unclear about the details of what G is and hence how to get it, then the sensible thing to do is discover more about G before setting out on one's project. For example, suppose we think that it is a good thing to avoid ingesting any prussic acid, but we don't know exactly what the chemical constitution of prussic acid is and we know that its presence, although sometimes obvious, is also sometimes difficult to detect. In this situation the sensible thing to do would be to analyse further what prussic acid is so that we know exactly what to look for and can devise better tests for it. It may seem that analogously given that we want to treat the mentally disordered with respect for their autonomy, we need first to work out by philosophical reflection what autonomy is and then apply that insight to seeing what we should look for to find whether autonomy is or is not present in the varying situations of the mentally disordered. And this is the form of thought which is implicit in some discussions of how to respect autonomy in dealings with the mentally disordered.

But what I shall suggest in this paper is that this form of thought may be methodologically inappropriate given the particular kinds of unclarity and dispute we have about autonomy. A pattern of thinking which proceeds on the assumption that there is some one thing which is real or true autonomy, and that we can identify it by philosophical discussion, may well be in order, particularly in some contexts of constructive and hopeful ethical or political debate. But in the context of other debates, particularly ones about how in practice things should go for the mentally disordered, the pattern is, I shall argue, potentially unhelpful.

Accepting this suggestion does not mean that there can be no fruitful interchange between philosophical speculation about the nature of autonomy and practical thought about how to treat those suffering from mental disorder. Each kind of thinking can and should influence the other. The claim defended here is only that a more realistic sense of the shape of the concepts used, in particular 'autonomy', and hence what issues are really in play at various points, could be helpful in preventing various styles and strands of thought from getting confusingly intertwined.

The structure of the paper is as follows. Section 1.2 will discuss the shape of the concept of 'autonomy'. It will sketch the agreed surface of its logical form, consider some of the disagreements lurking beneath that surface, and suggest an explanation of these things in terms of our historical context. Sections 1.3, 1.4, and 1.5 will then explore some implications of that account for the use of the word 'autonomy' in discussions of right interaction with the mentally disordered. The argument will proceed via consideration of three recent papers by philosophers—Silver (2002), Jaworska (1999), and van Willigenburg (2005)—all of which concern, in one way or another, the idea of respecting autonomy in the treatment of the mentally disordered. The aim in discussing these papers is not to take issue with what I take to be the central ethical recommendations advanced by these authors. On the contrary, there may well be much of value in what they say. The aim is rather to consider how certain ways of proceeding in those discussions, in particular the practice of using the word 'autonomy' as if there were one right account of it to be given, may not be the best way of presenting those ideas.

Before embarking on any of that, it may be useful to indicate how 'mental disorder' is to be understood in what follows. 'Mental disorder' is, like 'autonomy', a confusing expression, the right understanding of which is much debated. For the purposes of this paper we will evade these complexities by understanding 'mental disorder' in a weak and inclusive sense. Central examples for application of the term are provided by the kinds of condition from which those who appear in mental health clinics suffer and for which mental health professionals offer such individuals help and support. 'Mental disorders' thus include certain kinds of anxiety and depression, bipolar disorder, autistic spectrum disorders, schizophrenia, obsessive–compulsive disorder, and many others, as found in the diagnostic manuals. These conditions are marked by patterns of thought, feeling, decision, and action which make difficulties for the sufferers in interacting with other people and in carrying on ordinary life.

The suggestions made in this paper are also, however, relevant to consideration of how to cope with other conditions in which the same or similar difficulties are present but which tend not to be labelled 'mental disorders'; for example, the depression sometimes associated with Parkinson's disease, the confusion and loss of memory in

Alzheimer's disease, or the cognitive and emotional impairments arising from brain damage through blows to the head, brain tumours,
strokes, etc. So for purposes of this paper, these also will be included as
'mental disorders'.

Thus, for the purposes of this paper, the 'mental' in 'mental disorder' characterizes only symptoms, namely certain kinds of difficulty-
inducing patterns of thought, feeling, decision, and action. We are
therefore sweeping under the carpet interesting and important issues
raised by common but more restrictive uses. For example, it is often the
case that applying 'mental' to a condition signals that there is something 'mental' in the nature of its causes. And there is another possible
use on which the term would apply because of the 'mental' nature of
possible treatments. (There are also, of course, possible uses in which
these criteria are combined.) To the extent that we do not distinguish
these three ways of logically connecting 'mental' with 'disorder', or
assume unreflectively that they must line up with each other, we risk
using the phrase 'mental disorder' with no clear meaning. This potential unclarity is compounded by our lack of real grip on what a 'mental
cause', as opposed to a '(merely) physical' or 'organic' cause, might be.
This lack of grip is, in turn, a corollary of our lack of understanding of
whether and to what extent we can rightly think of the mental aspects
of a person as an, at least in part, autonomous system ('the mind'), in
which causes and effects might be in some sense 'located' and the structure and functioning of which can be studied in its own terms.

The slew of difficulties just sketched has to do with the 'mental' part
of 'mental disorder'. They crosscut with yet other contentious issues
about how the 'disorder' part of the phrase is to be understood, in
particular how the standards for fixing 'non-disordered' mental functioning are to be set. The upshot of these various unclarities is that the
term 'mental disorder' remains a minefield, planted with ambiguities
and possibly false presuppositions. (Bolton (2008) offers a helpful discussion of some of these issues.)

It is also the case that knowledge of empirical facts, about the complex multifactorial aetiology of the many different kinds of symptoms
and syndromes and also about the possible effectiveness of various
treatments or ways of managing things, is still painfully lacking.

As Hacking remarks (Hacking 1999, pp. 108–9) 'Each [psychopathology] is to some extent a dreadful mystery, a veritable pit of human ignorance'. It is salutary and important, even if depressing, to remind ourselves how little we can be confident of with respect to 'mental disorders', either as to the appropriate way of conceptualizing them or as to the empirical facts of origins and prognoses.

1.2 'Autonomy' and its complexities

It takes only the smallest amount of delving to reveal that the literature on autonomy is vast and that there are many competing accounts of how 'autonomy' ought properly to be understood. Here are a couple of attempts, from those well versed in the field, to say what the common thread of the various accounts is:

> [A] theory of autonomy is simply a construction of a concept aimed at capturing the general sense of 'self-rule' or 'self-government' (ideas which obviously admit of their own vagaries) and which connects adequately with the other principles and norms typically connected to those notions. (Christman 2003)
>
> The conceptual thread which links these different uses of the notion of autonomy is the idea of self-determination or self-government, which is taken to be the defining characteristic of free moral agents. Notions of autonomy as individual choice or as a political right, flow from, and are derivative of, this defining characteristic. (Mackenzie and Stoljar 2000, p. 5)

Taking off from the orientation provided by these remarks, and calling also on helpful points brought out by Feinberg (1986) in his classic discussion, I offer here a way of schematizing some main features of (at least one strand of use of) the concept 'autonomy'.

In brief outline, it is generally taken that talk of autonomy is appropriate because there is a capacity, which most normal people have and exercise to some degree, to be 'self-governing'. Norms and principles are linked to this in two ways. First it is assumed that possession and exercise of this capacity demands respect. Secondly other normative commitments arise insofar as it is also taken that it would be valuable if the capacity were further developed and/or exercised. We may develop this outline as follows.

(A) We start with what is, in one sense, the basis of the notion, the idea of a capacity for self-government. The idea is that (most) people, at least to some extent, have the capacity to engage in critical reflection on the actions open to them, together with the reasons for which they might do them. People's exercise of this capacity results not only in their choosing between actions but also in their endorsement of some reasons for action as against others. They thus lay down for themselves their own principles of action and are in that sense, 'self-governing'. The word 'autonomous' can, given this picture, be applied in an easily intelligible way to many different but related categories of item—persons who have the capacity, persons who exercise the capacity, decisions reached through the exercise of the capacity, principles of action endorsed in such decisions, etc.

(B) Next we have the core principles and norms associated with autonomy. An autonomous person should be allowed to exercise his or her autonomy and should not be coerced or manipulated into subserving another's projects. This negative value of non-interference and non-coercion may also be presented as or developed into a more positive value of respectful and supportive appreciation of individual autonomous choice.

(C) There are also further and more aspirational norms and principles associated with autonomy. It is supposed that we may be able to develop and/or apply the capacity for critical reflection further, that in doing this we would become more autonomous, and that this kind of change would be a good thing. In short, there are lines of human development which, in valuing autonomy, we ought to identify and promote in ourselves and others.

So much for the surface agreement. Underneath it, however, is much disagreement, particularly about (A) and (C). Just to remind ourselves, here are some of the kinds of claims which are debated.

As to (A), the nature of critical reflection and how it works, there are many models, some Kantian, some Millian. Kant takes it that there are constraints (roughly, those of the moral law) on the kind of action which practical reason can coherently endorse. Hence agents who resolve the question of what to do by clear-eyed exercise of practical reason will thereby come to acknowledge and abide by these constraints.

The capacity to embrace a way of living in which one reflectively (and so rationally and freely) acts in accordance with the moral law is something which practical reason itself shows must be allowed to flourish, in that it is a moral imperative that those who have the capacity be allowed and encouraged to exercise it. Hence it is a corollary of embracing the life of reflective practical reason that we treat with respect others who have the capacity to do the same. We do not enslave them, or demean them, or manipulate them by telling them lies, or overbear their wills by subordinating their projects to our own. Rather we work with them to create the harmonious and rational Kingdom of Ends. This, on the Kantian view, is how (B) arises from (A).

But there are also non-Kantian packages, of a Millian and utilitarian kind, which may be invoked in spelling out (A). These highlight the idea that, as a matter of fact, people are happier in important ways when they are able to decide for themselves what to do and are encouraged to make such decisions reflectively. This is because they are likely to know better than others what will yield them a satisfactory life, given tools and opportunity to reflect on what they really value. Moreover having the power to make decisions about one's life in this way is itself a significant source of a sense of worth. On the Millian view, it is these consequences for individual fulfilment which mean that (A) mandates (B).

Given differences in ways of filling out (A), it is not surprising to find that there are differences in filling out (C). The aspirational values associated with autonomy are the ones we commit ourselves to by thinking that it would be good if we were more autonomous, i.e. if more of what (A) describes occurred. So differences about (A) result in proliferating differences about (C). What good things would there be more of if we were more autonomous? Would there be more rationally chosen morality? Or would there be more creativity and authenticity? Would there be more rational and articulated planning? Or might there still be much spontaneity and change of mind? Would there be less vulnerable dependence on others, less reception of influence from them? Or might there be deeper ties and greater integration? These are the kinds of things about which theorists of autonomy debate, in ethics and political philosophy.

Standing back from all this, what may we conclude? In one sense the foundation of the notion is (A), the capacity for critical reflection in which the idea of self-government is grounded. Unless there is something to play this role the whole construction collapses. But if by 'foundation' we mean that in which we have most confidence, (B) is what underpins the package. Our (i.e. Western, liberal, democratic) current ethical and political culture gives great prominence to the idea that people ought to treat others with respect, ought not to demean them, overbear their wills, or treat their projects as subordinate. Slavery, serfdom, rigid hierarchical social structures, and the like are unacceptable. People ought to be provided with access to information and resources and then allowed to develop their own lives as they choose. These are views on which there is much more public agreement than there is on any account of why this way of relating to others is appropriate or how it should be worked out in detail.

Why is this so? I would like to suggest that it is not surprising that the notion of autonomy has the shape we have just seen, given its emergence in the context of Enlightenment political and intellectual repudiation of restrictive traditional regimes, and its role in attempts to articulate what ought to replace them. It is often easier for human beings to agree that something is wrong and needs changing than to agree on exactly why it needs changing or what in detail should replace it. The kinds of concepts deployed in movements of social and ethical change will, in consequence, often have the kind of tripartite shape outlined. They will evoke the idea of something(s) we do not like and which must be done away with. At the same time they will tend to be employed as if there were some agreed reason(s) why those things must be done away with and as if there were also some agreed longer term goal(s) at which we aim, since that way of using them makes them more useful rhetorical tools. In practice, however, often only the first element comes into any sort of sharp focus and the other two elements remain cloudy.

It does not follow from this that the word 'autonomy', or any other word with conceptual backing of this shape ('freedom', 'democracy', 'authenticity', etc.), ought to be discarded as too unclear to be fit for any use in ethical and political discussion. Concepts do not have to be sharp-edged to be useful. Employment of a concept which embodies presuppositions of ultimate agreement but tolerates current unclarity about how those presuppositions are to be fulfilled may help in the emergence of the very agreement its users desire. Discussion conducted in terms of such a concept may contribute to the creation of ways of thinking, and also ways of feeling and acting, in which the aspirations to agreement at which the concept gestures are in fact realized. The discussion may result in the resolution or purging of the conflicts and debates endemic at the earlier stage of use of the concept.

One way of looking at current theorizing about 'autonomy', in political and ethical thought, is as aiming at such emergence of an improved detailed concept. Discussion is conducted in the hope that we will hit on a way of articulating (A) which we all find compelling and which thus reveals to us why (B) is so important and at the same time points us in the right direction in developing (C). Any account of this kind which is to have real plausibility will need to incorporate harmoniously a fair number of the proposed valuable features which appear in discussions of (A) and (C) and which currently seem to us to be in tension. The account will need to show that, when understood rightly, important elements of most of these seemingly attractive but competing things can be combined. (Perhaps the route to deep self-fulfilment is via commitment to Kantian moral reasoning. Perhaps self-reliance and independence of judgement, when we really understand what matters about them, turn out to be compatible with loving interdependence in enterprises and relationships.) If discussion does not do this, but rather convinces us that we ought to discard one or other side in many or all of the apparent clashes, then whatever ethical or political consensus emerges will not be on 'the real nature of autonomy' but will rather show that the current notion is incoherent and needs to be replaced.

As one illustration of the kinds of thinking gestured at earlier in this section, we may contrast two strands in feminist thought. For one group of feminist philosophers certain of the aspirational goals associated with autonomy are both centrally entwined into the notion and thoroughly objectionable. The goals are objectionable because they present as ideals things which are incoherent (e.g. total self-transparency and total rationality) or positively bad (e.g. not being in any relationships of love and dependency). If it is right that these things are incoherent and/or objectionable and also part of the centre of gravity of 'autonomy', then continuing to give the notion an important role in normative political and ethical thinking will be a poor move.

But other feminists do not share this view. (A way into both these outlooks would be through a recent wide-ranging collection (Mackenzie and Stoljar 2000).) These feminists think that, as an anti-oppression and exploitation device, invocation of the notion of autonomy is useful, perhaps indispensable. They think it may be possible to purge the notion of embroilment with these incoherent or objectionable goals. In pursuing this strategy these thinkers are (as I read them) trying to articulate a clarified and purged concept of autonomy, adoption of which will enable a way of living in which the bathwater of rigidity and exploitation is thrown out, but in which the baby of rootedness and care is preserved. The upshot at which they aim is the emergence of new and better ways of conceiving of ourselves and our possible actions, ways which we can honestly adopt and employment of which would enable us to live lives in which current difficulties and conflicts over autonomy are resolved. This enterprise may not work out, conceptually and/or empirically, but it is not fatuous or ignoble.

Suppose that this sketch of the logical shape of 'autonomy' is correct, what are the implications for invocation of the notion in consideration of how things should go for the mentally disordered? Here are three things which it may be helpful to consider further. First is the fact that (B) is at present the only solid common element and, apart from that, there is much disagreement about what 'autonomy' is. Second is the fact that autonomy is nevertheless a heavyweight moral notion, and use of the word is a powerful rhetorical tool. Third is the fact that using the word as if there were one thing which is true autonomy is part of a hopeful project of conceptually engineering new ways of living. The following three sections will consider what pitfalls exist if we overlook these facts in debates about how things should go for the mentally disordered.

1.3 The benefits of cutting out the middleman

In this section we shall consider three interesting papers which are concerned in making suggestions about how things should go for the mentally disordered and present their proposal via presenting an account of how 'autonomy' should be understood.

Our first example is Mitchell Silver's suggestions about when a patient should be deemed competent to refuse treatment (Silver 2002). His claims are, in very brief summary, the following. A patient should be deemed competent to decide on his/her treatment if he/she is capable of autonomous action. A person's performance of some action should be deemed autonomous if the person's choosing that action can be seen as a meaningful continuation of the story of that person as a self. A self exists where a plausible story can be found linking the actions of that self across time. Therefore, says Mitchell our respect for autonomy means that when determining competency 'we must engage in a collaborative effort, with colleagues, family members and the patient to create the autonomy, to find an interpretation of human behaviour that recognises a self in it' (Silver 2002, p. 468). The conclusion about refusal of treatment, which is implicit is that if a patient's refusal of treatment can be interpreted (by the clinician, patient, family, etc.) as a meaningful continuation of the patient's life story then the patient's refusal should be respected.

Our second example is Agnieszka Jaworska's consideration of the margins of agency (Jaworska 1999). She is not considering consent to treatment but rather what respect for autonomy demands in further aspects of the life of a mentally disordered person. Her view (again in extreme brevity—we shall return to other aspects of it in the next section) is that a person is autonomous if he/she has 'critical interests' as well as merely 'experiential interests'. Jaworska also argues, on empirical grounds, that Alzheimer's patients are capable of having critical interests. The conclusion, which she draws explicitly, is that respect for the autonomy of such patients should lead carers to seek to help the patients realize their critical interests.

Leaving aside the detailed content of these views and operating at a merely schematic level, we see that, formally speaking, both arguments have roughly this shape: the correct account of autonomy is that an autonomous person is one who is F. A mentally disordered person can be F. We should give very high priority to respecting autonomy. Therefore the right thing to do vis-à-vis a mentally disordered person who is F is to respect her decisions and enable her to carry out her projects.

Our third example has a slightly different shape. Theo Van Willigenburg, writing on pre-commitment directives (van Willigenburg 2005), argues as follows. There are two ways in which a person at a later time may carry out an intention formed earlier. A person may enforce an earlier decision on himself, as Ulysses did by having himself bound to the mast as his ship was rowed past the singing sirens. Ulysses was able to carry out his earlier resolution not to yield to the lure of the sirens only because at the critical point he was under irresistible pressure, from the ropes which bound him, to behave as he did. Alternatively a person may carry out an earlier decision even when such strong further pressures are lacking, through acknowledging again the force of the reasons recognized earlier. A person who acts the latter way is a 'self-legislator', whereas one who acts as Ulysses does is a 'self-enforcer'. A self-enforcer does not act autonomously. It is only the self-legislator who has true autonomy. Nevertheless, it is right to carry out the pre-commitment directives of those who are mentally disordered. Since self-enforced action is not autonomous the justification for this cannot be that it supports autonomy. An alternative and preferable way of articulating the justification is that carrying out pre-commitment directives enables the agent to continue to be authentic, i.e. to have his/her life develop in a way which respects his/her deepest identity conferring concerns.

Van Willigenburg's argument has a different form from that of Silver and Jaworska. Reduced to the same level of abstraction it goes like this: the correct account of autonomy is that it is being G not that it is being F. It is right to carry out pre-commitment directives. But carrying them out is a matter of sustaining a person in being F and not in being G. So respecting pre-commitment directives cannot be justified by respect for autonomy and we must look for another justification. A better justification is found in the fact that being F is a good ground for respecting the wishes of those who are F.

The disputed nature of autonomy is immediately evident in a comparison of the arguments. Silver stresses narrative unity. Jaworska thinks the possession of critical interests is the crucial thing. (Indeed for Jaworska an interesting and important thing about autonomy, as she conceives it, is precisely that it can survive a person's loss of grip on narrative unity of his or her life.) For Van Willingenburg it is self-legislation. What is agreed by all is that autonomy is linked to the need to respect the wishes of the autonomous person. This combination of dispute and agreement is just what we would expect in the light of the previous section.

Each author can thus be seen as presenting two kinds of claim. One kind is about the 'real nature of autonomy', that it should be understood in terms of F and should not be understood in terms of G or whatever. The other kind is about what should be taken as being a ground for having your wishes respected, and is a substantive ethical proposal that being F or G is such a ground.

These two kinds of claims are intertwined in the expositions, in that the substantive ethical proposal is presented as supported via an argument (of the different outlined structures in the different cases) in which the favoured account of autonomy plays some role. But has anything been gained by this intertwining? We can pose the following dilemma. One possibility is that the favoured F stands up on its own, as providing us with good grounds for respecting the wishes of those who are F. If this is so, all that is achieved by taking a detour via identifying (or not identifying) it with autonomy is risk of alienating those who favour a different way of unpacking that notion, but who might otherwise be sympathetic to the proposal about F. The other possibility is that F does not stand up as a ground for respecting the wishes of those who are F. And in that case the practical proposal is no good. So the conclusion is that, whichever horn we take, invocation of autonomy has not served to clarify matters or to strengthen the case for the substantive ethical claim.

We should note also that the arguments are only valid if further strong assumptions about the logical shape of the concept of autonomy are added. In the case of Silver and Jaworska, they need to assume that the condition they point to is not merely a necessary condition for autonomy but is also sufficient for it. If their proposed F is not sufficient then the argument that the decision of one who is F should be respected because such a person is autonomous will fail. In the case of van Willigenburg, if ability to self-legislate and ability to self-enforce were both elements of autonomy, each coming into play in different circumstances to enable the subject to be autonomous, then his conclusion does not follow. So he needs to assume that the concept does not have a disjunctive structure, with alternative sets of necessary conditions. (A further example of the kind of tangle produced by lack of attention to the exact logical shape of claims is found in the fact that van Willigenburg both argues that only the self-legislator is really autonomous, but is also happy to use the phrase 'autonomy as authenticity' in the title of his article and in a section heading. This latter usage seems to presuppose that talk of autonomy is likely to be appropriate where we find grounds for respecting wishes. So if an authentic wish attracts respect, and is worthy of self-enforcement or fulfilment via a pre-commitment directive, then there is 'autonomy' somewhere. But if that is sufficient for autonomy, what is at stake in the debate between self-legislation and self-enforcement?)

But none of the articles mentioned addresses questions about the logical shape of the concept of autonomy, or not explicitly at any length. In addition to questions about necessity and sufficiency or whether the concept might be disjunctive, other interesting issues are whether we should expect autonomy to be a rich and demanding matter or a simple and undemanding one, also whether it comes in degrees and what the degrees are. What the neglect of these questions suggests is that giving an account of autonomy is not really the main purpose of any of the discussions. Rather the point using the word 'autonomy' is to alert us to the fact that it is questions about respecting wishes which are going to be at issue, and that recommendations are going to be made about when we should show such respect. Invocation of 'autonomy' is, in effect, a rhetorical flourish.

This is not to say that the word 'autonomy' ought not to appear in discussions of this kind. It is effective in signifying and evoking a certain stance when approaching practical issues. It puts in place reminders about the importance of not patronizing or pressurizing people, of not being overbearing, of being sensitive and respectful. The ethical weight of the notion of autonomy is shown by the way in which the use of the word tends to set this orientation.

But doing this is may be the limit of what invocation of autonomy can contribute in these contexts. With the orientation in place, what is needed next is a description of the situation of the various sufferers in terms more specific and less controversial than 'autonomy'. We need to know about their abilities and circumstances, so that we can think whether certain ways of proceeding are or are not acceptable. Thus Silver's proposal stands or falls with the defensibility of the implicit conclusion of his discussion, namely that if a sufferer's decision to refuse treatment can be seen as part of an intelligible narrative of his life, then it should be respected. Similarly for the other proposals. For all of them what we need to think about is the exact F being brought to our attention, its varieties and complexities, and whether it will take the weight being put on it. This is where thought needs to go, rather than into those more abstract and idealistic philosophical debates about the real nature of autonomy, into which the form of the discussion might tempt us.

1.4 **The risk of overshoot**

'Autonomy', as just noted, is a word which has a powerful ethical charge. A consequence of this is that using it in a way which presupposes that it has a real nature and that this can be identified opens up a space for drawing heavyweight conclusions about the right treatment of the mentally disordered, conclusions which reflection might well be uneasy about. My claim is not that anyone does draw these conclusions. The point is rather to illustrate again how little invocation of the concept does, given that its presence does not in fact signal support for these conclusions. In pursuing these thoughts I will consider further elements of the interesting paper by Jaworska, already mentioned in Section 1.3.

Jaworska starts her discussion (and illustrates her argument at later points also) by offering detailed and sensitive descriptions of some sufferers from Alzheimer's disease, their capacities, and responses.

Following Dworkin, she then distinguishes 'experiential' interests, i.e. interests having to do with the quality of one's immediate experience, from 'critical' interests, i.e. interests having to do with promoting what one understands to be valuable independent of one's immediate experiences. She makes a powerful case for taking it that some patients with Alzheimer's continue to have critical interests, despite their being in many ways confused and having lost grip on the narrative of their lives as a whole. To take a particular case, one sufferer expressed a desire to help her fellow human beings and was willing to volunteer for tests and experiments, and also to assist in a day-care centre, understanding that by doing so she was helping her fellow human beings. Another sufferer was a man, a mild case of dementia, for whom knowing himself to be the owner of a pick-up truck conferred an important element of status in his life.

For Jaworska, it is having critical interests which is 'fundamental' for being autonomous. She writes:

> [T]he capacity for autonomy ought not to be thought of as the capacity to carry out one's convictions into action without external help, a capacity that requires reasoning through complex sets of circumstances to reach the most appropriate autonomous decisions; rather . . . the capacity for autonomy is first and foremost the capacity to espouse values and convictions, whose translation into action may not always be fully within the agent's mastery. (Jaworska 1999, p. 127)

Bringing out the implications of this, she adds:

> On my analysis, these patients [i.e. the Alzheimer's patients described] are still capable of the fundamentals of autonomy. Accordingly, a caregiver committed to respect for autonomy must respect these patients' contemporaneous autonomy. (Jaworska 1999, p. 133)

So, according to her, respect for autonomy requires that patients with critical interests should be assisted by their carers to carry out actions by which these interests are realized, even when the patients are not capable of planning or executing such actions on their own. An example of this would be enabling the patient who values helping others to assist in taking part in the experiments or in helping at the day-care centre.

In proposing her account, Jaworska is in dispute with Dworkin. Jaworska agrees with him in making the possession of critical interests central to autonomy. But she disagrees with him over whether grip on the narrative of one's life as a whole is necessary for having critical interests. For Dworkin it is, for Jaworska it is not. Given Dworkin's view, for sufferers from dementia the only critical interests which could be in play are the ones they had before becoming demented. So for him respect for a patient's autonomy points in the direction of considering what, if anything, is required in the light of their previous critical interests. For Jaworska, by contrast, respect for autonomy requires noting also what current critical interests may be in play.

So for Jaworska, a patient might have both current critical interests and previous critical interests. How should these be weighed if they conflict? It is part of Jaworska's project to raise the possibility that the current critical interests might trump other interests. But what does Jaworska really want to say about this? And what do we think plausible?

There are three kinds of interests which may be in play in a sufferer's situation at a time:

1 Certain pre-dementia critical interests—e.g. in the future plans of particular children or the long term financial position of the family. These are interests a person can possess only while he or she has memory and grip on the narrative of life as a whole, i.e. only if not demented to any significant extent.

2 Current critical interests—e.g. in helping fellow human beings, in having the status of owning a pick-up truck. These are interests a person may continue to have even when memory and other cognitive capacities have diminished considerably.

3 Experiential interests—e.g. in food, warmth, not feeling stressed. These are interests a person will have as long as he or she remains sentient.

We should note to start with that in the cases where Jaworska implies clear views as to what carers should do, there is no conflict between interests of these various kinds. So taking part in the experiments or helping in the day-care centre are presented as congenial for the patients concerned, so not conflicting with their experiential interests. Moreover there is no hint in Jaworska's description of the cases that doing these things threatens any pre-dementia critical interest, e.g. is harmful to the future of their children.

But what happens if we build in some conflicts? One kind of conflict, between previous and current critical interests, occurs in the case already mentioned of the moderate dementia sufferer who wants to own a truck. ('A man needs his truck' Jaworska quotes him as saying.) Because he values this status, he goes and buys a truck, oblivious of the fact, which he previously remembered and cared about, that the purchase adversely affects the long-term financial position of his family.

Does respecting his autonomy mean that the family must put up with his truck buying? Jaworska raises this as a possibility, but does not say straight out that this is what should be done. Rather she says that the family's decision is difficult. So it is plain that she does not think that the current critical interests of this patient evidently outweigh his pre-dementia critical interests. It is consistent with what she says that it might (depending on the exact circumstances) be right to coax the patient away from his truck, to arrange that it is likely that he forgets the purchase, and to manoeuvre behind his back to undo it.

By contrast, with a non-demented person who reverses a previously expressed judgement on priorities and makes what, by previous criteria is a rash purchase, we would not think it right to do these things.

Another kind of possible conflict is between current critical interests and experiential interests. Consider a patient who has volunteered to take part in an experiment, conceiving it as a way of allowing the discovery of knowledge which will help others. Suppose that the experiment becomes boring or otherwise somewhat unpleasant for the patient, who now wants to give up. Would it be right for the carer to pressure the patient to continue—e.g. by saying 'But don't you care about helping others? This is an important experiment and you promised to take part'. Many of us would have qualms about that.

By contrast we would not have such qualms about those who are in robust mental health. If some wholly healthy person has knowingly and freely volunteered for a worthwhile experiment, taking part in which then becomes mildly unpleasant, encouragement to carry on seems the right thing. Of course cases will vary, depending on the value of the experiment and the degree of unpleasantness. But the point is that with a competent adult some degree of pressure to continue with the important project is in order, especially if the experiential interest to which it is being sacrificed is comparatively minor. With a mentally disordered person, however, one might well be unhappy with any degree of pressure to continue.

Consideration of these possible conflicts shows that current critical interests of an Alzheimer's patient play out, both vis-à-vis their previous critical interests and also vis-à-vis their current experiential interests, in a very different way from that in which the current critical interests of non-demented persons play out. A corollary of this is that the Alzheimer's patients do not, after all, have 'autonomy', in a heavyweight sense which would give their 'autonomous' projects serious standing vis-à-vis other possible claims on their or their carer's resources, for example, the claims of their pre-dementia interests or the claims of their current experiential interests. Jaworska's argument does not support the attribution of autonomy in such a heavyweight sense and her handling of the examples does not suggest that she believes in it. So (picking up again on the point from the previous section about the logical shape of 'autonomy') perhaps having critical interests is necessary but not sufficient for autonomy? Or perhaps 'autonomy' of its nature comes in various strengths and we need to distinguish various versions of it? Until these things are sorted, all that emerges clearly from the discussion is a recommendation about how the lives of dementia sufferers should go.

This recommendation is that the richness of their lives and their sense of self-worth should be fostered by calling on whatever concepts and awarenesses they still have which enable them to take part in projects where they can see themselves as contributing to something important or having some worthwhile status. They should not just be fed, kept warm and clean, and otherwise ignored, but should be drawn in as cooperators, enabled to feel valued.

Has the recommendation gained force by being presented via a claim about autonomy? It is difficult to see that it has, since the logical shape of the concept remains as murky and disputable as ever. Moreover the recommendation stands entirely on its own feet, as eminently humane, attentive, and respectful. It is a recommendation we can all endorse, even if we think Jaworska wrong to link autonomy with critical interests or wrong to think that one can have the kinds of critical interests needed for autonomy in the absence of grip of the narrative structure of one's life. The problem with carrying out the recommendation is not that family, physicians, and carers have had mistaken views about autonomy and therefore have not bothered to think of doing the kinds of things pointed out. The problem is that family, physicians, and carers are pressed for time, have limits to their patience, find the Alzheimer's patients boring, embarrassing, etc.

In summary, the thrust of Sections 1.3 and 1.4 is this. It looks as if the discussions we have considered have been significantly shaped by what we might call 'the prussic acid model'. The discussants proceed on the assumption that there is some element in the situation, the patient's (possible) autonomy, the nature of which we start off being unclear about and the presence or absence of which is initially unclear. The aim of the discussion is then to give us a better grip on what autonomy really is, thereby enabling us to work out an appropriate test for it, through application of which we shall get guidance on what to do. But this model is, I have suggested, not appropriate for the cases in question. The idea that there is some one thing which is autonomy is a philosophers' hope, not a given fact. In our current state of philosophical muddle about autonomy, the only things we can be sure we agree about are: (1) that we should bring a general orientation of respect and care to our deliberations and (2) that will we find various complex and distressing details in each particular case.

It is true that philosophical thought inspired by discussion of autonomy in other contexts may suggest things to look for in these sufferers' lives (narrative coherence, critical interests, ability to self-legislate, possession of deep identity-conferring interests, etc.) and looking to see whether these things are present and to what extent, may help us to a more sympathetic appreciation of the complex situations of those who are mentally disordered. But philosophical thought, in its current state, has no agreed insight to deliver on what real autonomy is, an insight on which we can call and in the light of which we can make decisions. It is more likely that thinking about what is humane, respectful, and decent in dealing with the mentally disordered will help us to see the complexities of 'autonomy' than that theorizing about autonomy is going to show us how to treat the mentally disordered.

1.5 **Balancing hope and realism**

It was earlier allowed that, despite the unclarity and dispute over the nature of autonomy, it is defensible to go on using the word on the assumption that some agreed account of its nature may emerge. So one might press the question of why thinking about 'the autonomy of the mentally disordered' should not invoke this same optimistic usage. The previous sections have brought out some of the confusions and dangers of proceeding in that way, given our current state of disagreement. But another reason for separating issues about how things should go for the mentally disordered from the work of attempting to construct a future and better notion of 'autonomy' is that, even if the hoped-for future agreed concept does emerge, it might not solve difficult questions in this area. This is the possibility we shall address in this section.

Acquiring the hoped-for future concept is a matter of discussion and practice leading to the emergence of new ways of acting, feeling, and thinking, ways which are appropriately structured and enabled by the use of the future concept. In the pattern of living we then come to adopt, at least some of the kinds of conflict which now present themselves will have been overcome, since we shall find ourselves able to combine refined versions of the genuinely valuable, but seemingly incompatible, things which the current concept confusedly gestures at.

Ways of acting, feeling, thinking which are structured by elaborated and culturally evolved concepts of this kind typically require the robust workings of complex psychological and social structures in which emotions, habits, thoughts, etc. intertwine in an intricate way. Take sport as an example. Our present institutions of sporting clubs, leagues, regular fixtures, etc. enable a variety of pleasures, among them those of competition, securing dominance, experiencing the excitement of risk, enjoyment of the exercise of extreme physical strength and skill. These are pleasures which in other social settings are or have been provided by sporadic warfare, by expeditions to raid and steal from neighbouring communities, and the like. Sporting contests enable participants to enjoy these pleasures while at the same time providing the benefits of reduced risk of death, destruction of property, or injury to uninvolved bystanders. In a social setting which provides conceptually and materially for sporadic minor warfare but not for sporting contests, life is either boring but safe or exciting but seriously dangerous. In that kind of social setting people cannot combine safety with a particular kind of competitive excitement because the needed concepts and social institutions do not exist.

Sporting contests make the combination of excitement and (comparative) safety possible because: (1) serious things hang on the contest which make defeat a really bad thing, (2) there are sufficient inducements to keep all the players more or less observing the rules, and also (3) there are sufficient inducements to keep potential losers in the competition. To provide for these things the structure builds in rewards for winning and shame for losing, but at the same time rewards for being a fair player and also chances of reversing the tables in later contests. If all these elements are to come together in the right way to sustain the practice, the relative strength of the various motivations (to compete at all, to win, to abide by the rules, to come back for a second contest, etc.) need to be appropriately and stably balanced. And complex structures of cognition and habit (understanding the rules, being able to rely on oneself and others to follow them, grasping the consequences for oneself and others of cheating, knowing the time and structure for further contests etc.) need to be in place to channel these motivations into appropriate action (really strenuous play, but within the rules).

Failure or maladjustment of any part of this complex psychological structure (not being able to internalize habits of following rules, caring too much about winning, not grasping the time structure of the contest, not being amenable to being motivated by the idea of being approved as a fair player, etc.) will make it difficult if not impossible for a person to engage in sporting contests. For those who enjoy excitement and physical competition but whose psychological make-up does not enable them to realize the structure (as with some mentally disordered people) the choice may be back to boring but safe or exciting but dangerous.

The imagined future concept of autonomy will, in some roughly analogous way, allow us to combine at least some of the advantageous things which are invoked in the current discussions but which now seem to conflict—rational future planning versus spontaneity, reliance on oneself versus deep caring for others, or whatever. Any future society in which this concept has got a grip on us and is shaping our behaviour will be one which requires us to have achieved the appropriate psychological structures of habit, feeling, and thought. Suppose this to be achieved and the new way of living to be instituted, will the mentally disordered be capable of it and taking part in it? Perhaps. It will need looking at in each individual case. But the depressing probability is that mental disorder is just the kind of thing which will, one way or another, disrupt the capacity for such rich, elegantly balanced autonomy. And if so, for the mentally disordered the starker choices will be back.

References

Bolton, D. (2008). *What is Mental Disorder? An essay in philosophy, science and values*. Oxford: Oxford University Press.

Christman, J. (ed.) (1989). *The Inner Citadel: Essays on Individual Autonomy*. New York: Oxford University Press.

Christman, J. (2003). Autonomy in Moral and Political Philosophy. In E.D. Zalta (ed.) *Stanford Encyclopedia of Philosophy (Fall 2009 Edition)*. [Online] http://plato.stanford.edu/archives/fall2009/entries/autonomy-moral/

Feinberg, J. (1986). *Harm to Self. The Moral Limits of the Criminal Law*. Oxford: Oxford University Press. (Ch 18 on 'Autonomy' is reprinted in Christman (1989 pp. 27–43).)

Hacking, I. (1999). *The Social Construction of What?* Cambridge, MA: Harvard University Press.

Jaworska, A. (1999). Respecting the margins of agency: Alzheimer's patients and the capacity to value. *Philosophy and Public Affairs* 28: 105–38.

Mackenzie, C. and Stoljar, N. (2000). Introduction: autonomy reconfigured. In C. Mackenzie and N. Stoljar (eds.) *Relational Autonomy: Feminist Essays on Autonomy*. Oxford: Oxford University Press, pp. 3–31.

Silver, M. (2002). Reflections on determining competency. *Bioethics* 16: 455–68.

Van Willigenburg, T. (2005). Protecting autonomy as authenticity using Ulysses contracts. *Journal of Medicine and Philosophy* 30: 395–409.

Chapter 2

Autonomy and neuroscience

Alfred R. Mele

2.1 Introduction

Have neuroscientific experiments shown that there are no autonomous
human beings? That depends, of course, on what it means to say that
a human being is autonomous and on what neuroscientific experiments have shown about relevant properties or capacities of human
beings.

Even when philosophers apply the term 'autonomy' specifically to
individual human beings (as opposed to nations, for example), we
understand the term in a variety of different ways.[1] The root idea of
autonomy—from *autos* (self) and *nomos* (rule or law)—is self-rule or
self-government. My attempt to understand autonomous agency in
earlier work (especially Mele 1995) is an attempt to understand the
agency distinctive of self-ruled or self-governed individuals. 'Autonomy',
as I use the term there (as applied to individuals) is in the family of metaphysical freedom terms: 'free will', 'free choice', 'free action', and the
like. For my purposes in this chapter, it is enough that being an autonomous agent requires being able to perform some free actions—where
free actions are exercises of free will, the power or ability to act freely.

This last claim obviously raises the question what 'act freely' means.
My own view about this is non-committal on the issue that divides
compatibilists from incompatibilists (Mele 1995, 2006).[2] I offer two

---

[1] Joel Feinberg usefully distinguishes among four 'meanings' of the term 'autonomy' as
applied to individuals (1986, p. 28). Also see Arpaly (2003, pp. 118–25).

[2] Here is a gloss on the terminology for the uninitiated. Compatibilism (about free will and
determinism) is the thesis that the existence of free will is compatible with the truth of
determinism. Incompatibilism is the thesis that the existence of free will is incompatible
with the truth of determinism. And determinism is the thesis that a complete statement of

overlapping sets of sufficient conditions for acting freely, one for compatibilists and the other for incompatibilist believers in free will—that is, for *libertarians*. The main difference is that my incompatibilist conditions include indeterministic causation of actions, including actions of choosing or deciding to do something.

Whereas the laws that apply to deterministic causation are exceptionless, those that apply most directly to indeterministic causation are probabilistic.[3] Typically, events like *deciding* to help a stranded motorist—as distinct from the physical actions involved in actually helping—are counted as mental actions.[4] Suppose that your decision to help a stranded motorist is indeterministically caused by, among other things, your thinking that you should help. Because the causation is indeterministic, you might not have decided to help given exactly the same internal and external conditions. Some libertarians appeal to indeterministic causation to secure the possibility of doing otherwise that they require for free action (Kane 1996), and typical causal brands of libertarianism encompass a commitment to what may be termed *agent-internal indeterminism*—especially, indeterminism in internal processes that issue in decisions.

The claim that neuroscientists have shown that free will is an illusion is now very familiar; it even shows up in the popular press (Siegfried 2008; Youngsteadt 2008). If being an autonomous agent requires having free will and free will is an illusion, so is autonomous agency. Some scientists—neuroscientists and others—who argue for the illusion thesis about free will arrive at that conclusion by way of some empirical propositions that they infer from their data. For example, Benjamin Libet contends that, in experiments he conducted, the brain

---

the laws of nature together with a complete description of the entire universe at any point in time logically entails a complete description of the entire universe at any other point in time.

[3] So if the occurrence of x (at time $t1$) indeterministically causes the occurrence of y (at $t2$), then a complete description of the condition of the universe at $t1$ together with a complete statement of the laws of nature does *not* entail that U occurs at $t2$. There was at most a high probability that the occurrence of x at $t1$ would cause the occurrence of y at $t2$.

[4] For the record, as I understand 'deciding' to help a stranded motorist, it is an action of forming an intention to help; and, as I see it, many intentions are acquired without being actively formed (Mele 2003, chapter 9).

produces unconscious decisions to act about a third of a second before the person becomes aware of them (Libet 1985, 2004), and Daniel Wegner argues that 'conscious intentions' are never among the causes of corresponding actions (Wegner 2002, 2004, 2008). In Mele (2009), I review experiments (in neuroscience and social psychology) that are claimed to support empirical propositions such as these and I explain why the propositions are not justified by the data. Because these empirical propositions play a central role in the reasoning that leads such scientists as Libet and Wegner to their conclusions about free will, if my arguments that the propositions are not justified by the data hit their mark, they undermine the scientific arguments at issue about free will. For example, it may be plausible that a person whose conscious intentions never play a role in producing corresponding behaviour never acts freely; but if we lack good reason to believe that our conscious intentions never play a role of this kind, this particular line of argument for the thesis that free will is an illusion is out of the running (at least until powerful evidence for the claim about conscious intentions is produced).

In this chapter, I focus on two topics. One is a fall-back line of argument for the non-existence of free will that some scientists have offered. The other is a question about the bearing of neuroscientific studies of behaviour in one sphere on behaviour in another sphere. In Section 2.2, I sketch some background on Libet's work to set the stage for my discussion of both topics.

2.2 **Background: Libet's studies and more**

Azim Shariff and coauthors report (2008, p. 186) that 'almost all of the works involved in the deluge of anti-free will arguments have referenced' experiments by neurobiologist Benjamin Libet. Libet contends both that 'the brain "decides" to initiate or, at least, prepare to initiate [certain actions] before there is any reportable subjective awareness that such a decision has taken place' (Libet 1985, p. 536)[5] and that

---

[5] Elsewhere, Libet writes: 'the brain has begun the specific preparatory processes for the voluntary act well before the subject is even aware of any wish or intention to act' (1992, p. 263).

'If the "act now" process is initiated unconsciously, then conscious free will is not doing it' (Libet 2001, p. 62; see 2004, p. 136). Although these claims are based on results of experiments conducted in a very artificial setting, Libet is inclined to generalize: 'Our overall findings do suggest some fundamental characteristics of the simpler acts that may be applicable to all consciously intended acts and even to responsibility and free will' (Libet 1985, p. 563).

In some of Libet's studies, subjects are regularly encouraged to flex their right wrists whenever they wish. In subjects who do not report any advance planning of their movements, electrical readings from the scalp—averaged over at least 40 flexing actions for each subject—show a shift in 'readiness potentials' (RPs) beginning about 550 ms before the time at which an electromyogram shows relevant muscular activity to begin (Libet 1985, pp. 529–30). These are type II RPs (p. 531). Subjects who are not regularly encouraged to aim for spontaneity or who report some advance planning produce RPs that begin about half a second earlier—type I RPs. The same is true of subjects instructed to flex at a prearranged time (Libet et al. 1982, p. 325).

Subjects are also instructed to recall where a revolving spot was on a special clock when they first became aware of something, x, that Libet variously describes as a decision, intention, urge, wanting, will, or wish to move (1985, p. 529). (The spot on this Libet clock makes a complete revolution in about 2.5 seconds.) On average, the onset of type II RPs preceded what the subjects reported to be the time of their initial awareness of x (time W) by 350 ms. So time W preceded the beginning of muscle motion by about 200 ms. Libet's findings for type II RPs may be represented as follows:

−550 ms	−200 ms	0 ms
RP onset	time W	muscle begins to move

One inference that Libet makes on the basis of these findings is that the brain produces a proximal decision or intention to flex—that is, a decision or intention to flex *now*—about a third of a second before the subject becomes aware of that decision or intention. On the basis of a variety of data, including Libet's, I have argued elsewhere that it is more plausible that what the brain produces around −550 ms is a potential cause of a subsequent proximal decision or intention to flex and that the decision or intention emerges significantly later (Mele 2009, chapters 3 and 4). Someone who is persuaded by my argument can claim that, even so, all that really matters is that what initiates the process that results in a flexing action is unconscious brain activity; in that case, as Libet puts it, 'conscious free will is not doing it' (2001, p. 62).

How might this claim about what really matters be supported? Some scientists have claimed that because conscious proximal intentions to flex in Libet's experiment arise later than the onset of the type II RP, they are not causes of flexings. If this claim were true, it might provide some support for the idea 'conscious free will' has no place in the production of the flexing actions.

I criticize the claim at issue in Mele (2009, pp. 70–76). So I will be brief here. To take just one example, Patrick Haggard writes: 'The seminal studies of Benjamin Libet . . . suggested that conscious intention occurs *after* the onset of preparatory brain activity. It cannot therefore cause our actions, as a cause cannot occur after its effect' (2005, p. 291; also see Banks 2006, p. 237; Pockett 2006, p. 21; Roediger et al. 2008, p. 208; Shariff et al. 2008, p. 186). One might think that Haggard is claiming that 'conscious intention' cannot cause actions because it occurs after the actions with which it is associated. But he is not. Haggard finds it plausible that, in these studies, conscious intentions arise before the associated actions (Haggard 2006, p. 83; see 2005, p. 291). His claim is that because 'conscious intention occurs after the onset of *preparatory brain activity*' (emphasis altered), it 'cannot . . . cause our actions' (Haggard 2005, p. 291).

The observation that unconscious preparatory brain activity precedes conscious proximal intentions to flex is entirely consistent with its being true that the brain activity is a more remote cause of an action that has the acquisition of a conscious proximal intention among its less remote causes. Of course, even if the acquisition of the conscious intention is a less remote cause of the action, it is a further question whether the intention plays a role in producing the action that depends on its being a *conscious* intention (see Mele 2009, pp. 30–40 and chapter 7). The point to be noticed here is that from the datum that some 'preparatory brain activity' begins before a conscious proximal intention emerges, one cannot legitimately infer that any of the following play no role in producing the movement: the acquisition of the proximal intention, the agent's consciousness of the intention, the physical correlates of either of these items. After all, when the lighting of a fuse precedes the burning of the fuse, which in turn precedes a firecracker's exploding, we do not infer that the burning of the fuse plays no causal role in producing the explosion. Notice also that the neural events that precede the emergence of a conscious intention in Libet's studies may be intrinsically indistinguishable from neural events that occur in cases in which Libet's subjects spontaneously veto conscious urges and then wait for a subsequent urge before flexing (see Libet 1985, pp. 530, 538). If that is so, the occurrence of the 'preparatory brain activity' leaves it open whether the agent will or will not flex very soon and open that he would not have flexed about half a second later if he had not acquired a conscious proximal intention to flex before flexing.

2.3 **Arguing about free will**

I have just explained why we should reject one attempted line of support for the claim that, regarding the threat that Libet's studies pose to free will, all that really matters is that what initiates the process that results in a flexing action is unconscious brain activity. How else might the claim be supported?

After describing the threat that he believes Libet's work poses to free will, C.M. Fisher writes:

> Somewhat the same conclusion may be reached on the basis of rather elementary observation. Every thought, feeling, inclination, intention, desire . . . must be created by nervous system activity. How else could they arise? Ideas would have to arise without a physical basis. Nervous system activity must always precede. . . . If one has the experience of 'willing' the nervous system to do something, the impression of willing must have been preceded by nervous system activity. Otherwise there would be no source and we are in the realm of the supernatural. (2001, p. 56)

Fisher's claim seems to be that because all mental events are produced by brain events, free will is an illusion—that the Libet-style thesis that free will is an illusion is entailed by the fact that all mental events are produced by brain events.[6] He seems to assume that free will has to be 'supernatural'.

P. Read Montague takes a similar position:

> Free will is the idea that we make choices and have thoughts independent of anything remotely resembling a physical process. Free will is the close cousin to the idea of the soul – the concept that 'you', your thoughts and feelings, derive from an entity that is separate and distinct from the physical mechanisms that make up your body. From this perspective, your choices are not caused by physical events, but instead emerge wholly formed from somewhere indescribable and outside the purview of physical descriptions. This implies that free will cannot have evolved by natural selection, as that would place it directly in a stream of causally connected events. (2008, p. 584)

Here Montague represents free will as something that depends for its existence on the truth of substance dualism—a view that includes a commitment to the idea that 'associated with each human person, there is a thinking thing . . . not composed of the same kinds of stuff as . . . nonmental things' (Zimmerman 2006, p. 115; Zimmerman describes the 'thinking thing' as a soul, but some substance dualists prefer to use the word 'mind'). And as I pointed out in Mele (2009, pp. 67–68, 110–13), there are similar dualistic elements in Libet's and Wegner's thinking about free will.

The passages I quoted from Fisher 2001 and Montague 2008 suggest the following argument (Argument *A*):

1 No human being has free will unless he or she has supernatural powers.

2 There is excellent neuroscientific evidence that no human being has supernatural powers.

3 So there is powerful support for the thesis that no human being has free will.

---

6 Libet himself believes that free will is possible in a limited domain. He asserts that 'if the "act now" process is initiated unconsciously, then conscious free will is not doing it' (2001, p. 62; see 2004, p. 136). But he also claims that once we become aware of our decisions or intentions, we can exercise free will in *vetoing* them (2004, pp. 137–49). Some people follow him part of the way. They accept the thesis about when and how decisions to act are made but reject the window of opportunity for free vetoing as an illusion (Wegner 2002, p. 55; Hallett 2007).

In Mele (in press), I challenge a premise that does the work of premise 1 in a related argument. That premise reads as follows: 'A conscious decision is freely made (or is an exercise of free will) only if it has no neurological antecedents'. The fact that the great majority of living philosophers who work on free will would reject premise 1 and this related premise about conscious decisions might not make much of an impression on Fisher and Montague. They might believe that their own opinions about what 'free will' means are at least as deserving of acceptance as philosophers' opinions about this. They might also believe that their own opinions are in line with common usage whereas philosophers' opinions about what 'free will' means are polluted by untestable theories. The challenge I mentioned from Mele (in press) is based partly on survey studies of non-specialists. There is good evidence (some of which is discussed shortly) that 'free will', as most people use that expression, does not entail that only beings with supernatural powers can exercise free will and does not require that free conscious decisions have no brain events among their causes (see Mele in press). To the extent to which the dispute is about the meaning of 'free will', this evidence should count for something. And, of course, there is no reason to think that neuroscientists are in a better position than philosophers and lay folk to understand what the expression 'free will' means.

At times, Anthony Cashmore writes as though he would endorse Argument A. For example, he asserts that 'if we no longer entertain the luxury of a belief in the "magic of the soul," then there is little else to offer in support of the concept of free will' (Cashmore 2010, p. 4499). But he also makes the following claim:

> In the absence of any molecular model accommodating the concept of free will, I have to conclude that the dualism of Descartes is alive and well. That is, just like Descartes, we still believe (much as we pretend otherwise) that there is a magic component to human behavior. Here I argue that the way we use the concept of free will is nonsensical. (Cashmore 2010, p. 4503)

Cashmore seems to suggest here that if there were a molecular model that accommodates 'the concept of free will', people who believe that free will exists would not be committed thereby to a belief in substance dualism.

Here is an obvious point: our current lack of a molecular model that accommodates free will does not entail that there will never be a model of this kind. Obviously, Cashmore believes that substance dualism is false. And if the claim I quoted about the absence of a molecular model is to be taken seriously, part of his reason for holding that belief in free will implies belief in substance dualism is that we now lack a molecular model of free will. It is noteworthy in this connection that although Cashmore grants that we now lack a molecular model of consciousness (2010, p. 4502), he does not conclude that belief in consciousness depends on belief in substance dualism. Nor does he contend that consciousness is an illusion. Indeed, he holds that 'consciousness acts on behavior' (p. 4502).

Why is Cashmore a substance dualist about free will but not about consciousness even though he believes that we lack molecular models of both? He describes a belief in free will as 'a belief that there is a component to biological behavior that is something more than the unavoidable consequences of the genetic and environmental history of the individual and the possible stochastic laws of nature' (2010, p. 4500). And he contends that although stochasticity 'may remove the bugbear of determinism, it would do little to support the notion of free will: I cannot be held responsible for my genes and my environment; similarly, I can hardly be held responsible for any stochastic process that may influence my behavior!' (p. 4500). Now, Cashmore evidently is open to the possibility of a non-dualistic solution to the mind–body problem that is consistent with the truth of his assertion that 'consciousness acts on behavior' (p. 4502). An attractive non-dualistic solution would presumably allow for conscious deliberation about what to do, conscious decisions about what to do, and the like. Suppose that some episodes of practical deliberation and some decision-producing processes are stochastic processes. Why should it be thought that we cannot have any responsibility for them? Cashmore might claim that we cannot have any responsibility for them because what they result in is 'unavoidable'. But given that the processes at issue are, by hypothesis, stochastic, this claim about results would be very puzzling. Other things being equal, a stochastic process that results in *x* might not have—precisely because it is stochastic.

It may be claimed that all causation occurs at too low an ontological level for deliberation about what to do to have an effect on what one does. But this is not Cashmore's view: again, he asserts that 'consciousness acts on behavior' (p. 4502). In his view, 'there must be a mechanism by which consciousness does influence behavior. There must be a flow of information from consciousness to neural activity'. So, for Cashmore, some relatively high-level events do have effects.

Cashmore apparently understands free will in such a way that, necessarily, we exercise it only if our 'will' is uncaused (2010, p. 4501). He seems to understand free will in such a way that, necessarily, any free decision is an uncaused decision. But what puts him in a position to be confident that this theoretical proposition is true? It is not as though research in biology—Cashmore's field—tells us what 'free will' means. Even if there is no way to gain widespread agreement about the meaning of 'free will', it may be that attention to common usage of the expression would motivate the idea that free decisions do not have to be uncaused.

Eddy Nahmias, Justin Coates, and Trevor Kvaran conducted a study designed to test, among other things, how the kind of causation featured in a probe affects lay judgements about free will (Nahmias et al. 2007). In some of the probes decisions are 'completely caused by the specific chemical reactions and neural processes' occurring in a person's 'brain', whereas in other, parallel probes decisions are 'completely caused by the . . . thoughts desires, and plans' occurring in the person's 'mind' (Nahmias et al. 2007, p. 223). This difference had the biggest effect when the probe was 'abstract' (that is, did not mention specific actions) and featured scientific hypotheses about the actual universe.

Bracketed material in the following extract appeared in a parallel probe:

Many respected neuroscientists [psychologists] are convinced that eventually we will figure out exactly how all of our decisions and actions are entirely caused. . . . If these neuroscientists [psychologists] are right, then once specific earlier events have occurred in a person's life, these events will definitely cause specific later events to occur. For instance, once specific chemical reactions and neural processes [thoughts, desires, and plans] occur in the person's brain [mind], they will definitely cause the person to make the specific decision he or she makes. (Nahmias et al. 2007, p. 224)

Participants were asked to indicate their degree of agreement or disagreement with the following statement: 'If the neuroscientists [psychologists] are right, then people make decisions of their own free will' (p. 225). When the probe featured causation by 'thoughts, desires, and plans', 82.9% agreed with the statement; and when it featured causation by 'chemical reactions and neural processes', 38.3% agreed (p. 227). This is a huge difference, of course. But for present purposes it is noteworthy that the overwhelming majority of respondents to the probe featuring causation by thoughts, desires, and plans apparently do not require decisions made of one's own free will to be uncaused. And it is interesting that 38% of the participants count even decisions that are 'entirely caused [by] specific chemical reactions and neural processes' as being made of the person's own free will. Such participants would seem to see no need for a non-physical mind or soul to be at work in the production of free decisions and no need for free decisions to be uncaused.

It also is interesting that when the setting is switched from the actual universe to a possible universe and the probes involve an agent who performs a good or a bad action, most participants regard the decisions as being made of the person's own free will. The results were as shown in Table 2.1 (N indicates causation by 'chemical reactions and neural processes' and P indicates causation by 'thoughts, desires, and plans'):

Table 2.1 Of one's own free will: agree

	Bad	Good
N	59.8	57.4
P	66.1	61.1

Apparently, when they entertain these probes—including the *N* probes—a *majority* of people see no need for a non-physical soul or mind to play a role in the production of decisions made of the person's own free will and no need for free decisions to be uncaused.

I conducted two survey studies of my own that bear on these issues. Participants in the first study were 69 students in a basic philosophy class at Florida State University. Free will and moral responsibility were not on the course agenda. About half of the participants (33) were presented with the following text:

> First answer the question on page # 1. Then turn the sheet over and answer the question on page # 2.
>
> We're interested in how you understand free will. Please read the following sentences and answer the question by circling your answer.
>
> In 2019, scientists finally show exactly where decisions and intentions are found in the brain. Our decisions are brain processes, and our intentions are brain states.
>
> In 2009, John Jones saw a 20-dollar bill fall from the pocket of the person walking in front of him. He considered returning it to the person, who did not notice the bill fall; but he decided to keep it. Of course, given what scientists later discovered, John's decision was a brain process.
>
> Question: Did John have free will when he made his decision?

On page 2, the participants read an expression of our interest in how they understand 'deserved moral blame', the same probe as on page 1, and the following question: 'Does John deserve to be blamed for what he does?'. The other participants (36) were presented with the same material in the opposite order. (Order did not have a significant effect.)

The results were as follows. About 90% (89.85%) of the participants answered yes to the question about free will and about 87% (86.95%) answered yes to the question about deserved blame. Apparently, for the overwhelming majority of participants, viewing a person's decisions as brain processes was compatible with regarding the person as having free will (and as deserving blame).

I conducted a second study with another group of students in basic philosophy courses at Florida State University. Again, free will and moral responsibility were not on the course agendas. Because the responses to the questions about free will and moral responsibility in the first study were so similar, I decided to ask about just one this time—free will. I used a version of the initial probe that was augmented to include the idea that 'our decisions and intentions are caused by other brain processes'.[7] There were 86 participants; 74 of them (86%) said that John had free will when he made his decision. For the over-whelming majority of participants, viewing a person's decision as 'a brain process that was caused by other brain processes' was compatible with regarding the person as having free will.

Whether or not free will is an illusion depends on what 'free will' means. Even if free will would be an illusion if Cashmore were right about what 'free will' means, free will might exist. Cashmore may contend that anyone who does not require free decisions to be uncaused is conceptually confused. For a pair of ways of understanding how caused decisions can be free—one for compatibilists and the other for incompatibilists—see Mele (2006). I do not regard the proposals there as conceptually confused; others are free to make up their own minds about that.

2.4 **Generalizing**

Libet is inclined to generalize, as I mentioned, from his findings in the sphere he studied—wrist flexings under the conditions I described in Section 2.1—'to all consciously intended acts and even to responsibility and free will' (1985, p. 563). As I also mentioned, I have argued elsewhere that we lack good reason to believe that, even in the sphere of actions Libet investigates, the brain makes proximal decisions before the

---

[7] This probe read as follows:

In 2019, scientists finally show exactly where decisions and intentions are found in the brain and how they are caused. Our decisions are brain processes, and our intentions are brain states. Also, our decisions and intentions are caused by other brain processes.

In 2009, John Jones saw a 20-dollar bill fall from the pocket of the person walking in front of him. He considered returning it to the person, who did not notice the bill fall; but he decided to keep it. Of course, given what scientists later discovered, John's decision was a brain process and it was caused by other brain processes.

The survey also asked whether students were taking their first philosophy class after high school. The breakdown was 58 yes and 28 no. This difference did not have a statistically significant effect on their answers about free will. About 88% of the first group and 82% of the second group answered yes to the question about free will.

person becomes aware of them (Mele 2009). But let that pass. Even if Libet were right about proximal decisions in this sphere, what would that tell us about practical decisions—decisions to do things—in general? Would we be entitled to infer that they are all made unconsciously or that 'conscious free will' cannot do anything more than 'veto' decisions or intentions once we become conscious of them (see Libet 2004, pp. 136–49)?

In Mele (2009), I compared the situation of subjects in a Libet-style study to people in 'Buridan's ass' scenarios (pp. 83–87). The key point of comparison is the agents' indifference regarding the relevant options. Suppose you take a shopping list to a supermarket. One item on your list is a 16-ounce jar of Planters peanuts. When you get to the relevant part of the peanut display (assuming normal conditions), you simply grab a 16-ounce jar of Planters peanuts, and you are indifferent between that jar and each of the two jars adjacent to it. You do not see yourself as having a reason to prefer the jar you pick to these others. Similarly, subjects in a Libet-style experiment do not see themselves as having reasons to prefer certain potential moments to begin flexing over other 'nearby' moments. The 'selection' of a moment to begin flexing is arbitrary.

How similar is our behaviour in scenarios in which we are indifferent between or among the relevant options to our behaviour in scenarios in which we put a lot of thought into which option to select? And is either kind of behaviour more closely associated with—or more central to—autonomy? I take up the second question first.

The assertion that a subject in a Libet-style experiment autonomously—or non-autonomously—decided to flex his wrist now is not particularly jarring, but the philosophical literature on autonomous action pays little attention to relatively trivial actions. That literature focuses on the deliberative sphere, not the sphere of indifference. To the extent to which it is reasonable to take our lead on the present question from what aspects of our lives philosophers tend to focus on when they investigate autonomy, it is reasonable to believe that deliberative conduct is more central to autonomy than is conduct in the sphere of indifference.

One difference between actions in these two spheres is reflected in what agents will tend to say when asked for their reasons for doing what they did. Compare questions 1 and 2 with questions 3 and 4:

Q1. (Addressed to a subject in a Libet-style experiment.) What was your reason for flexing just then?

Q2. (Addressed to me in the supermarket.) What was your reason for taking that particular jar of Planters peanuts?

Q3. (Addressed to Al after he thought long and hard about whether to accept a job offer.) What was your reason for rejecting that offer?

Q4. (Addressed to Ann after she thought long and hard about whether to attend law school or a Ph.D. program in philosophy.) What was your reason for accepting admission to the philosophy program?

In the case of the first two questions, we would be surprised if we were given a reason.[8] In the case of the last two questions, we expect to hear statements of reasons. Of course, it is possible for Al and Ann to be stumped after weighing lots of factors. They might resort to tossing a coin. But receiving thoughtful statements of reasons is in line with ordinary expectations.

Why does this matter? Because one path from Libet's alleged finding about decisions in his scenario to a general autonomy-threatening thesis features the following claim: just as unconscious processes result in particular proximal decisions or intentions to flex independently of any conscious assessment of reasons at the time, unconscious processes result in all decisions or intentions independently of any conscious reasons-assessment that may accompany those processes. In the case of Libet's subjects, there are no reasons to flex at any particular time, and it is not at all surprising that unconscious tie-breaking mechanisms are at work (see Mele 2009, p. 83). For this very reason, it is extremely difficult to generalize from Libet's alleged finding to the claim at issue about all decisions and intentions. Some decisions and intentions are at least preceded by serious, protracted thought about reasons. And the finding that in a scenario in which there are no reasons for agents to

---

[8] Sometimes, in related scenarios, agents can be induced to provide a reasons explanation. See Nisbett and Wilson (1977).

assess, reasons-assessment has no effect on their intentions and decisions carries little weight when we move to scenarios in which there are reasons for and against the relevant options and agents are seriously involved in assessing or weighing them. Moving from this finding to the general claim about decisions and intentions is rather like moving from the finding that, in certain situations, people communicate with one another in the absence of cell phones to the claim that all communication is accomplished without cell phones.

Is there a better path from Libet's alleged finding to an autonomy-threatening thesis? Consider the following claim: (*C1*) Just as subjects make their proximal decisions to flex before they are aware that the decision has been made, we make all of our decisions before we are aware they have been made. Someone who endorses *C1* may conjoin it with the following claim to threaten autonomy: (*C2*) Any decision we make before we are aware of the decision is not made freely and therefore is not made autonomously; freely making a decision requires consciously making it.

Again, although I have argued elsewhere that Libet has not shown that his subjects make unconscious proximal decisions to flex (Mele 2009), I let that pass. What is supposed to justify the move made in *C1*? Even if unconscious proximal decisions are made in a Libet-style setting, in which agents have no relevant reasons to assess, how do we get from this alleged finding to the claim that we make all of our decisions before we are aware they have been made? If there is evidence that consciously assessing reasons with a view to making a decision about what to do does not increase the probability of the reasoner's making a conscious decision, I am not aware of it. Libet's studies certainly produce no direct evidence of this. In his studies, subjects are not assessing reasons with a view to making decisions about when to flex.[9]

---

[9] Claim *C2* raises a number of questions that cannot be pursued here, including the following. What are decisions to act (practical decisions)? Can such decisions be made unconsciously? Do people who claim that there are unconscious practical decisions really mean only that some intentions are acquired unconsciously? Can any unconscious decisions be free decisions? Can any actions that are executions of unconscious decisions be free actions?

2.5 **Conclusion**

I opened this chapter with the question whether neuroscientific experiments have shown that there are no autonomous human beings. In my opinion, the answer is *no*. I have not argued for that answer here, of course. Doing so is much too grand a project for a single chapter. Instead, I attacked one line of argument for the claim that neuroscientific experiments have shown that human autonomy is an illusion and I discussed an important difficulty in moving from an alleged finding about proximal decisions in a common experimental setting to an autonomy-threatening thesis about all decisions.

Acknowledgements

This chapter was made possible through the support of a grant from the John Templeton Foundation. The opinions expressed in this chapter are those of the author and do not necessarily reflect the views of the John Templeton Foundation.

References

Arpaly, N. (2003). *Unprincipled Virtue*. Oxford: Oxford University Press.

Banks, W. (2006). Does consciousness cause misbehavior? In S. Pockett, W. Banks, and S. Gallagher (eds.) *Does Consciousness Cause Behavior? An Investigation of the Nature of Volition*. Cambridge, MA: MIT Press, pp. 235–56.

Cashmore, A. (2010). The Lucretian swerve: The biological basis of human behavior and the criminal justice system. *Proceedings of the National Academy of Sciences of the United States of America* 107: 4499–504.

Feinberg, J. (1986). *Harm to Self*. Oxford: Oxford University Press.

Fisher, C.M. (2001). If there were no free will. *Medical Hypotheses* 56: 364–66.

Haggard, P. (2005). Conscious intention and motor cognition. *Trends in Cognitive Sciences* 9: 290–95.

Haggard, P. (2006). Conscious intention and the sense of agency. In N. Sebanz and W. Prinz (eds.) *Disorders of Volition*. Cambridge, MA: MIT Press, pp. 69–86.

Hallett, M. (2007). Volitional control of movement: The physiology of free will. *Clinical Neurophysiology* 118: 1179–92.

Kane, R. (1996). *The Significance of Free Will*. Oxford: Oxford University Press.

Libet, B. (1985). Unconscious cerebral initiative and the role of conscious will in voluntary action. *Behavioral and Brain Sciences* 8: 529–66.

Libet, B. (1992). The neural time-factor in perception, volition and free will. *Revue de Métaphysique et de Morale* 2: 255–72.

Libet, B. (2001). Consciousness, free action and the brain. *Journal of Consciousness Studies* 8: 59–65.

Libet, B. (2004). *Mind Time*. Cambridge, MA: Harvard University Press.

Libet, B., Wright, E., and Gleason, C. (1982). Readiness potentials preceding unrestricted 'spontaneous' vs. pre-planned voluntary acts. *Electroencephalography and Clinical Neurophysiology* 54: 322–35.

Mele A. (1995). *Autonomous Agents: From Self-Control to Autonomy*. Oxford: Oxford University Press.

Mele A. (2003). *Motivation and Agency*. Oxford: Oxford University Press.

Mele A. (2006). *Free Will and Luck*. Oxford: Oxford University Press.

Mele A. (2009). *Effective Intentions*. Oxford: Oxford University Press.

Mele A. (in press) Another scientific threat to free will? *The Monist*.

Montague, P.R. (2008). Free will. *Current Biology* 18: R584–85.

Nahmias, E., Coates, J., and Kvaran, T. (2007). Free will, moral responsibility, and mechanism: Experiments on folk intuitions. *Midwest Studies in Philosophy* 31: 214–42.

Nisbett, R. and Wilson, T. (1977). Telling more than we can know: Verbal reports on mental processes. *Psychological Review* 84: 243–44.

Pockett, S. (2006). The neuroscience of movement. In S. Pockett, W. Banks, and S. Gallagher (eds.) *Does Consciousness Cause Behavior? An Investigation of the Nature of Volition*. Cambridge, MA: MIT Press, pp. 9–24.

Roediger, H., Goode, M., and Zaromb, F. (2008). Free will and the control of action. In J. Baer, J. Kaufman, and R. Baumeister (eds.) *Are We Free? Psychology and Free Will*. Oxford: Oxford University Press, pp. 205–25.

Shariff, A., Schooler, J., and Vohs, K. (2008). The hazards of claiming to have solved the hard problem of free will. In J. Baer, J. Kaufman, and R. Baumeister (eds.) *Are We Free? Psychology and Free Will*. Oxford: Oxford University Press, pp. 181–204.

Siegfried, T. (2008). The decider. *Science News* 174: 28–30.

Wegner, D. (2002). *The Illusion of Conscious Will*. Cambridge, MA: MIT Press.

Wegner, D. (2004). Frequently asked questions about conscious will. *Behavioral and Brain Sciences* 27: 679–88.

Wegner, D. (2008). Self is magic. In In J. Baer, J. Kaufman, and R. Baumeister (eds.) *Are We Free? Psychology and Free Will*. Oxford: Oxford University Press, pp. 181–204.

Youngsteadt, E. (2008). Case closed for free will? *ScienceNOW Daily News* 14 April.

Zimmerman, D. (2006). Dualism in the philosophy of mind. In D. Borchert (ed.) *Encyclopedia of Philosophy* (2nd edn. vol. 3). Detroit, MI: Thomson Gale, pp. 113–22.

Chapter 3

Three challenges from delusion for theories of autonomy

K.W.M. (Bill) Fulford and Lubomira Radoilska

3.1 Introduction

The main ambition of this chapter is to identify and explore a series of challenges that the phenomenology of delusions poses to our systematic thinking about autonomy. For the sake of the argument, we shall understand autonomy in terms of intentional agency over time (see, for example, Bratman 2007) and will not expand on the possible interactions between this and alternative conceptions, which either take an ahistorical perspective and define autonomy as a distinctive relationship to one's motives at the time of action (Frankfurt 1971), or integrate further criteria, such as responsiveness to reasons (Watson 1975) and accordance with particular values (Hill 1991).[1] An implication of this methodological choice is that the challenges at issue will have no immediate bearing to emancipatory accounts which define autonomy as a particular social-relational status and therefore have no apparent reason to take delusions as likely failures of autonomy per se, independently of specific institutional contexts (Mackenzie and Stoljar 2000).[2] In other words, the following discussion is primarily aimed at theories

---

[1] For a comprehensive analysis of these alternatives, see Buss (2008).

[2] This is because such accounts take interpersonal dynamics to be a constitutive part rather than a circumstance only of autonomy. A partial parallel from the phenomenology of delusion is *folie à deux* in which people living with someone who has delusions (e.g. within a family) get caught up in their delusional world but only so long as they remain in close and largely exclusive proximity with the person concerned (e.g. Gelder et al. 2001, p. 394).

which conceive autonomy as an agency rather than a status concept.[3] The central claim is that in order to avoid circularity, such theories should be able to address the subsequent challenges from delusion. This becomes clear if we consider the compelling intuition according to which 'insanity' is an obvious case where autonomy as just specified has broken down (see, in particular, Wolf 1987). What seems to be implied in it, however, is that 'insanity' is definable independently of whether it compromises autonomy or not. Psychosis as a central mental disorder and delusion, its central symptom, seem to provide the required theoretical leverage. The thought is that, unless delusion is conceived as theoretically independent from autonomy, we would end up with a vicious circle: defining 'insanity' as lack of autonomy and then turning back to clarifying autonomy as a state where autonomy is not lacking.

Yet, as we shall argue drawing on Fulford (1989)[4] the following challenges from delusion suggest that delusions are implicitly understood in terms of various kinds of breakdowns of intentional agency.[5] Hence, in order to avoid circularity both in defining autonomy and delusions, we need to explicitly address the putative failures of autonomy as presented by the logical topography of delusions, encompassing: their centrality (Challenge 1), their diverse logical range (Challenge 2), and non-pathological instances (Challenge 3). We take these challenges in turn, first setting out and illustrating the relevant features of delusions and then expanding on the implications for theories of autonomy. We conclude by spelling out several caveats that emerge from the discussion and briefly indicating the relevance of the analysis to contemporary policy and practice in mental health.

---

[3] See the Introduction to the volume, p.xxix.

[4] Fulford (1989) develops an agentic account of the experience of illness in general and of mental illness in particular. This account is further developed in a number of publications, including Fulford (1996, 1998). Many of the cases described in this chapter are derived from these sources (see Acknowledgements).

[5] See, however, Chapter 5, this volume, where Bortolotti et al. discuss possible cases of delusions which enhance rather than undermine intentional agency.

3.2 **Challenge 1**

3.2.1 **The centrality of delusions**

Our first challenge from delusions for theories of autonomy is to address their central legal and ethical significance consistently with their correspondingly central place among other kinds of psychopathology. In this section we fill out this challenge with an illustrative series of brief case examples starting with the central place of delusions in the map of mental disorders.

3.2.1.1 The central psychopathological significance of delusions

Delusions are the paradigm symptoms of the most serious forms of mental disorder, the psychotic disorders. These disorders include both organic psychoses, such as the dementias and other conditions caused by gross pathology affecting the brain (brain tumours, brain infections, etc.) and non-organic or, as they are called, 'functional' psychoses, such as schizophrenia and the affective psychoses (including hypomania, some forms of depression, and bipolar disorder). We will be giving examples of these and of a variety of other disorders in the course of this chapter. As these examples will illustrate, the psychoses as a whole are characterized by the presence of delusions and of related symptoms, such as hallucinations.

Psychotic disorders (and with them delusions) are the most serious kinds of mental disorder in two senses: contingent and constitutive. Contingently, the psychotic disorders carry the highest risk of premature death (by suicide or, far more rarely, homicide). Constitutively, psychotic disorders are the most serious mental disorders in the sense that the delusions and related symptoms by which they are defined are in turn characterized by a particularly profound disturbance of rationality called in descriptive psychopathology, 'loss of insight'.

Like many other psychopathological concepts, psychotic loss of insight, although identifiable with a high degree of reliability in the form of delusions and related symptoms (Wing et al. 1974), remains a much contested concept (Lewis 1934; Perkins and Moodley 1993; Amador and David 2004). Essentially, what loss of insight means in this context is that people with psychotic disorders (characteristically) fail to recognize that there is anything (mentally) wrong with them. We can see this by comparing the *delusions* of guilt arising typically in people with severe depression with the *obsessions* of guilt that occur in people with obsessive–compulsive disorders.

Case 1: Delusions of guilt in depressive disorder—Mr SD, 50-year-old shop keeper

Mr SD went to see his family doctor asking for 'something to help me sleep'. He looked depressed, however, and he had 'biological' symptoms (early waking, weight loss, and fixed diurnal variation of mood) consistent with a serious form of depressive illness. Questioned further about why he was not sleeping, he was initially reticent but finally admitted that he was worried sick with guilt because he was responsible for causing the (then) recent war in the Balkans. Asked how he (a local shop keeper) could be responsible for what was going on in the Balkans he turned away saying in a quiet voice 'you know' and then refused to talk about it further.

Case 2: Obsessions of guilt in obsessive–compulsive disorder—Mr OC, age 27, solicitor's clerk

Mr OC was referred by his general practitioner (GP) to a psychiatrist with a 3-year history of progressive slowness. He had a recent history of moderate depression and anxiety following suspension from his job (as a result of his increasing failure to get through his work) but was otherwise well and showed no neurological signs (e.g. of Parkinsonism). The problem he said was that he had been experiencing increasingly intrusive feelings of guilt combined with compulsive checking (it took him, for example, often 20 minutes to leave his house because of repeated urges to return to check that he had locked the door). He was unable to resist these urges even though he regarded them as 'completely ridiculous' and said that he knew perfectly well that he had nothing to feel guilty about 'any more than the next man'.

In both these cases the person concerned was troubled by what most people would regard as irrational feelings of guilt. Mr SD (Case 1) however, with his *delusions* of guilt, really believed he was guilty of causing a war and he rejected attempts to reassure him (we return to the features of delusion later under Challenge 2). Mr OC (Case 2), by contrast, with his *obsessions* of guilt, recognized that his feelings of guilt were irrational (he described them as 'completely ridiculous') and he resisted them albeit unsuccessfully (an obsession is like a bad case of getting a tune 'stuck in your head' and a compulsion is its behavioural counter-part—as in this case with Mr OC repeatedly returning to check he had locked his front door).

Mr OC (Case 2) then (with obsessions of guilt) had preserved insight: he recognized along with everyone else that his feelings of guilt though persistent and intrusive were irrational and he asked for help because there was *something (mentally) wrong with him*. Mr SD (Case 1) how-ever (with delusions of guilt), had 'lost insight': far from recognizing that there was anything (mentally) wrong with him he believed that what was wrong was *what he had done* (caused a war) and for this he felt (justifiably) guilty.

3.2.1.2 The central legal and ethical significance of delusions

Both senses in which psychotic disorders are serious disorders are relevant to their central legal and ethical significance. The contingently increased risks (to the person themselves and to others) with which the psychotic disorders are associated mean that the stakes are high in man-aging them. A *laissez faire* attitude won't do. Decisions *have* to be made. But the 'loss of insight' by which delusions and related psychotic symp-toms are defined carries with it the implication that those concerned are not capable of making decisions for themselves in a fully autono-mous way. The following two cases illustrate the consequences of this for the status of psychotic disorders respectively as excusing conditions in law and as conditions justifying the use of involuntary psychiatric treatment.

Case 3: Not guilty by reason of insanity—Daniel McNaughton

On 20 January 1843 in the Charing Cross area of London, Daniel McNaughton was arrested by a police constable, James Silver, who witnessed him firing a pistol into the back of Edward Drummond who died a few days later. McNaughton was accordingly arraigned on a charge of murder. However, it soon transpired that McNaughton killed Drummond, the Prime Minister's Secretary, by mistake for the Prime Minister, under the delusion that the government was persecuting him. When he came to trial his coun-cil, Alexander Cockburn, argued that although McNaughton had indeed killed Drummond he was 'the victim of a fierce and fearful delusion, which, after the intellect has become diseased, the moral sense broken down, and self-control destroyed, has led him on to the perpetration of the crime with which he now stands charged'. The argument was successful. The jury found McNaughton 'not guilty, by reason of insanity' and instead of being hung as a murderer he was admitted as a patient to Bethlehem Hospital.

This vignette is based on a classic 19th-century case from which the eponymous McNaughton Rules defining the grounds for the 'insanity defence' in England are derived (8 ER 718, [1843] UKHL J16).[6] The vignette illustrates the intuitive link between delusion as the defining symptom of what we would now call a psychotic disorder and the legal intuition that disorders of this kind amount not merely to mitigating factors, such as 'guilty but under duress' but to a full-blown legal excuse as 'not guilty (at all) by reason of insanity'.

The 'insanity defence', as it is nowadays called, builds on a long history: the intuition that people who are insane are not responsible for their actions and hence that they are 'mad not bad' dates back to pre-classical times and is evident in a wide variety of both Western and non-Western cultures (Robinson 1996). A similar intuition underpins the central place of delusion-defined psychotic disorders in involuntary treatment.

Case 4: Justified involuntary psychiatric treatment—Mr AB, age 48, bank manager

Mr AB was brought into casualty by his wife complaining of head and facial pains. His wife, however, explained to the casualty officer that the reason she had persuaded her husband to come to casualty was because she believed he was becoming depressed. This was not the first time and she recognized the warning signs. When her husband gets depressed 'he always imagines he has some dreadful disease' and on one occasion he had made a sudden and nearly successful attempt to kill himself. Mr AB certainly looked depressed to the casualty officer although he denied this. On further questioning Mr AB said that 'there was no point in all this because he had a brain tumour and was dying'. After examining him carefully, the casualty officer explained to Mr AB that he had found no signs of a brain tumour but that he believed Mr AB was becoming depressed again and that he needed to be in hospital for a while so that they could go into everything properly. Mr AB reacted angrily to this saying that he had agreed to

---

6 Further accepted spellings include: McNaughten and M'Naughten (see West and Walk 1977).

come to casualty only so that he could get 'something stronger for the pain'. He remained adamant that he would not come into hospital and, given the clear risk of suicide, he was admitted as an involuntary patient under the Mental Health Act.

Most administrations around the world have legislation in place that allows people with mental disorders to be admitted to hospital and/or treated against their wishes if this is considered to be necessary in their own interests or for the protection of others. In contrast with the McNaughton rules and other similar criteria for the use of the insanity defence what is meant by mental disorder is generally left essentially undefined in legislation covering involuntary psychiatric treatment (Fulford and Hope 1996). Involuntary treatment could thus in principle be used for anyone with a mental disorder who presents a risk to themselves or others. In practice, though, as in Mr AB's case, the use of involuntary treatment is mainly restricted to the psychotic disorders (Sensky et al. 1991; Fulford and Hope 1994).

Challenge 1: the centrality of delusions
The first challenge presented by delusion for theories of autonomy is thus to address its autonomy-impairing nature consistently with its central legal/ethical and psychopathological significance as the characteristic symptom of psychotic mental disorders.

3.2.2 Autonomy and the centrality of delusions

Drawing on the preceding discussion of the insanity defence and theory and practice of involuntary psychiatric treatment, it is compelling to infer they both presuppose the idea that mental disorder in general and delusions in particular are forms of internal obstacles to autonomy.[7] In extremis, these obstacles lead to loss of autonomy, where an agent can no longer be treated as the source of at least some of his or her actions. This is particularly clear in the case of the insanity defence understood

---

[7] This notion builds on the distinction between internal and external obstacles to freedom which Feinberg (1980) sets apart from the distinction between positive and negative obstacles to freedom or obstacles to positive and negative freedom that was originally set out by Berlin (1958).

as grounds for full excuse rather than a mitigating factor. For, in order to make sense of this notion, we have to think of delusion-motivated behaviour as resulting in outcomes or states of affairs that are merely caused by a delusional agent but are not actions attributable to him or her (Davidson 1980).

The underlying intuition could be clarified with reference to Aristotle's account of voluntariness developed in the *Nicomachean Ethics* 3.1–5.[8] There, Aristotle contrasts voluntary actions not only with involuntary or coerced ones (external constraint to intentional agency), but also with non-voluntary actions which although initiated by the agent are not up to him or her (internal constraint to intentional agency). Examples are physiological processes, such as digestion that do not allow for direct volitional control. In contrast, Aristotle shows that choice not only offers unambiguous evidence for the voluntary character of an action but also has significance of its own for the appraisal of the agent's involvement. This suggestion opens up space for an important category of actions which are voluntary but not done out of choice. Instances of weakness of will offer the paradigm for this kind of behaviour within the original Aristotelian framework.

Following this line of thought, we are able to explain the distinction between compulsion- and addiction-motivated behaviours which could allow for mitigation but not full excuse, on the one hand, and on the other, delusion-motivated behaviours which as outlined earlier are eligible for full excuse (Watson 1999; Morse 2000). Whilst the former class of behaviours undermine intentional agency over time but are compatible with voluntary individual actions, the latter seem to exhibit a deeper mismatch between effective intentions and resulting actions which locates them at the margins of voluntariness and beyond.

The contrast with addiction and compulsion indicates that the centrality of delusions has to do with the idea of a breakdown of, rather than mere impediment to, intentional agency and confirms the initial account in terms of internal obstacles to autonomy. However, as soon

---

[8] For a discussion of this notion of voluntariness within the context of Aristotle's philosophy and its relevance to current debates in theory of action, see Radoilska (2007, pp. 153–290).

as we take into consideration the implicit social context of human action, it becomes apparent that the idea of delusions as internal obstacles to autonomy could provide a vehicle for oppression from outside. For it is open to misuse as a putative rationale for interventions limiting a person's negative freedom whilst at the same time concealing the restrictive or liberty-diminishing character of these interventions.[9] Berlin's critique of positive freedom illustrates well the underlying concern:

> The perils of using organic metaphors to justify the coercion of some men by others in order to raise them to a 'higher' level of freedom have often been pointed out. But what gives such plausibility as it has to this kind of language is that we recognise that it is possible, and at times justifiable, to coerce men in the name of some goal . . . This renders it easy for me to conceive of myself as coercing others for their own sake, in their, not my, interest. I am then claiming that I know what they truly need better than they know it themselves. What, at most, this entails is that they would not resist me if they were rational and as wise as I and understood their interests as I do. But I may go on to claim a good deal more than this. I may declare that they are actually aiming at what in their benighted state they consciously resist, because there exists within them an occult entity – their latent rational will, or their 'true' purpose – and that this entity, although it is belied by all that they overtly feel and do and say, is their 'real' self, of which the poor empirical self in space and time may know nothing or little; and that this inner spirit is the only self that deserves to have its wishes taken into account. Once I take this view, I am in a position to ignore the actual wishes of men or societies, to bully, oppress, torture them in the name, and on behalf, of their 'real' selves. (Berlin 1958, pp. 179–80)

This concern could provide a plausible motivation for attempts to define delusions as involving some form of cognitive impairment instead of a breakdown of intentional agency. As we note under the second challenge later, much empirical research effort has gone into attempts (thus far inconclusive) to identify one or more particular kinds of cognitive impairment specific to delusion. An account of delusions in terms of cognitive malfunctioning (if such were to prove possible) would apparently warrant the kind of theoretical independence from an implicit conception of autonomy brought up in the Introduction. In turn, this would arguably help construe a notion of

---

[9] See footnote 7. We return to this issue in Sections 3.3.2 and 3.4.2, with reference to the notions of objectivity as non-arbitrariness and agential success.

delusion as an internal obstacle to autonomy that is resistant to coercive uses like that identified in the earlier quotation from Berlin.

The appeal of this approach stems from a particular understanding of cognitive performances as objectively measurable and, in this respect, safer to assess than other aspects of the life of the mind, deemed to be merely subjective and, therefore, arbitrary. As we note in the next section, Anthony Flew (1973) relied on just this kind of supposed objectivity in his account of delusion as an excuse in law. However, even if we assume that this way of thinking about cognition is correct, it cannot help avoid the intuition that delusions are breakdowns of intentional agency. This becomes clear, if we take into consideration recent work in virtue epistemology the central claim of which is that knowledge is an apt, creditable performance (Zagzebski 2001; Greco 2003; Sosa 2007). This analysis clarifies and expands upon our ordinary intuitions, according to which cognitive tasks are something we do, a category of actions subject to appraisals to which mere physiological processes, such as digestion, are not. Following this line of thought, it is persuasive to interpret even the simplest cases of cognition where we merely 'get things right' as instances of intentional agency (Radoilska 2010). Therefore, even if delusions could be defined as cognitive failures, this would not get us away from the conclusion that they present breakdowns of intentional agency but merely specify where these breakdowns are likely to occur. At all events, the significance of intentional agency for understanding delusions becomes even clearer if we look in a little more detail at just what exactly delusions are. This brings us to our second challenge.

3.3 Challenge 2

3.3.1 The logical range of delusions

Textbook definitions of delusion often take them to be a particular kind of false belief. For instance, the *Encyclopedic Dictionary of Psychology* defines delusion as:

> A false belief, held despite evidence to the contrary, and one which is not explicable in terms of the patient's educational and cultural background. It is held with complete conviction and cannot be shaken by argument. (Harré and Lamb 1987, p. 142)

3.3.1.1 Delusion as false belief

This way of defining delusions certainly covers many instances. Here is an example from a person with schizophrenia, though similar delusions may occur in other psychotic disorders.

Case 5: Thought insertion in schizophrenia—Mr S, aged 18, student

Mr S was admitted as an emergency from the college where he was a student. The story was that he had been behaving in what his friends and tutors regarded as an increasingly odd way. He had started to accuse people of talking about him and had taken to wandering about the university playing fields on his own apparently talking to himself. He told the admitting doctor that people were getting at him. It was not anyone at the university, however. The problem was that Mike Yarwood (a well known popular entertainer at the time) was 'getting into' his thinking. Mr S became angry and tearful as he tried to describe this. 'My mind is not my own anymore. Thoughts come into my head but they are not my thoughts. It is this Mike Yarwood using my mind for his thinking. It's like I'm just a receiving station for his thoughts'.

To all appearances Mr S's belief that anyone could be using his mind for his thinking in this way is clearly false and as the standard definition further requires, it is a culturally atypical belief which (on further questioning) proved to be resistant to argument and appeals to evidence. The evident falsity of this and other delusions furthermore ties in with their legal and ethical significance as outlined under Challenge 1. For instance, Flew (1973) argued that the objective falsity of delusions is the one sure defence against the (ab)use of psychiatric authority for the sake of social control rather than medical treatment.

The problem, though, is that the standard definition although indeed covering some kinds of delusion is very far from covering them all. In the first place, many (perhaps most) delusions are not culturally atypical: delusions of guilt, for example as in Case 1 described earlier, are culturally consonant as are other common delusions (Mr AB's hypochondriacal delusion of brain cancer in Case 4 is a further example). Then again, the resistance to argument and appeals to evidence shown by delusions are features also of other strongly held but non-delusional beliefs (political and religious beliefs, for example). Worse still though, from the perspective of the standard definition, delusions may not even be false beliefs at all, at least not in the 'objectively false' sense required by Flew.

3.3.1.2 Delusion as true belief

Case 6: Othello syndrome—Mr A, age 47, publican

Mr A was seen by his GP initially because his wife was depressed. Mr A, however, had symptoms of his own: he complained of anxiety and impotence and his GP suspected that he was drinking far more than was good for him. Some way into the interview, Mr A suddenly announced that the real problem behind all his difficulties was that his wife was 'a tart'. Once started, he went on at length about her infidelity, drawing on a wide range of evidence, some of it bizarre (that she did her washing on a different day; that the pattern of cars parked in the street had changed). A subsequent psychiatric opinion confirmed the diagnosis of Othello syndrome. The Othello syndrome is defined by the presence of delusions of infidelity. Neither the GP nor the psychiatrist were in any doubt that Mr A had delusions of infidelity. Yet both knew at the time they made their diagnosis of Othello syndrome that Mrs A had become depressed following the break-up of an affair.

Notice then, that this is not a case of a delusion that turns out to be true as, for example, a patient with delusions of persecution who later turns out to have been persecuted. In Mr A's case the diagnosis of Othello syndrome based on delusions of infidelity was made notwithstanding the fact that those making the diagnosis were aware *at the time they made the diagnosis* that Mr A's beliefs far from being false were as to the essential fact true.

That delusions may be true beliefs in this sense was pointed out many years ago in a series of detailed case reports of cases of the Othello syndrome (Shepherd 1961). But the logical point that delusions are not essentially false beliefs as to matters of fact is shown perhaps even more decisively by the occasional variant of hypochondriacal delusion, the paradoxical delusion of mental illness.

3.3.1.3 Paradoxical delusion of mental illness

Case 7: Hypochondriacal delusion of mental illness—Mr MI, age 40, labourer

Mr MI was brought to casualty by ambulance following an overdose. He had tried to kill himself, he said, because he was mentally ill and people who are mentally ill get 'put away'. He was seen by an experienced duty psychiatrist who confirmed a diagnosis of hypochondriacal disorder with delusions of mental illness.

If delusions really were *essentially* false beliefs, then Mr MI's delusion of mental illness would be a belief that if false would be true and if true would be false. Mr MI's diagnosis would thus have been strictly undecidable. Yet there was no doubt about the diagnosis in the minds of those who saw Mr MI. Indeed so clear were they that he was deluded they would have treated him under the Mental Health Act had he not accepted ordinary reassurance that people who were mentally ill did not get 'put away' and was thus no longer considered to be at risk of suicide.

3.3.1.4 Delusions as value judgements

Cases of delusions as true beliefs are unusual (though no less conceptually significant for that). Mr MI's story is not a philosophical thought experiment but rather based on the story of a (biographically disguised) real patient. There is, though, a further kind of delusion that runs counter to the false belief of the standard definition and that is entirely commonplace, namely evaluative delusions (Fulford 1991). One example of such a delusion is the evaluative delusion of guilt. Delusions of guilt may take the form of beliefs as to matters of fact. We had an example of such a delusion with Mr SD in Case 1: Mr SD you will recall thought he was responsible for starting a war. But delusions of guilt may also take the form of value judgements.

Case 8: Delusions of guilt (negative evaluation)—Mr ED, age 40, postman

Mr ED was seen at a local psychiatric hospital on a Monday evening as an emergency admission from his GP. The story was that he had become increasingly depressed in the course of the preceding few weeks with a sudden deterioration in his condition over the weekend. The admitting doctor noted severely depressed affect and Mr ED's partner confirmed that he had been sleeping badly and had lost weight. When asked if anything particular had happened over the weekend Mr ED became tearful explaining that he had forgotten to give his children their pocket money. His partner confirmed that this was so but added that he seemed to have gone 'completely over the top about it'. He seemed to think that it was 'some terrible sin', 'going on about being useless as a dad', and, which really frightened her, saying that 'they would all be better off if he was dead'.

The delusional content of Mr ED's thinking in this case thus differs critically from that of Mr SD in Case 1. Mr SD (factual delusion) delusionally believed that he had caused a war and felt (justifiably) guilty as a consequence. Mr ED (evaluative delusion) had forgotten to give his children their pocket money and it was the way he evaluated this (as a deeply wicked sin, etc.) that was delusional.

Delusions may also take the form of positive value judgements, notably in hypomania (the elevated mood counterpart of depression). The following case illustrates how factual and evaluative delusions of grandeur may often be combined in this condition.

Case 9: Grandiose delusions (positive evaluation)—Miss HM, age 25, a novice nun

Miss HM was brought by two of her superiors for an urgent outpatient appointment. The story was that she had started to show bizarre and sexually disinhibited behaviour that was completely uncharacteristic of her and that they were unable to contain. She had not been sleeping. She showed pressure of speech (ideas rushing out one after the other) and became irritable when questioned about her behaviour. She was, she said, Mary Magdalene and was trying to do God's work. She also had 'all this poetry to write'. The nuns who came with her reported that she believed she was writing a great mystical text but that her poetry, although showing some imaginative 'flashes', was rambling and largely incoherent.

3.3.1.5 Different logic, same practice

The gap between the standard definition of delusion as a false belief and the actual range of logical forms of delusion that we find in practice could thus hardly be more dramatic. Delusions as our examples illustrate may certainly take the form of false beliefs; but they may also take the form of true beliefs; and they may not be beliefs at all at least as to matters of fact, but value judgements, negative and/or positive in sign. Delusional value judgements furthermore unlike delusional true beliefs are as we have indicated entirely commonplace. And there is a further twist to the story here in the fact that all these different kinds of delusion have the *same implications for practice*. A delusion is a delusion as it were, regardless of its logical form, when it comes to treatment (Fulford 1989, chapter 10). This extends to the legal and ethical significance of delusions. Mr SD (Case 1), for example, with his factual delusions of guilt and Mr ED (Case 8) with his evaluative delusions of guilt would have been equally eligible to have been treated as involuntary patients.

Faced with these difficulties with the standard definition some have sought to define delusion not as a false but as an unfounded belief.[10] This approach, however, begs the question 'in what sense are delusions unfounded?'. Clearly it is right that in some sense delusional beliefs being irrational beliefs are unfounded beliefs. This is at the heart of the ethical and legal as well as psychopathological significance of delusions. But people with delusions may reason intellectually at a very high level and despite some promising early results and credible ideas for certain kinds of delusion, no disturbances of cognitive functioning unique to and covering the full range of delusions has yet been identified.[11] We come back then to the question we raised at the end of Challenge 1 as to the precise sense in which psychotic disorders disturb intentional agency over time, but now with the added challenge of accommodating the full range of logical forms of delusion.

Challenge 2: The logical range of delusions
Delusions may take the form of true or false factual beliefs, of positive or negative evaluations, and of the paradoxical delusion of mental illness. The second challenge for theories of autonomy is thus to take

---

[10] For example, Gelder et al. (2001, p. 13) define delusion as 'a belief that is firmly held on inadequate grounds, is not affected by rational argument or evidence to the contrary, and is not a conventional belief that the person might be expected to hold given his educational and cultural background'. The authors go on to spell out some of the problems with this definition including the fact that delusions may occasionally not be false beliefs.

[11] Jolley and Garety (2004) reviews recent psychological theories of delusion including motivational and perceptual as well as cognitive approaches. Martin Davies, Max Coltheart, and others (e.g. Davies and Coltheart 2000; Davies et al. 2001) have developed fruitful cross-disciplinary approaches to some of the monothematic delusions such as the Capgras syndrome (the delusion of doubles).

into account this logical range consistently with the status of delusion as the paradigm case of autonomy-impairing mental disorder.

3.3.2 Autonomy and the logical range of delusions

The diverse logical types of delusions pose a problem for accounts of delusions in terms of objective falsehood and resistance to facts. Such accounts could be seen as a follow-up of the attempts to confine delusions to problems with cognitive functioning in order to avoid subjectivity. However, the variety of delusions covering both factual inaccuracies and evaluative distortions puts into question the effectiveness of this follow-up strategy.[12] For it would be able to account only for the former but not the latter cluster of delusions. This is essentially why Fulford (1989), pointing to the parallel between the logical range of delusions and the corresponding logical range of reasons for action, argued for an agentic rather than narrowly cognitivist account of delusions.[13]

We can take this argument still further though in recognizing that leaving aside evaluative delusions, even some instances of the latter, factual type of delusion may be difficult to accommodate to an 'objective falsehood' account. Examples include cases, such as the Othello syndrome (Case 6) where a delusion is known to be true by those making the diagnosis. This kind of delusion is similar to Gettier cases of true justified belief that nevertheless does not amount to knowledge, to the extent that in order to explain what goes wrong in both instances, we need to tap into richer conceptual resources than the notion of facts or objective reality as being 'out there' independently of our epistemic endeavours (Gettier 1963; Zagzebski and Fairweather 2001). As indicated in the previous section, virtue epistemology offers the required conceptual resources; however, they lead to re-interpreting cognitive functioning in terms of intentional agency, an outcome that the accounts of delusions at issue apparently aim to avoid.

---

[12] A related point has been made by Richard Gipps in Gipps and Fulford (2004).

[13] Thus, the reasons we (as agents) give for our actions mirror the logical range of delusions in taking the forms respectively of factual beliefs (true or false) and of value judgements (positive or negative). The parallels here are set out in Fulford (1989, chapter 10).

Where does this leave us with respect to concerns about the coercive potential of an account of delusions in terms of inner obstacles to autonomy? In fact, the diversity of delusions may not be bad news about objectivity, understood as non-arbitrary application of the concept. As pointed out in the context of Challenge 1, the interest of confining delusions to instances of cognitive malfunctioning comes from the prospect of avoiding arbitrariness in defining what counts as a delusion. For arbitrariness could easily lead to employing redress of internal obstacles to autonomy as pretence for introducing external obstacles to it.

This valid concern seems misinterpreted by approaches which present delusions as involving objective falsehood and resistance to facts as opposed to subjective viewpoint and evaluative judgement. The root of the problem is that these approaches do not deliver objectivity as non-arbitrariness which is at the heart of the valid concern about coercion but go after a different kind of objectivity that turns out to be both superfluous and unfit for the task, namely, objectivity as mind-independence. For the sake of clarity, this critical point will be broken down into constitutive steps:

1 It is possible to first merge the two conceptual pairs 'objectivity–subjectivity' and 'fact–value' into one, and then redefine the poles of the resulting pair as mutually exclusive, only if it is assumed that objectivity means mind-independence. This is because on alternative conceptions of objectivity, such as non-arbitrariness the expression 'objective value' is not an oxymoron and the predicates 'subjective' and 'objective' could be compatible.[14]

2 Accounts of delusions in terms of objective falsehood and resistance to facts do take objectivity and facts to be on the same side of a conceptual gap, on the other side of which are located subjectivity and values.

3 Hence, these accounts are committed to a conception of objectivity as mind-independence.

4 This conception of objectivity implies that values are by their very nature outside the realm of objectivity for they do not partake in the

---

[14] A more detailed discussion of this point can be found in Radoilska (2007, pp. 39–57). See also Langton (2007); Railton (1995) and Wiggins (1995).

'fabric of the world' (Mackie 1977). Instead, it is up to us to endorse or reject any particular values. Hence, they are bound to remain arbitrary.

5 Another direct implication of defining objectivity as mind-independence is that along with values, mental states as such also fall outside the realm of objectivity. They only make a proper subject of inquiry in so far as they are stripped from their subjectivity and reduced down to underlying physiological processes, which are part of the 'fabric of the world'.

6 As argued earlier, the task that a quest for objectivity in defining delusions is meant to fulfil is to identify non-arbitrary criteria for the application of this concept. Accounts in terms of objective falsehood and resistance to facts fail to carry out this task. What is more, they implicitly deny its possibility. This is because they posit delusions as objectively inexplicable over and above the cognitive or other physiological malfunctioning that delusions may involve. In other words, by substituting the ideal of objectivity as non-arbitrariness with that of objectivity as mind-independence, some accounts of delusion deprive themselves of means to investigate the putative breakdowns of intentional agency which are central aspect of the phenomenology of delusions. For such accounts end up obfuscating the very idea of intentional agency.[15]

An important consequence of this analysis is the acknowledgement that the logical diversity of delusions does not pose a greater challenge to our systematic thinking because some delusions have evaluative rather than factual content. For, as outlined earlier, either would be just as mysterious if we opt out of the vernacular of intentional agency.

3.4 Challenge 3

3.4.1 Non-pathological delusions

From everything that we have said under Challenges 1 and 2 it may seem that this third challenge involves a contradiction in terms. How it

---

[15] See Chapter 2, this volume, in which Alfred Mele addresses a related confusion in some neuroscience-based arguments for the nonexistence of free will.

may be said can delusions be, on the one hand, constitutive of the paradigmatically autonomy-impairing psychotic mental disorders, and, on the other hand, *non*-pathological? We will return to 'how?' later. First, as in earlier sections, we will start by letting the stories of real people (one particular person in this instance) speak for themselves.

Case 10 (Part I): Primary delusions—Simon, aged 40, lawyer

Simon was a senior, black, American lawyer from a middle-class, Baptist family. Although not a religious man he had had occasional relatively minor psychic experiences that had led him from time to time to seek the guidance of a professional 'seer'. Otherwise his career and life generally were going well.

Then, out of the blue, he was threatened by a malpractice legal action from a group of his colleagues. Although he claimed to be innocent, mounting a defence would be expensive and hazardous. He responded to this crisis by praying in front of an open bible placed on a small altar that he set up in his front room. After an emotional evening's 'outpouring' he found that wax from two large candles on the altar had run down onto the bible marking out various words and phrases (he called these wax marks 'seals' or 'suns'). He described his experiences thus. 'I got up and I saw the seal that was in my father's bible and I called my friend John and I said, you know, "something remarkable is going on over here". I think the beauty of it was the specificity by which the sun burned through. It was . . . in my mind, a clever play on words'.

From this time on, Simon received a complex series of 'revelations' largely conveyed through the images left in melted candle wax. They meant nothing to anyone else including Simon's Baptist friends and family. But for Simon they were clearly representations of biblical symbols particularly from the book of Revelations (the bull, the 24 elders, the arc of the covenant, etc.) signifying that 'I am the living son of David . . . and I'm also a relative of Ishmael and . . . of Joseph'. He was also the 'captain of the guard of Israel'. He found this role carried awesome responsibilities: 'Sometimes I'm saying "O my God, why did you choose me", and there's no answer to that'. His special status had the effect of 'increasing my own inward sense, wisdom, understanding, and endurance' which would 'allow me to do whatever is required in terms of bringing whatever message it is that God wants me to bring'. When confronted with scepticism, he said simply: 'I don't get upset, because I know within myself, what I know'.

Simon's story is one of a number of similar accounts collected by Mike Jackson in a study of the differences between psychosis and spiritual experience (Jackson 1997; Jackson and Fulford 1997). So what should we make of Simon's experiences? Are they delusional?

One way to answer this question is by reference to psychiatry's standard diagnostic tools. Among these, the PSE (Present State Examination) provides a carefully developed diagnostic schedule for identifying key psychiatric symptoms (Wing et al. 1974). The PSE covers over a hundred such symptoms including a wide variety of delusions. Among these we find what is called a 'primary delusion' the description of which fits Simon's case like a glove. The PSE defines this as a delusion which is:

> Based upon sensory experiences (delusional perceptions) [Simon's wax seals in this case] in which a patient suddenly becomes convinced that a particular set of events has a special meaning. (Wing et al. 1974, pp. 172–73)

Simon therefore according to best practice in psychiatric diagnosis has a primary delusion. But delusions, as we indicated earlier, are the constitutive symptoms of psychotic mental disorders. Correspondingly then, when we turn to the World Health Organization's International Classification of Diseases (ICD), we find that such delusions persisting, as in Simon's case, for longer than a month are sufficient for a diagnosis of a psychotic disorder, including schizophrenia, hypomania, etc. (1992, p. 88).

QED, then, you may think. But this is where our third challenge bites. For Simon showed no signs of being ill, still less of suffering from a severe psychotic illness.

Case 10 (part II): Non-delusional primary delusions?

Simon's 'seals' as we indicated empowered him. But more than this they guided him first to take on his accusers and then over how to run his case (as a lawyer he defended himself). To cut a long story short, the result was that he won his case (it was shown to be a racially motivated attempt to undermine his growing practice), his reputation as a lawyer was further enhanced, he went on to make a great deal of money, and when last heard of was setting up a trust fund to support research not on schizophrenia but on religious experience.

Presented with the outcomes of Simon's story, psychiatrists (and others) have a split reaction. Some insist that Simon's story should be understood as an illness, albeit one that in his case ran an unusually benign course. Others take Simon's story at face value (and as Simon himself took it) as a story of religious (if idiosyncratic) experience. Both interpretations are possible. As to the illness interpretation, Simon would have strongly rejected the idea that his experiences, which were so formative in his life, should be written off as some kind of pathology, however 'benign'. Such a rejection, though, of there being 'something (mentally) wrong', is, you will recall from Challenge 1, fully consistent with the 'loss of insight' by which delusions are characterized.

As to the religious experience interpretation of Simon's story on the other hand, there is support for this from a perhaps surprising quarter, the main competitor to the ICD diagnostic classification, the American Psychiatric Association's Diagnostic and Statistical Manual (2000). The DSM, as it is called, is closely similar to the ICD in the symptoms, including primary delusions that it takes to be diagnostically significant. But the DSM differs from the ICD in requiring in addition to symptomatic criteria for psychiatric diagnosis what it calls 'criteria of clinical significance'. Simon in experiencing primary delusions satisfies the DSM's symptomatic criteria for a diagnosis of schizophrenia or other psychotic disorder just as he does the corresponding criteria in the ICD. But it turns out that he fails to satisfy the DSM's additional criterion of clinical significance. The so-called Criterion B for schizophrenia reads as follows:

> Social/occupational dysfunction: For a significant portion of the time since the onset of the disturbance, one or more major areas of functioning such as work, interpersonal relations, or self-care are markedly below the level achieved prior to the onset. (American Psychiatric Association 2000, p. 285)

Criterion B then, is as it says a criterion of 'social/occupational dysfunction'. For a diagnosis of schizophrenia in the DSM Simon must show not only primary delusions or other relevant symptoms but also deterioration in his social and/or occupational functioning. His story is silent on his social functioning. But it is clear that his occupational functioning far from deteriorating was actually enhanced.

3.4.1.1 Delusions normal and pathological

How should this be understood? With Challenges 1 and 2 we set up delusion as the constitutive symptom of the paradigmatically autonomy-impairing psychotic mental disorders. Challenge 3 now suggests that delusions although indeed sometimes symptoms of mental disorder may at other times not be pathological at all. This suggestion moreover comes not from a critique of delusion that is external to psychiatry but from the story of a real person (biographically disguised as Simon) interpreted through one of psychiatry's most influential diagnostic manuals, the DSM.

Simon's story is not a one-off exception that proves the rule. It is, as we said earlier, one of a series of similar stories collected originally by Mike Jackson. Jackson and others have subsequently carried out wider epidemiological studies confirming that non-pathological psychotic experiences are widespread in the general population (Jackson 1997; Johns and Van Os 2001). The British Psychological Society has indeed gone on to publish a platform statement arguing that psychotic experiences as such should be regarded as the basis of a problem solving capacity (2000). There are perhaps resonances here of traditionally recognized links between madness and creativity (Jamison 1993). To be clear, there is no suggestion that psychotic disorders are a fiction. Like any other capacity, the capacity for psychotic experience may sometimes 'go wrong'. But there is no necessity here, contingent or analytic. Delusions and other psychotic experiences for all their significance as symptoms of mental disorder may also be not only normal but positively life enhancing.

Challenge 3: Non-pathological delusions
The third challenge for philosophical theories of autonomy is thus to clarify how pathological (autonomy-impairing) delusions are different from non-pathological (autonomy-preserving) delusions.

3.4.2 Autonomy and non-pathological delusions

Non-pathological delusions offer a critical perspective onto the first two challenges which build upon the idea that there is a strong link between delusions and different kinds of breakdowns of intentional agency. In particular, they prompt us to look again into the notion of internal obstacle to autonomy we introduced earlier. This is not to say that in so far as delusions turn out to be beneficial for a person, they cannot present internal obstacles to his or her autonomy. For good luck is compatible with a breakdown of intentional agency.

This becomes clear if we consider a thought experiment set out by Linda Zagzebski (2001) in which a benign manipulator ensures that a prospective knower believes only truths. In this scenario, the manipulator monitors the belief formation of the manipulated agent and intervenes, unbeknown to her, only if she is on the verge of acquiring a false belief. The prospective knower ends up holding only true beliefs. Yet, her epistemic agency is undermined by the implicit manipulation of her reasoning. Hence, fortunate end results could be brought about by internal obstacles to intentional agency.[16]

In light of these observations, it is more promising to interpret the challenge from non-pathological delusions as an indication that there is an implicit success criterion at work in the previous two challenges and in particular that effective intentional agency over time is the reference point when defining what goes wrong with delusions. Having ruled out cases in which things just happen to work out well for delusional agents, it is important to clarify whether an underlying success criterion adds to the legitimate concerns about coercion we identified earlier or, on the contrary, could help to address them. Practically, it may be thought, a sufficient response to any concerns raised by the recognition of an implicit success criterion is the development of more effective ways of balancing complex and conflicting values in decision making (as in the model of values-based practice[17]). But the very effectiveness of this practical move in turn points us back to the need for a more robust theoretical understanding of how values come in to judgements of autonomy if we are to avoid it being used for abusive ends. The following discussion will not aim to provide anything in the way of a comprehensive theory but rather to identify and briefly comment upon three prima facie plausible interpretations of the agential success which seems to distinguish non-pathological delusions from pathological ones: conventionalist, particularist, and universalist.

As its name suggests, the first alternative proposes to construe agential success in conventional terms. To put it crudely, an agent is successful on this view in so far as he or she manages to secure the kind of goods that are generally considered as enviable by his or her society or

---

[16] This point is developed in more detail in Radoilska (2010).

[17] See, for example, Fulford (1994), Woodbridge and Fulford (2004), and Fulford et al., (2012) on values-based practice.

social group. This interpretation is consistent both with a notion of mental disorder as involving significant impairment of social or occupational functioning and diagnostic guidelines advising to pay particular attention to the cultural backgrounds of prospective psychiatric patients. The plausibility of a conventionalist approach to agential success in the context of delusions stems from its ability to provide an additional perspective onto putative clinical cases. The thought is that this extra viewpoint could act as a corrective to potentially coercive applications of clinical authority in deciding which delusions are pathological. However, the conventionalist interpretation leaves unattended concerns about societal rather than medical arbitrariness in defining mental disorder. In doing so, a conventionalist understanding of agential success may offer a platform for the resentment of majorities by inadvertently allowing them to discredit unpopular conceptions of the good and penalize dissenters. That this is no merely theoretical possibility is indicated by for example attributions of mental disorder to political dissidents on the basis of 'delusions of reconstruction' in the former USSR (Fulford et al. 1993).

The second, particularist interpretation of agential success could be seen as an improvement on the latter issue. This is because the success criterion it employs is the set of goals that an agent endorses, independently of the ways in which the projects at issue are seen from an observer's perspective. This would be closer to Simon's case. However, both the appeal and the limitations of the particularist approach stem from an instrumental conception of practical rationality, with its strict distinction between facts and values, means and ends (Foot 1972).[18] Like accounts of delusions in terms of objective falsehood and resistance to facts, the particularist interpretation locates the relevant questions about intentional agency at the level of beliefs and handling of evidence. The crucial question however is not whether they reflect correctly an external reality conceived as independent of the human mind. What matters instead is whether an agent's set of beliefs and overall reasoning promote rather than impede the pursuit of objectives

---

[18] See also Radoilska (2007, pp. 109–28) for a critical analysis.

he or she has set for him or herself. An apparent advantage of the particularist interpretation is that the notion of internal obstacle of autonomy becomes directly linked to a fist-person perspective.[19] This could be seen as a reliable barrier to coercive uses of this notion aiming to impose a third-personal perspective on delusional experiences as ultimately authoritative. However, this advantage comes at a rather unexpected price: the final ends of action are assigned beyond the confines of practical rationality. In this sense, they are made irrelevant to ascertaining either agential success or possible breakdowns of intentional agency. For these ought to be conceived in purely executive as opposed to evaluative terms[20] in order to forestall coercive uses of the notion of internal obstacle to autonomy as specified by the particularist strategy. The distinction between the two kinds of failures of intentional agency is helpfully brought out by the following illustration:

> There is no doubt but that there are different kinds of cases of contrary-to reasonness, and not surprisingly it is possible to contravene rationality in more than one way at the same time. I once read of a burglar who was caught because he sat down to watch television in the house he was burgling, thus adding the contrary-to-reasonness of imprudence to that of dishonesty. Because his actions were faulty in that he did not hurry away with the swag, we can say, if we like, that he should have done so. (Foot 1995, p. 7)

The particularist interpretation of agential success considers as problematic only the 'contrary-to-reasonness' due to imprudence or in terms of the distinction we introduced earlier executive rather than evaluative failures of intentional agency. As pointed out at the start of the discussion, this may be considered as an advantage for the particularist strategy since it rules out a moralized account of agential success. In doing so, it seems to avoid the danger of facilitating external obstacles to autonomy under the guise of redressing internal ones. Unfortunately, there is good reason to doubt that this danger has been avoided. By choosing to treat the ultimate ends of action as tangential

---

[19] On the significance of distinguishing first-personal from third-personal considerations about autonomy, see Chapter 9, this volume, by Hallvard Lillehammer.

[20] This contrast draws on the distinction between executive and evaluative practical commitment introduced by Mele (1995, p. 71).

to a person's success as an agent, the particularist interpretation becomes unable to track down a central case of obstacle to autonomy which has external origins but internal manifestation: the internalization of oppressive social norms (Stoljar 2000). The underlying worry is that by focusing merely on how an agent carries out his or her plans the particularist interpretation lets inappropriate influences in the formation of these plans to slip under the radar. Yet these kinds of influences grossly undermine a person's intentional agency, for the affected plans are not up to him or her in the required sense for voluntariness as spelt out in the context of Challenge 1.

The third, universalist interpretation is in a position to address not only executive, but also evaluative obstacles to autonomy. This is because it conceives agential success as a twofold achievement: not only is an agent's plan brought to fruition, the plan itself also has to be worth undertaking in a sense that cannot be fully reduced to the agent's endorsement. However, the latter requirement seems open to the objection that it peddles a moralized view of intentional agency and could easily serve the purposes of coercion. For if agential success applies to instances where the ends of action are worthwhile, not merely effectively implemented, a third-person or observer's perspective becomes as important as the first-person or agent's perspective.

A possible way of addressing this worry is to impose stringent conditions on the kinds of third-personal considerations that could be given such weight. For instance, it is plausible to argue that non-arbitrary third-personal considerations about agential success should stop at the formal as opposed to substantive features of the plans under consideration. The idea is to be able to locate unobvious obstacles to autonomy, such as self-loathing and related effects of internalized oppression, and to make sure that the plans the agent pursues are sufficiently up to him or her in order to qualify as voluntary. Yet, the underlying theoretical objective cannot be achieved unless the features of a plan for action yield themselves to a neat distinction to formal, on the one hand, and substantive, on the other. In light of our earlier observations about fact and value, and means and ends, there is good reason to doubt that this strategy would be entirely successful. For the kind of voluntariness implicit in the notion of a plan being up to the agent may not be easily separable from a notion of reasonableness. This becomes clear if we take into consideration an intuitive test for discovering whether a particular option has been freely chosen or imposed. In this respect, the inherent choiceworthiness of the option offers just as valuable an indication as the availability of possible alternatives. This outcome sends us back to the initial concern about non-arbitrariness in defining both agential success and possible breakdowns of intentional agency.

3.5 Concluding remarks

The three challenges that we identified and explored in this chapter point to an inescapable yet elusive association between delusions on the one hand and various kinds of breakdowns of intentional agency on the other. In particular, the centrality of delusions helped clarify both the appeal and the coercive potential of thinking about delusions in terms of internal obstacles to autonomy, in the presence of which an action is no longer up to the agent but merely caused by him or her. In turn, the parallel between the logical diversity of delusions and the corresponding logical diversity of reasons for action led us to the need to distinguish between two separate conceptions of objectivity that may be at work in existing accounts of delusions. This distinction is significant, for it suggests that the difficulty in defining delusions is not due to the evaluative as opposed to factual content of some delusions but to a potentially misleading conception of objectivity as mind-independence. Finally, non-pathological instances of delusions enabled us to put a spotlight on a success condition that is implicit in the notion of a breakdown of intentional agency. Yet, none of the three initially plausible interpretations of agential success that we looked into could satisfy the legitimate ideal of objectivity as non-arbitrariness that emerged from the discussion. This outcome is not entirely aporetic as it opens up a promising line of inquiry for clarifying putative breakdowns of intentional agency within a viable objectivity conception. Such a line of inquiry would both draw critically on the features of delusion and, in turn through such initiatives as values-based practice aim to inform policy and practice relative to this most challenging symptom of mental disorder.

Acknowledgements

Case 3 (Daniel McNaughton) is based on *R v McNaughton* [1843] 4 St Pr 847, 8 ER 718 and West and Walk (1977), and Case 10 (Simon) is based on case materials collected by Jackson (1997). The remaining cases, including Case 7 (paradoxical delusion of mental illness) are adapted from examples published in various forms in Fulford (1989, 1991, 1996, 1998). More detailed accounts of these and other forms of psychopathology, including first personal accounts together with detailed reading guides and philosophical annotations (provided by Richard Gipps) are given in chapter 3 'Experiences good and bad: an introduction to psychopathology, classification, and diagnosis for philosophers' of *The Oxford Textbook of Philosophy and Psychiatry* by Fulford et al. (2006).

References

Amador, X.F. and David, A.S. (eds.) (2004) *Insight and Psychosis* (2nd edn.). Oxford: Oxford University Press.

American Psychiatric Association. (2000) *Diagnostic and Statistical Manual of Mental Disorders. Fourth Edition with Text Revision.* Washington, DC: American Psychiatric Association.

Aristotle. (1995). *Nicomachean Ethics.* In J. Barnes (ed.). *The Complete Works of Aristotle.* Vol. 2. Princeton, NJ: Princeton University Press; pp. 1729–867.

Berlin, I. (1958). Two concepts of liberty. In Berlin, I. *Liberty* (Hardy, H. ed. 2002). Oxford: Oxford University Press, pp. 166–217.

Bratman, M. (2007). *Structures of Agency.* Oxford: Oxford University Press.

British Psychological Society. (2000) *Recent Advances in Understanding Mental Illness and Psychotic Experiences.* Leicester: The British Psychological Society, Division of Clinical Psychology.

Buss, S. (2008). Personal autonomy. In E.N. Zalta (ed.) *The Stanford Encyclopedia of Philosophy* (Winter 2008 Edition) [Online] http://plato.stanford.edu/entries/personal-autonomy/

Davidson, D. (1980). Freedom to act. Reproduced in Davidson, D. (2001). *Essays on Actions and Events.* Oxford: Clarendon Press, pp. 63–81.

Davies, M., Coltheart, M., Langdon, R., and Breen, N., (2001) Monothematic delusions: Towards a two-factor account. *Philosophy, Psychiatry, & Psychology* 8(2/3): 133–58.

Davies, M. and Coltheart, M. (2000) Introduction: pathologies of belief. In M. Coltheart and M. Davies (eds) *Pathologies of Belief.* Oxford: Blackwell, pp. 1–46.

Feinberg, J. (1980). The idea of a free man. In *Rights, Justice and the Bounds of Liberty: Essays in Social Philosophy.* Princeton, NJ: Princeton University Press, pp. 3–29.

Flew, A. (1973) *Crime or Disease?* New York: Barnes and Noble.

Foot, P. (1972). Morality as a system of hypothetical imperatives. *Philosophical Review* 81: 305–16.

Foot, P. (1995). Does moral subjectivism rest on a mistake? *Oxford Journal of Legal Studies* 15(1): 1–14.

Frankfurt, H. (1971). Freedom of the will and the concept of a person. *Journal of Philosophy* 68(1): 5–20.

Fulford, K.W.M. (1989) *Moral Theory and Medical Practice.* Cambridge: Cambridge University Press (later editions 1995; 1999).

Fulford, K.W.M. (1991) Evaluative delusions: their significance for philosophy and psychiatry. *British Journal of Psychiatry* 159: 108–112 (Suppl. 14: Delusions and Awareness of Reality).

Fulford, K.W.M. (1996) Value, illness and action: delusions in the new philosophical psychopathology. In G. Graham and G.L. Stephens (eds.) *Philosophical Psychopathology* Cambridge, MA: MIT Press.

Fulford, K.W.M. (1998) Completing Kraepelin's psychopathology: insight, delusion and the phenomenology of illness. In X.F. Amador and A.S. David (eds.) *Insight and Psychosis* (2nd edn.). Oxford: Oxford University Press.

Fulford, K.W.M. (2004) Ten principles of values-based medicine. In J. Radden (ed.) *The Philosophy of Psychiatry: A Companion.* New York: Oxford University Press, pp. 205–34.

Fulford, K.W.M. and Hope, R.A. (1994) Psychiatric ethics: a bioethical ugly duckling? In R. Gillon and A. Lloyd (eds.) *Principles of Health Care Ethics.* Chichester: Wiley, pp. 681–95.

Fulford, K.W.M. and Hope, T. (1996) Control and practical experience. In H.-G. Koch, S. Reiter-Theil, and H. Helmchen (eds.) *Informed Consent in Psychiatry: European Perspectives on Ethics, Law and Clinical Practice.* Baden-Baden: Nomos, pp. 349–77.

Fulford, K.W.M., Peile, E.P., and Carroll, H. (2012). *Essentials of Values-based Practice: Clinical Stories Linking Science with People.* Cambridge: Cambridge University Press.

Fulford, K.W.M., Smirnov, A.Y.U., and Snow, E. (1993) Concepts of disease and the abuse of psychiatry in the USSR. *British Journal of Psychiatry* 162: 801–10.

Fulford, K.W.M., Thornton, T., and Graham, G. (2006). *The Oxford Textbook of Philosophy and Psychiatry.* Oxford: Oxford University Press.

Gelder, M., Mayou, R., and Cowen, P. (2001) *Shorter Oxford Textbook of Psychiatry* (4th edn.) Oxford: Oxford University Press.

Gettier, E. (1963). Is justified true belied knowledge? *Analysis* 23: 121–23.

Gipps, R.G.T. and Fulford, K.W.M. (2004) Understanding the clinical concept of delusion: from an estranged to an engaged epistemology. In M.R. Broome and P. Bebbington (eds.) *International Review of Psychiatry: Special Issue on the Philosophy of Psychiatry* 16(3): 225–35.

Greco, J. (2003). Knowledge as credit for true belief. In M. DePaul and L. Zagzebski (eds.) *Intellectual Virtue: Perspectives from Ethics and Epistemology*. Oxford: Clarendon Press, pp. 111–34.

Harré, R. and Lamb, R. (eds.) (1987). *The Encyclopedic Dictionary of Psychology*. Oxford: Blackwell.

Hill, T.E. (1991). *Autonomy and Self-Respect*. Cambridge: Cambridge University Press.

Jackson, M.C. (1997) Benign schizotypy? The case of spiritual experience. In G.S. Claridge (ed.) *Schizotypy: Relations to Illness and Health*. Oxford: Oxford University Press, pp. 227–50.

Jackson, M. and Fulford, K.W.M. (1997). Spiritual experience and psychopathology. *Philosophy, Psychiatry, & Psychology* 4(1): 4–66.

Jamison, K.R. (1993). *Touched With Fire: Manic Depressive Illness and the Artistic Temperament*. New York: Free Press Paperbacks.

Johns, L.C. and van Os, J. (2001) The continuity of psychotic experiences in the general population. *Clinical Psychology Review* 21(8): 1125–41.

Jolley, S. and Garety, P.A. (2004) Insight and delusions. In X.F. Amador and A.S. David (eds.) *Insight and Psychosis* (2nd edn.). Oxford: Oxford University Press, pp. 89–100.

Langton, R. (2007). Objective and unconditioned value. *Philosophical Review* 116(2): 157–85.

Lewis, A.J. (1934) The psychopathology of insight. *British Journal of Medical Psychology* 14: 332–48.

Mackenzie, C. and Stoljar, N. (eds.) (2000). *Relational Autonomy: Feminist Perspectives on Autonomy, Agency and the Social Self*. New York: Oxford University Press.

Mackie, J.L. (1977). *Ethics: Inventing Right and Wrong*. New York: Harmondsworth, Penguin.

Mele, A. (1995). *Autonomous Agents*. New York: Oxford University Press.

Morse, S. (2000). Hooked on hype: addiction and responsibility. *Law and Philosophy* 19(1): 3–49.

Perkins, R. and Moodley, P. (1993) The arrogance of insight. *Psychiatric Bulletin* 17: 233–34.

Radoilska, L. (2007). *L'Actualité d'Aristote en morale*. Paris: Presses Universitaires de France.

Radoilska, L. (2010). An Aristotelian approach to cognitive enhancement. *Journal of Value Inquiry* 44: 365–75.

Railton, P. (1995). Subject-ive and Objective. *Ratio* 8(3): 259–76.

Robinson, D. (1996). *Wild Beasts and Idle Humours*. Cambridge, MA: Harvard University Press.

Sensky, T., Hughes, T., and Hirsch, S. (1991). Compulsory psychiatric treatment in the community, Part 1: A Controlled study of compulsory community treatment with extended leave under the mental health act: special characteristics of patients treated and impact of treatment, *British Journal of Psychiatry* 158: 792.

Shepherd, M. (1961). Morbid jealousy: some clinical and social aspects of a psychiatric syndrome, *Journal of Mental Science* 107: 687–704.

Sosa, E. (2007) *A Virtue Epistemology. Vol. 1: Apt Belief and Reflective Knowledge.* Oxford: Clarendon Press.

Stoljar, N. (2000). Autonomy and the feminist intuition. In C. Mackenzie and N. Stoljar (eds.) *Relational Autonomy: Feminist Perspectives on Autonomy, Agency and the Social Self.* New York: Oxford University Press, pp. 94–111.

Watson, G. (1975). Free agency. *Journal of Philosophy* 72(8): 205–20.

Watson, G. (1999). Excusing addiction. *Law and Philosophy* 18: 589–619.

West, D.J. and Walk, A. (1977). *Daniel McNaughton: his Trial and the Aftermath.* London: Gaskell Books.

Wiggins, D. (1995). Objective and subjective in ethics with two postscripts about truth. *Ratio* 8(3): 243–58.

Wing, J.K., Cooper, J.E., and Sartorius, N. (1974) *Measurement and Classification of Psychiatric Symptoms.* Cambridge: Cambridge University Press.

Wolf, S. (1987). Sanity and the metaphysics of responsibility. Reprinted in Watson, G. (ed.) (2003). *Free Will.* Oxford: Oxford University Press, pp. 372–87.

Woodbridge, K. and Fulford, K.W.M. (2004) *'Whose Values?' A Workbook for Values-Based Practice in Mental Health Care.* London: The Sainsbury Centre for Mental Health.

World Health Organization (1992) *The ICD-10 Classification of Mental and Behavioural Disorders: Clinical Descriptions and Diagnostic Guidelines.* Geneva: World Health Organization.

Zagzebski, L. (2001). Must knowers be agents? In A. Fairweather and L. Zagzebski (eds.) *Virtue Epistemology: Essays on Epistemic Virtue and Responsibility.* Oxford: Oxford University Press, pp. 149–52.

Zagzebski, L. and Fairweather, A. (2001). Introduction. In A. Fairweather and L. Zagzebski (eds.) *Virtue Epistemology: Essays on Epistemic Virtue and Responsibility.* Oxford: Oxford University Press, pp. 3–15.

Part II

Autonomy in light of mental disorder

Chapter 4

Does mental disorder involve loss of personal autonomy?

Derek Bolton and Natalie Banner

4.1 Introduction: mental disorder and the meanings of autonomy

The problem of defining mental disorder has long vexed philosophers and psychiatrists keen to distinguish conditions warranting healthcare from those variations and eccentricities of human experience that, whilst negative, are considered normal and not illness. Two broad approaches are identifiable in the contemporary literature: naturalism, and characterizing in terms of distress and disability. Considering the naturalist approach, the highly successful disease paradigm in 19th-century biomedicine expressed non-self-consciously the idea that illness is a disruption of a natural bodily function: the disease was observable as lesion or cellular pathology. This paradigm and its implicit naturalist view of illness transferred into the new psychiatry and its notion of mental illness, which, in the 1960s, was attacked ferociously by the social science constructionist/deconstructionist critiques of psychiatry (Clare 1976). Since then the disease paradigm has lost some of its prominence and naturalist theories of illness have had to seek foundations elsewhere. Two explicit versions of naturalism have been proposed: Boorse's biostatistical theory (Boorse 1976, 1997), and Wakefield's evolutionary theoretic naturalism (1992, 1999). Both of these forms of naturalism have been much criticized in the literature (e.g. Cosmides and Tooby 1999; Bolton 2000, 2008; Kingma 2010). A recent criticism of Wakefield's evolutionary theoretic version is that it presumes separation of the 'natural' and the 'social' in psychological and behavioural phenotypes which is invalid in terms of the current biobehavioural science, particularly genetics and recent advances in gene–environment interactions and epigenetic mechanisms: in this new scientific paradigm what is 'natural' is interwoven with what is 'social', and indeed both with what is 'individual' (Bolton 2008, 2010). We will not repeat the arguments here but will consider further options from this point. The main implication is that insofar as this kind of criticism of naturalism as applied to mental disorder is correct, we have to move beyond the naturalism versus social construction/ deconstruction debate, and consider other ways of understanding what mental disorder is.

An alternative approach, embedded in healthcare, takes *distress* and *disability* to be fundamental to illness. The standard psychiatric diagnostic manuals, the *International Classification of Diseases* (ICD; World Health Organization 1988) and the *Diagnostic and Statistical Manual of Mental Disorders* (DSM; American Psychiatric Association 1994), both contain explicit definitions of 'mental disorder', and in both *distress* and *disability* are taken to be primary. The DSM-IV, for example, has (p. xxi):

> Each of the mental disorders is conceptualized as a clinically significant behavioral or psychological syndrome or pattern that occurs in an individual and that is associated with present distress (e.g., a painful symptom) or disability (i.e., impairment in one or more important areas of functioning).

However, as is well known, the notions of 'distress' and 'disability' are too broad to define illness. Such difficulties can arise in many ways, such as in response to normal life challenges and losses; so we have to narrow the domain. One way of narrowing the domain conceptually is, of course, by invoking naturalism; as in recent attempts to distinguish normal sorrow from depressive illness (Horwitz and Wakefield 2007). If, however, this naturalist solution is unviable and unavailable—as is being assumed for the sake of argument here—then we have to take a more explicitly personal and social approach.

We can go some way to restricting the kind of 'distress' that is relevant to mental disorder by noting that distress brought to the clinic typically is becoming experienced as *unmanageable* (or *intolerable*)—and this in turn begins to involve impairments of functioning. Distress and impairment of functioning are not the same, in that someone may be very distressed (depressed or excessively anxious, say) and still be able to function well enough in work or childcare, for example; nevertheless, in conditions in which people are inclined to seek healthcare, the level of distress typically is at least bordering on the unmanageable, and functioning is or is becoming difficult. These points are intended to be obvious rather than controversial, but they are not elaborated on in the psychiatric diagnostic manuals, which have other aims, in particular describing and classifying symptoms and syndromes. On the other hand it can be seen that while 'distress' appears somewhat factual and straightforward, the qualification of 'unmanageability' signals the person's experience of their distress, and of coping, which are complex matters, highly personalized, and also highly socialized, because what we can or cannot cope with is typically dependent on what we or others expect us to do, and often on what support we can elicit. In brief, 'unmanageable distress' is a complex judgement made by the person involved within their social context, not a simple matter of medical fact.

This point about distress echoes the familiar point made about disability from the perspective of the social model of disability (e.g. Disability Awareness in Action campaign, 2007). It is pointed out by advocacy groups that disability is not an absolute category but is relative to environments and expectations typically imposed by majority social groups. Such-and-such a condition would not give rise to disability, it is argued, if the environments and task-demands were not incompatible with the condition, in which case diagnosis of disorder is actually a cover for discrimination and social exclusion (e.g. Oliver 1990). This line of thought, which can be applied to both physical and mental disabilities, emphasizes among other things that the judgement of disability has to be made by the person concerned, not by society or the doctor alone.

We suggest that the broad alternative to naturalism is the view that unmanageable distress and/or disability are constitutive of illness, and in this context it is critical to investigate and understand these phenomena more clearly. We will examine the extent to which mental disorder understood in these terms involves a loss of personal autonomy. The potential gain to be made by viewing mental disorder through the lens of personal autonomy is primarily conceptual: the concept of personal autonomy has been extensively explored in the philosophical literature, while distress and impairment of functioning have hardly been addressed as concepts in the psychiatric literature.

The term 'autonomy' connotes self-determination but beyond this obvious point, as is often commented, the term has many contentious uses in a large literature or sets of literatures. In the course of the chapter we will consider two general kinds of autonomy in relation to the concept of mental disorder, in brief as follows. One approach to explicating autonomy highlights the conditions under which a person's desires, beliefs, reasons, and action can be considered as originating in or belonging to the self, as authentic in this sense— as opposed to having some other origin. In this approach, autonomy is fundamentally a relational property of mental states and associated behaviour, linking them to the self. This view of autonomy as authenticity has a complex history in Kant, in Heidegger and Sartre, and has been proposed more recently by such authors as Frankfurt and Dworkin. Several versions of this view can be distinguished in the literature, ranging from the idea of agent-autonomy as a kind of self-control and endorsement of one's actions, to autonomy as authenticity or being true to oneself, grounded in one's volitional essence (Arpaly 2002). All such accounts hinge on the idea that what makes an action autonomous is a particular kind of motivational pedigree within the agent's own internal psychology.

While the philosophical details have proven difficult to work out satisfactorily, some such notion is apparently relevant in the present context when we say colloquially that a person is not being himself, for example, when intoxicated—or when otherwise mentally disturbed. This idea in turn is connected, in serious cases in which the person is thought to be in harm's way, with provisions of mental health legislation that permit over-ruling of the person's expressed wishes at a particular time, if necessary compulsory detainment in hospital, for reasons of mental illness. In brief, a person's mental states and behaviour, when mentally ill, may not be considered a true expression of themselves, but rather as expressions of the illness, and therefore as lacking autonomy in this sense. While we may be sceptical about the possibility of a general philosophical theory of autonomy as authenticity, nevertheless some such idea is apparently required if the intuitions behind these aspects of mental disorder discourse and of mental health legislation are to be accommodated.

Another approach to autonomy belongs with liberal political philosophy, in which context it means freedom of the individual citizen to carry on with his or her own affairs, in particular freedom of the individual from state control, provided this does not interfere with the freedom of others. Autonomy here refers not to an authentic psychological pedigree of action, but to freedom of action—it signifies a political value. This is more akin to what Arpaly (2002) refers to as normative, moral autonomy, and it requires that individuals be free of intervention by others or by the state in their actions. While this political concept of autonomy has complex connections with the idea of autonomy as authenticity, one clear difference is that it emphasizes freedom of action—it is in this sense a pragmatic concept. The political, pragmatic approach to autonomy interacts with the concepts of illness in general and mental illness in particular in two major ways. First, as already mentioned, mental health legislation permits deprivation of liberty for reasons of mental illness. Second, while the primary concern of the political, pragmatic approach to autonomy is protection of the individual's freedom to act from external interference, we will propose that the notion of illness signals a different kind of threat to individual freedom: threats to action that lie within the person, in the mind and body, rather than outside the person, in the sociopolitical arena. In brief, we will propose that our notion of illness refers to internal breakdowns of pragmatic autonomy.

4.2 The varieties of disorder, distress, and disability

The linkage between illness and disability is apparent in the fact that illness attribution typically excuses the person from normal social role obligations, serving as a defence against being blamed for inaction. The idea is simple enough, that the person when ill cannot do certain things for reason of illness—he is really unable—and this explanation can be compared and contrasted with lack of desirable activity due to such factors or excuses as laziness, immaturity, eccentricity, or moral defect. This way of thinking works reasonably straightforwardly for us in many kinds of case of physical illness or disorder, as with a broken leg or high fever, but the question arises whether this whole mode of understanding and, if necessary, excuse, transfers to mental illness. In the case of mental illness we suppose that the body is able—there is no broken leg, no general muscle weakness—but 'the mind is unable'. But what does this mean: 'the mind is unable?'. If one surveys the broad domain of mental disorder, as compiled in psychiatry textbooks or the diagnostic manuals, the responses to this question splinter into many kinds. The mind is many things, and different components become non-operational for normal purposes in many ways.

For example, in post-traumatic stress reaction, the person suffers from intrusive, persistent, distressing thoughts or images of the traumatic event, tries to put them out of mind but typically cannot, or cannot for long, and this has a highly adverse impact on the ability to concentrate. This means that people commonly cannot continue their previous work, for example, for the duration of the episode. Or another kind of example: a child suffering from obsessive–compulsive disorder finds that he has to, because of compulsion or to avoid distress that he finds entirely unmanageable, spend 3 or 4 hours cleaning himself before going to school, to which he therefore arrives late, or not at all. The person in a severe depressive episode is energy-less, a phenomenon that spans the mind–body divide, and feels despair and hopelessness, sees no point in getting up. The child with severe attention-deficit hyperactivity disorder cannot sit still for longer than a few minutes at a time, or attend to what the teacher says, or to the task he is meant to be doing, but wanders around, often getting into trouble, but in any case not learning either school work or how to get on with his peer group. These cases involve inability—as usual in disability: these matters are not under the person's control—or at least they are only to some extent, to a point only, for some of the time at best, beyond which and otherwise the person cannot help it.

Let us press further the question of how disability arises, examining some of the issues here from a philosophical and psychiatric point of view, concerning not having sufficient control of one's action, and bringing in the related notion of distress. So far as we are aware, the connection between mental disorder and disruption of the person's control over their activity has not been much explicitly discussed in the philosophical or psychiatric literature, although recent research on the assessment of mental capacity is beginning to ask important questions in this regard (e.g. Owen et al. 2009).

It is more or less standard philosophy of mind and psychology that action results from interplay between processes in various mental faculties: perception, interpretation and belief, emotion and desire, combination into reason for action, and the will to act. In each of these states and processes, normative distinctions apply. Perception of reality can be veridical or mistaken, or in an extreme, hallucinatory. Beliefs may be true or false, reasonable or unreasonable, based on good evidence or otherwise. Desires are reasonable or otherwise depending on their relation to the person's needs. Emotions may be understandable reactions to events, for example, anger is an understandable response to being hurt, or not understandable, being angry for no reason; and so on. The will may fail to control action. Action may be reasonable or otherwise, depending on whether it follows from beliefs and desires, or on whether those beliefs and desires are themselves reasonable. Behaviour may be random, without any relation to the achievement of goals, without method, and in this sense may fail to be real action. A further issue is that we expect people to be able to give an account of their significant actions, to be able to explain why they are doing what they are doing, by citing beliefs and desires, reasons for action, and this capacity is intimately linked to the attribution of agency and responsibility for actions. These observations indicate the range of psychological functioning and dysfunction: there may be problems in the relation between perception and reality, in the rationality of belief, in the appropriateness of emotions and desires, and in the role of reasons in the regulation of action.

As well as having roots in medicine, modern psychiatry has developed within this broadly psychological thought space. The manuals for psychiatric diagnosis of 'mental disorders' explicitly and inevitably operate with normative terms of the above kinds, such as 'rational', 'reasonable', 'meaningful', 'appropriate', 'proportionate', and their opposites.

There is probably no single word which ideally fits all these various kinds of standards for the variety of kinds of mental functioning, but some may be used as a cover for them all, such as 'normal', or, following Jaspers (1913/1963), 'meaningful'.

In relation to current philosophical terminology, while we may say that the norms involved in evaluating belief are 'epistemic', we are not sure there is a technical philosophical term for the norms involved in evaluating affective states. Affective states are world-directed intentional states triggered by particular experiences, involving physiological responses, and potentiating a certain characteristic range of behavioural responses. Fear, for example, is triggered by threat-perception, involves the autonomic arousal system, and potentiates responses such as escape or aggression. Anger is a response to the experience of being hurt, again involves physiological arousal, and prompts revenge, returning hurt for hurt. Sadness is triggered by experience of loss, typically involves physiological and behavioural suppression, potentiating withdrawal or comfort-seeking. The norms involved in these cases are complex, being broadly matters of the affective state having an appropriate object (threat, being hurt, loss), being proportionate in degree (e.g. much threat, much anxiety, etc.), and proportionality of response (e.g. extent of aggression proportionate to extent of threat). These norms for the evaluation of affective states are presumably not well or adequately captured by the term 'epistemic', which refers primarily to evidence or other justification for belief. Folk psychology uses such terms as 'reasonable', 'meaningful', 'appropriate', 'proportionate', and folk psychiatry their opposites.

The main point for the present purpose is that when these norms are apparently broken the question of 'mental disorder' arises. It should not be put stronger than that; we have still to settle whether apparent rupture is what it seems, and the cases have to be important for us, not trivial. Criteria for diagnosis of mental disorder highlight this last feature by specifying that there should be 'clinically significant' distress and impairment, where 'clinically significant' means something like: severe enough for the person to find their way to the clinic (Spitzer and Williams 1982). The point about seriousness or severity being made, rupture of meaningful linkages in affective states is typically and intrinsically both disabling and distressing. Affective states take up mental and behavioural resources, orientating the living being to actual or potential problems in the environment that require more or less urgent attention and solving (e.g. Power and Dalgleish 1997). As such, strong affective states, whether appropriate or otherwise, direct attention and resources away from daily activities and the person typically has difficulty sustaining what is, for the person or for the peer group, normal social role functioning and obligation, at school, work, and in family life.

Negative emotional states such as anxiety, depression, and anger are inherently distressing, but breakdown of meaningful connections adds further distress: incomprehension brings with it confusion, feeling overwhelmed, not knowing why they are as they are, or what to do about it. Failure of mutual intelligibility brings with it further distress for families and friends. Disability brings further distress: failure to meet up to expectations of normal or desirable functioning—for apparently no good reason—is itself likely to be (though is not invariably) a further cause of distress. Distress and disability here interact and exacerbate one another.

These issues raise the question of self-control. There is a general question of what degree of control do we have, or normally expect to have, over affective states. We are often capable of suppressing or modifying our ordinary affective states, whether for the sake of keeping to social norms or ensuring one's actions are appropriately directed towards one's goals. But the stronger the intensity of the state, the more control over action it assumes. One clear way in which the state may be overcome, or not acted upon, is by being over-ruled by another, contrary, affect, such as loyalty, love, or fear of consequences. This refers to matters familiar in daily life, ethics, and law. In cases that come to the clinic, however, there are apparently no reliably effective counteraffective states: attempts to overcome anxiety have not worked, or have not worked reliably, attempts to become happier and to engage with the world again have failed, resulting in further feelings of hopelessness and helplessness; and so on. However, breakdown of meaningful connections raises further problems. In these cases mental states and associated behaviour appear as alien to the self, and not under the control of the self. In psychiatric conditions the intense affective state—anxiety, depression, or anger—is typically out of order, lacking an appropriate kind of object, and being too intense for its object if it has one. The emotion and the behavioural response it leads to are not understandable in relation to normal causes and regulators, therefore not predictable, and so far not controllable either.

A different though related kind of case is the so-called addictions. Individuals with addictions to psychoactive substances generally show dereliction of normal (for us or them) social role obligations, because of spending so much time and resources obtaining the desired substance, and because of being in no fit state once they have. The social jury is probably out on the question whether people with addictions really can or really cannot help it (e.g. Heyman 2009). In law the situation is complex, as addictions may be construed as wilful misconduct, entailing criminal responsibility for one's actions (Miller 2010). On the other hand in another main institution, healthcare, addiction (substance dependence) is recognized as a medical/psychiatric condition, as a mental disorder; and this pathologizing carries the implication that the person cannot help it and is not in control of his/her behaviour in relation to the substance.

The intentionality of distress in affective disorders includes distress about the appropriateness of the states themselves, and one's lack of control over them. Distress associated with having a particular cognition appears, however, qualitatively different. In disorders of cognition, of which delusional belief is a core symptom, the person is not distressed about the appropriateness (i.e. the epistemic status) of his belief. As far as we can see, belief—having a belief—is not itself distressing or otherwise. What I believe to be the case may well upset me, be more or less catastrophic so far as I am concerned, but it is the facts in the world that I am upset about, not the fact that I believe it. Beliefs aim to track the truth, and if they do so I am so far happy to have them. Further, if I believe that p, then I believe that p is true, so I always believe my beliefs have tracked the truth. I am never dissatisfied with—upset by— the epistemic status of my beliefs; if I am, this merely subtracts from my belief, from my conviction in the belief, from the fact that I do believe (as opposed to suspect, guess, or wonder whether).

The feature of belief that we are seeking to identify here is perhaps related to the paradox identified by Moore, namely, that while 'I believe that p' does not entail 'p' (and the speaker knows that), nevertheless the proposition 'I believe that p, but not-p' is odd (Moore 1942; Shoemaker 1995). The analogue in the feature of belief that we are trying to identify is as follows. 'I believe that p' does not entail 'the epistemic status of my belief is valid', but the proposition 'I believe that p, but the epistemic status of my belief is invalid', is nevertheless odd. This being the case, while I can have an emotional state which (I believe) ought to have an appropriate object or intensity, but which apparently (so far as I can see) does not, I cannot have a belief which (I believe) ought to have an appropriate epistemic basis, but which apparently (so far as I am concerned) does not.

This feature of belief is connected to controversies surrounding the important but slippery notion of 'insight' in psychiatry, specifically in application to delusional beliefs in psychosis (e.g. Saravanan et al. 2004). The clinician believes that there is something radically wrong, epistemically, with the delusional belief. The patient who has the belief, on the other hand, cannot, if the above argument is correct, believe this. The clinician supposes that the patient's belief is not epistemically well-founded, but is rather the symptom of an illness. If the patient can be persuaded to agree with this diagnosis, he is said to have 'insight'. Insight when achieved may indicate better prognosis, but it is often not achieved, and one reason for this may be connected to the particular logic of belief states, as sketched earlier.

What are the implications then for distress and disability in the psychoses and in particular in cases of delusional belief? As previously suggested, the person may well be distressed about what he believes to be the case, most obviously in paranoid delusions; and the person may be distressed because others do not agree with him and contradict him; and distressed by—if this happens—being taken away by force and locked up. There is plenty, then, to be distressed about. There is also disability, in the person's own terms: the person with a delusional belief may attempt to act in ways consistent with the belief but the action may fail because he is wrong about the way the world is. In this respect, he is indeed disabled as he is incapable of performing actions that result in the intended consequences. The person with delusional beliefs is also disabled from the point of view of other people, insofar as acting in accord with those beliefs is incompatible with behaviour we normally expect, such as giving priority to self-care, shopping and eating, conversation, and so on.

We have considered in this section distress and disability in the context of several kinds of mental disorder, especially disorders of affect and of cognition, and have seen that they involve different kinds of distress and disability. The class of mental disorders is diverse, however, and space does not allow adequate discussion of the diversity. We have omitted from detailed consideration, for example, serious problems of attention and concentration, which also give rise to distress and impairment in readily understandable ways. It is also difficult to do justice to the complexity and subtlety of presentations of mental disorder, known to the people involved and their families and in the clinic, but lost to broad diagnostic classifications and to faculty psychology. For example, severe or complicated depression may involve self-harming impulses or intentions, and associated beliefs such as 'I deserve to be punished', or 'I would be better dead', congruent with severely depressed mood, and with the self at the time. In these complex or severe presentations, depressed affect is not experienced as imposed upon the self, but rather as the self, involving beliefs, which border on—from the external point of view—the delusional.

4.3 Mental disorder and threats to autonomy

Among the many kinds of case and the complexities of mental disorder we may distinguish various themes that may be elucidated as threats to autonomy. There are cases in which the self experiences states of mind that interfere with what the person wishes to be doing, and that are in this sense alien to the self. The person may say, including at the clinic if they attend there: 'I cannot get up in the morning because I feel so low and hopeless and can hardly look after the children – and I want to be able to do this (or I want to because I need to)'. Or: 'I keep thinking of the assault, it replays in my mind over and over, and I try to distract myself but can't for long, and I can't get to sleep, and I'm exhausted, and can't concentrate at work, and I keep making mistakes, and I'm worried about losing my job'. These kinds of case apparently involve both alienation of states of mind from the self, and incapacity to carry out one's intended business—both of which imply threats to 'autonomy' in the general sense of self-determination.

In other kinds of case, usually brought under the broad heading of delusional belief, or complicated affective disorder with delusional features, the person has beliefs that—being beliefs—they do indeed endorse as theirs, as being the beliefs of the self. On the other hand, matters look different from the outside. To the family, friends, the clinician if attended, the beliefs appear paranoid, grandiose, or seriously depressive, and unwarranted. On the other hand, again, we tolerate differences often enough, happily or otherwise—so why do we worry so much about psychiatric delusions? Here the fundamental issue has to do with harm: such beliefs may imply significant risk of harm to self or harm to others. Mental health legislation is designed to manage these risks. Autonomy in the practical, political sense is lost if the person is compulsorily detained under mental health legislation for reasons of mental illness and risk to the safety of themselves or others. As a state sanctioned deprivation of political liberty, use of mental health legislation is liable to be much disapproved of within libertarian political thought (e.g. Bolton 2006; Szasz 2006).

Justification for the legislation refers straightforwardly to protection of the safety of other individuals, but what is the justification in the case of risk posed to the self? There is a paradoxical appearance in the notion of protecting the self against the self, the resolution of which presumably relies on some 'duality' in the self. In circumstances in which mental health legislation is typically applied, it is assumed that the person is in a temporary state of not being themselves, in an ill condition from which, all being well, with the passage of time, or with treatment, the person will recover. With this background assumption, deprivation of liberty for the protection of the self is for the protection of the future self, continuous with the past self; and it is difficult for this line of thought to avoid characterizing this self to be protected as something like the 'true' or 'real' self, while the current thinking, speaking self (the one ill-disposed) is not. Thus, for example, to consider one of the more straightforward kinds of case, let us suppose that a mother who has recently given birth to her third baby becomes seriously depressed and believes she deserves to die, and tries to throw herself under a bus; friends and family and neighbours say that hers is a happy family and she loves looking after the two children. The authorities diagnose a mental illness and she is compulsorily admitted to hospital, treated, and—to make a happy ending—let us suppose that she recovers and returns to her former way of life happily enough, and is grateful that she was not allowed to kill herself.

The notion of self that this line of thinking and practice presupposes is distributed through time, involving some degree of coherence and consistency. While coherence and consistency no doubt have blurred boundaries, there are clear enough cases in which they break down; they are likely to exclude, for example, loving one's children one week and wanting to die and not caring about leaving them dead the next. In brief, what is involved here is a narrative understanding of the self and agency, and the idea that illness disrupts the narrative (Kennett 2005).

It is important in the present context to emphasize that the discourse of breakdown of self and agency thought time in some instances of mental disorder, as outlined earlier, does not require notions of authenticity and inauthenticity applicable to a person's mental state at any one time. As previously referred to, one main philosophical approach to personal autonomy as authenticity involved the idea of a hierarchy of mental states such as desires (Frankfurt 1971; Dworkin 1976). The idea was that a person is autonomous with respect to a first-order desire if she endorses her possession of that first-order desire. Objections to these early approaches include that second-order desires may be manipulated in ways that apparently compromise autonomy, just as first-order desires may be, for example by deceptive information (e.g. Friedman 1986), and that it is unclear why second-order desires should be regarded as being any more authentic than first-order desires (e.g. Watson 1975). We may illustrate the difficulties in terms of, for example, the case of addiction already referred to. A person may want very much to smoke cannabis but not want to have this desire, yet his second-order desire is manipulated by threats of prosecution and punishment, rather than reflecting his own inclinations in the matter, and he may have a third-order desire, not to be intimated by the law, that may over-ride the second-order desire, and that in turn, may be over-ridden by a desire not to risk, for example, his social status and family life, or by fear of negative social evaluation. Which among these various conflicting, more or less hierarchical desires are to be valued as more authentically the person's, and as more autonomous, than the others? Much effort has been spent in the literature trying to resolve these kinds of objections and conundrums and to propose more viable accounts of autonomy as authenticity. Our purpose here is not to review these attempts—see, for example, Mackenzie and Stoljar (2000) and Taylor (2005). Our main point is rather that the notion of illness in general, and of mental illness in particular, has the connotation of an episode, being distinguished from personality or character, and that when ill the person may not be behaving mentally or physically as they usually do and 'as themselves'—this being understood as how they were before they became ill, and how they will be after they recover. In this there is no presupposition that there is a way of sorting out among conflicting mental states at a given point in time (whether in or out of an illness episode) the 'authentic' from the 'inauthentic'. Nor is there a presumption that the self understood in this way—as the person has been pre-episode, and hopefully will be after—is 'authentic' or 'autonomous' in any further psychological or metaphysical sense.

We introduce the term 'metaphysical' here to indicate a feature of the concept of autonomy which we believe has no role in explicating the concept of mental disorder—or indeed of mind in order. This feature can be characterized as the supposition that there is a self that exists independently of outside influences, this being the fundamental justification between mental states and actions that originate in the self as opposed to elsewhere. An a priori, metaphysical notion of this sort can be found in the strongest and clearest philosophical systems of autonomy and authenticity. The great Kantian concept of autonomy posited a rational will that was prior to and free of personal interest (Kant 1785). What was probably the last great metaphysics of self-determination, Sartre's existentialism, worked with an embodied, social self, developing through time, in which, one would suppose, the self is thoroughly muddled up with extraneous matter. However, Sartre's metaphysics of self-determination is formulated in this context by making no distinction between actions that are self-determined from those that were not: *all are of the self*—requiring Sartre to reject wholesale the alternative possibilities of biological or sociopolitical determinism of the sorts arguably proposed by Freud and by Marx (Sartre 1943, 1946). This idea did not last long, and insofar as the self tends now to be regarded as biologically conditioned and culturally involved, previous ideas of self-sovereignty, and associated notions of autonomy and authenticity, are undermined.

No such metaphysical view of autonomy, specifically no idea of an authentic self as opposed to a self involved in the body, family life, and culture, is required to understand that in states of illness a person may not be themselves and may need looking after, sometimes, in cases of danger, against their will. The concepts involved here are mundane, to do with continuity and narrative of the self through time, and its rupture by illness.

Interestingly in this connection the political sense of autonomy, fundamental to liberal political philosophy, has also been criticized for its reliance on a sense of self that is independent of culture, or which can set culture aside for the purposes of public political engagement—as, for example, in Sandel's criticisms of Rawls (Sandel 1982). Historical and conceptual linkages between the two senses of autonomy, the one to do with psychological and moral authenticity, and other political, and the parallel problems with both, are well reviewed by Christman and Anderson (2005).

On the other hand, notwithstanding these problems, the term 'autonomy' remains in judicial use in liberal democracies, used for example in interpreting Article 8, on the right to privacy, of the European Convention of Human Rights (Council of Europe 1950). Here 'autonomy' is used to signify the right to carry out one's 'private' business, broadly conceived, to include not only personal and family life but also, for example, activities in the workplace (see, e.g. ECHR 2007). Autonomy in this sense is a practical-political matter, not a psychological one. Indeed arguably the notion of autonomy in general has to include, as a necessary condition, the right to carry own one's intended action—it cannot be limited to a particular procedure in the mind only, otherwise it would be possible to have autonomy while chained in a cell, which we take to be an absurd proposition.

However exactly understood, 'autonomy' apparently requires being in sufficient control of one's own action—it is a practical matter. It can be threatened externally in many ways: in totalitarian regimes, in democracies in the absence of checks and balances, by imprisonment, legal or otherwise, by assaults on the person—most clearly in ways that limit bodily movement or that threaten violence unless the person submits. There are, however, more subtle ways in which autonomy is undermined, as noted by writers from feminist perspectives who emphasize its relational nature (e.g. Mackenzie and Stoljar, 2000). Individual identity is socially embedded and intersubjective, and thus the proper domain of autonomy is within the relations and dynamics one has with others and with the social and historical conditions in which one is embedded. For instance, the formation of one's motivational structures may be impeded by an oppressive social context or limitations imposed on what choices are available to one. Furthermore, autonomy is only possible if one's choices, decisions and desires are acknowledged and respected by others (Baier 1985). Socialization processes can also play a positive role in nurturing and encouraging the development of autonomy, and are not merely a source of suppression of a person's capacity to express free choices. This applies as much to whole social groups as it does to individuals. We agree with this shift of emphasis away from autonomy as involving inner processes, towards relational attitudes, but emphasize that social action and interactions need also to be considered. Autonomy is a practical matter and is denied to people in practical ways, by for example not listening, not respecting, not taking seriously, by also by exclusion from resources and power, and ultimately, by intimidation, physical violence, imprisonment, and murder. This view of autonomy, and how it is denied to minority groups by the various methods and mechanisms of social exclusion, we take to be compatible with feminist and related literature.

As indicated earlier, we suggest that 'illness' has a particular role in the conceptual space of autonomy as being an *internal limitation* to autonomy: there is nothing in the external environment to prevent the person having sufficient control of their own action, from going about their business—but internally, within the person, it doesn't work. This may be correct as far as it goes, though as generally with these matters of internal and external, it is complicated in various ways. Internal states of incapacity may be caused substantially by external factors, such as neglect or abuse. We also tend to internalize how are we are treated by others into our self-view. Or again, people who are ill have some degree of incapacity because of their illness, and still more on top because of the stigma and social exclusion that may go with the illness diagnosis (see, e.g. Thornicroft 2006). In various ways and contexts mechanisms of social advantage tend to promote a positive self-image of self-efficacy, while mechanisms of social exclusion foster self-doubt and incapacity.

Nevertheless, broadly speaking, and with complications as just described, 'illness' signifies breakdown of autonomous action because of an internal proximate cause or reason, within the person, as opposed to an external cause or reason. So what are the things that can go wrong internally? Can we specify the list, in effect defining the normal state of health? In considering the conditions of normal functioning that can break down, one may attempt to describe the physical case, referring to skeletal, muscle tone, respiratory features and functions—and we have to add, *and so on*. The mental case is more complex still, if that is possible. Is it possible to draw up a list of mental faculties that have to be in place—operating well enough, and well enough together—attention, concentration, absence of overwhelming emotion contrary to normal activities, beliefs that track the world accurately enough, etc.—such that, if these are not working well enough, rational agency becomes difficult or impossible? Can we draw up a full list? Interestingly, there seems to be no account of such a whole in the sciences such as psychology and the neurosciences.

Wittgenstein treats this general problematic in *On Certainty* (Wittgenstein 1969). In one place Wittgenstein considers circumstances in which a person makes not so much a mistake, but rather some apparently more fundamental error in judgement, and as usual, Wittgenstein doubts whether a rule (the expression of a rule) can define these cases. He then has at #27:

> If, however, one wanted to give something like a rule here, then it would contain the expression 'in normal circumstances'. And we recognise normal circumstances but cannot precisely describe them. At most, we can recognise a range of abnormal ones.

Interestingly in the present context it turns out that the more fundamental error in judgement (more fundamental than making a mistake) is something like mental disturbance, madness, dementia—variously called through *On Certainty*. But at present the point we wish to highlight is that the point in #27 apparently applies to conditions of agency, as much as to judgement (as one would expect); i.e. we recognize normal circumstances, but cannot precisely formulate them, and we recognize a range of abnormal cases. The abnormal cases include the conditions listed in the medical, psychiatric, and neurological textbooks.

Why is it not possible—if indeed it is not possible—to define the conditions necessary for action? Apparently the task is a philosophical one, perhaps a quasi-Kantian one: 'what are the conditions necessary for action to be possible?'. This question would seem to require for its solution an a priori account of the essence of the matter in question, but in the case of action, embodied agency, its conditions are indefinite. This suggestion would echo the line of thought discussed earlier in this section, that the notion of self-determination free of external influences (contexts and conditions), and of autonomy in this sense, is apparently not viable if the self is embedded developmentally in biology and culture. In this case we cannot define the conditions of health, which are limitless, but can recognize cases and kinds of case in which health is lost, and in which there are greater or lesser threats to the internal conditions of autonomy.

4.4 **Concluding remarks**

In the course of the chapter we have considered the nature and variety of the distress and disabilities involved in mental disorder and examined the extent to which these features may be helpfully explicated in terms of the various philosophical, psychological and political meanings of autonomy. Several main points relevant to this question have been identified. First, the notion of illness in general and of mental illness in particular refers to an episode in which normal functioning is disrupted or lost—'normal' including 'normal for the person'—as opposed to some lasting personality trait or character. In the case of mental illness in particular, mental states and the state of the self are disrupted. To the extent that the person speaking and acting identifies with these abnormal states, the person is not being themselves—for reasons of illness. This disruption of the states of the self could be described as a loss of autonomy as authenticity, but in our view this is unhelpful. This is mainly because the idea of autonomy as authenticity is itself problematic, quite possibly irredeemably so. But it is also because this formulation would stretch the meaning of authenticity too far. The central issue in this context is that people in an illness episode are not as they usually are; it is not that they are being inauthentic in any other sense, or that their usual self is authentic is any sense other than: the way they usually are. A second point is that the distress and disabilities fundamental to mental disorder typically involve loss of freedom to act. This idea of freedom to act is central to the political meaning of autonomy. Liberal political philosophy seeks to safeguard freedom of action, presupposing the autonomous, self-determined agent. This presupposition is interrogated by 'illness', among other things. When a person is ill, the person is not altogether themselves, and either or both of 'self' and 'determination' lose clarity. Illness typically involves not being able to do what one normally can, a loss of freedom, not because of any outside interference, but because of one's inner state.

References

American Psychiatric Association (1994) *Diagnostic and Statistical Manual of Mental Disorders* (4th edn.). Washington DC: American Psychiatric Association.

Arpaly, N. (2002). Varieties of autonomy. In *Unprincipled Virtue: An Inquiry into Moral Agency*. Oxford: Oxford University Press, pp. 117–48.

Baier, A. (1985). Cartesian persons. In *Postures of the Mind: Essays on Mind and Morals*. Minneapolis, MN: University of Minnesota Press, pp. 74–92.

Bolton, D. (2000). Alternatives to disorder. *Philosophy, Psychology, & Psychiatry* 7: 141–53.

Bolton, D. (2006). What's the problem? A response to "secular humanism and scientific psychiatry". *Philosophy, Ethics, and Humanities in Medicine* 2006, 1:6. http://www.peh-med.com/content/1/1/6 Reprinted in *Science and Ethics* (P. Kurtz ed. 2007) New York: Prometheus Books, 204–207.

Bolton D. (2008). *What is mental disorder? An essay in philosophy, science and values*. Oxford: Oxford University Press.

Bolton, D. (2010). Social, biological and personal constructions of mental illness. In D. Bughra and C. Morgan (eds.) *Principles of Social Psychiatry* (2nd edn.). Oxford: Wiley Blackwell, pp. 39–49.

Boorse, C. (1976). What a theory of mental health should be. *Journal of the Theory of Social Behaviour* 6: 61–84.

Boorse, C. (1997). A rebuttal on health. In J.F. Humber and R.F. Almeder (eds.) *Biomedical Ethics Reviews: What is Disease?* Totowa, NJ: Humana Press, pp. 1–134.

Christman, J. and Anderson, J. (2005) Introduction. In J. Christman and N. Anderson (eds.) *Autonomy and the Challenges to Liberalism*. Cambridge: Cambridge University Press, pp. 1–23.

Clare, A. (1976) *Psychiatry in dissent. Controversial issues in thought and practice*. London: Tavistock.

Cosmides, L. and Tooby, J. (1999). Toward an evolutionary taxonomy of treatable conditions. *Journal of Abnormal Psychology*, 108: 453–64.

Council of Europe (1950). European Convention on Human Rights. Current with Protocols at http://www.echr.coe.int/ECHR/EN/Header/Basic+Texts/The+Convention+and+additional+protocols/The+European+Convention+on+Human+Rights/Accessed 30/12/10.

Dworkin, G. (1976). Autonomy and behaviour control. *Hastings Center Report* 6: 23–28.

Frank, R. (1988) *Passions Within Reason: The Strategic Role of Emotions*. New York: Norton.

ECHR (European Court of Human Rights) (2007) Key case-law issues. The concepts of 'private and family life. http://www.echr.coe.int/NR/rdonlyres/F6DC7D2E-1668–491E-817A-D0E29F094E14/0/COURT_n1883413_v1_Key_caselaw_issues__Art_8__The_Concepts_of_Private_and_Family_Life.pdf

Frankfurt, H. (1971). Freedom of the will and the concept of a person. *Journal of Philosophy*, 68(1): 5–20; reprinted in Watson, G. (ed.) (2003) Free Will (2nd edn.). Oxford: Oxford University Press, pp. 322—36

Friedman, M. (1986). Autonomy and the split-level self. *Southern Journal of Philosophy* 24: 19–35.

Hill, Jr., T. (1989). The Kantian conception of autonomy. In Christman, J. (ed.) *The Inner Citadel: Essays on Individual Autonomy*. New York: Oxford University Press, pp. 91–105.

Horwitz, A.V. and Wakefield, J.C. (2007) *The loss of sadness. How psychiatry transformed normal sorrow into depressive disorder*. New York: Oxford University Press.

Heyman, G.M. (2009) *Addiction: A Disorder of Choice*. Cambridge, MA: Harvard University Press.

Jaspers, K. (1913/1963) *Allgemeine pychopathologie*, Berlin: Springer Verlag (3rd enlarged and revised edn., 1923). English translation of the 7th edn by J. Hoenig and M.W. Hamilton (1963) *General Psychopathology*. Manchester: Manchester University Press.

Kant, I. (1785). *Grundlegung zur Metaphysik der Sitten*. English translation J. Timmermann (2008). *Kant's groundwork of the metaphysics of morals. A Commentary*. Cambridge: Cambridge University Press.

Kennett, J. (2005). Mental disorder, moral agency and the self. In B. Steinbock (ed.) *The Oxford Handbook of Bioethics*. Oxford: Oxford University Press, pp. 90–113.

Kingma, E. (2010). Paracetomol, poison and polio: Why Boorse's account of function fails to distinguish health and disease. *British Journal for the Philosophy of Science*, 61(2): 241–64.

Mackenzie, C. and Stoljar, N. (eds.) (2000) *Relational Autonomy: Feminist Perspectives on Autonomy, Agency and the Social Self*. New York: Oxford University Press.

Miller, N.S. (2010) *Principles of Addiction and the Law: Applications in Forensic, Mental Health and Medical Practice*. London: Elsevier Academic Press.

Moore, G.E. (1942). A reply to my critics. In P.A. Schilpp (ed.) *The Philosophy of G. E. Moore*. New York: Tudor Publishing Company (2nd edn. 1952), 533–677.

Oliver, M. (1990). The cultural production of impairment and disability. In *Politics of Disablement*. Basingstoke: Macmillan, pp. 12–24.

Owen, G.S., Freyenhagen, F., Richardson, G., and Hotopf, M. (2009). Mental capacity and decisional autonomy: and interdisciplinary challenge. *Inquiry* 52: 79–107.

Power, M. and Dalgleish, T. (1997) *Cognition and emotion: from order to disorder*. Hove: Erlbaum.

Sandel, M. (1982) *Liberalism and the Limits of Justice*. Cambridge: Cambridge University Press.

Saravanan, B., Jacob, K.S., Prince, M., Bhugra, D., and David, A. (2004) Editorial. Culture and insight revisited. *British Journal of Psychiatry* 184: 107–109.

Sartre J.-P. (1943) *L'être et le néant*. English translation by H. Barnes (1958) *Jean-Paul Sartre, Being and Nothingness*, London: Methuen.

Sartre J-P. (1946). *Existentialisme est un Humanisme*. English translation by P. Mairet, Existentialism as a Humanism. In W. Kaufmann (ed.) (1956) *Existentialism from Dostoevsky to Sartre*. Cleveland, OH: World Publishing, Meridian Books, pp. 290–91.

Shoemaker, S. (1995). Moore's paradox and self-knowledge. *Philosophical Studies* 77: 211–28.

Spitzer, R.L. and Williams, J. B. (1982). The definition and diagnosis of mental disorder. In W.R. Grove (ed.) *Deviance and mental illness*. Beverly Hills, CA: Sage, pp. 15–31.

Szasz, T. (2006). Secular humanism and scientific psychiatry. *Philosophy, Ethics, and Humanities in Medicine* 1: 5. http://www.peh-med.com/content/1/1/5

Taylor, J.S. (2005). Introduction. In J.S. Taylor (ed.) *Personal Autonomy: New Essays on Personal Autonomy and Its Role in Contemporary Moral Philosophy*. Cambridge: Cambridge University Press, pp. 1–29.

Thornicroft, G. (2006) *Shunned: Discrimination against people with mental illness*. Oxford: Oxford University Press.

Wakefield, J.C. (1992). The concept of mental disorder: on the boundary between biological facts and social values. *American Psychologist* 47: 373–88.

Wakefield, J.C. (1999). Mental disorder as a black box essentialist concept. *Journal of Abnormal Psychology* 108: 465–72.

Watson, G. (1975). Free agency. *Journal of Philosophy*, 72: 205–20.

Wittgenstein, L. (1969) *On Certainty* (G.E.M. Anscombe and G.H. von Wright eds., D. Paul and G.E.M. Anscombe trans.). Oxford: Blackwell.

World Health Organization (1988) *Mental, Behavioral, and Developmental Disorders: Clinical Descriptives and Diagnostic Guidelines (ICD-10)*. Geneva: World Health Organization, Division of Mental Health.

Chapter 5

Rationality and self-knowledge in delusion and confabulation: implications for autonomy as self-governance

Lisa Bortolotti, Rochelle Cox,
Matthew Broome, and Matteo Mameli

5.1 Introduction

The main purpose of this paper is to explore the implications of the epistemic faults of delusions and confabulations for the autonomy of the people affected by these conditions. The issue whether autonomy is compromised and to what extent is of great practical relevance. Do people affected by psychiatric disorders that manifest with delusions and confabulations have capacity to consent to treatment? More generally, should they be allowed to make, and be deemed responsible for, significant decisions that affect their well-being?

We propose to look at autonomy as self-governance and to make a distinction between (a) whether one has the capacity to govern oneself and (b) whether one is successful at governing oneself. We argue that the capacity for self-governance depends on the capacity to develop a self-narrative which encompasses the capacity to endorse attitudes and actions on the basis of reasons. Success in self-governance depends on the coherence of self-narratives and on their correspondence to real life events.

Our thesis is that, in most cases, people with delusions or confabulations have the capacity for self-governance, but are unlikely to be successful at governing themselves. This is because they are likely to demonstrate failures of rationality and self-knowledge that impact on the coherence of their self-narratives and the correspondence between these narratives and real life events. The notion of rationality we use in this chapter is a comprehensive notion of rationality for beliefs, which encompasses procedural, epistemic, and agential considerations. It addresses whether there is consistency between a person's beliefs and other intentional states; whether a person's beliefs are well supported by, and responsive to, the evidence available to that person; and whether a person can defend her beliefs with reasons and act in accordance with her beliefs. By self-knowledge we mean knowledge of one's own present and past attitudes, dispositions, and actions, based on introspection, testimony, memory, self-observation, and inference from one's own behaviour.

Although in some cases the very capacity for self-governance may be compromised (e.g. in 'primary' delusions where no reasons are offered in support of the delusion or in delusions and confabulations which occur at advanced stages of dementia), our claim is that having delusions and confabulations does not *necessarily* imply a lack of capacity for self-governance. That said, delusions and confabulations interfere with the exercise of self-governance.

In Section 5.2, we argue that people with delusions and confabulations typically experience failures of rationality and self-knowledge. In Section 5.3, we sketch an account of authorship, a person's capacity to determine what to believe, intend, and do based on what she thinks are her best reasons for those beliefs, intentions, and actions. This capacity is important as it allows people to take responsibility for their own attitudes and integrate them in a personal narrative that underlies the conception of themselves as autonomous agents. In Section 5.4, we suggest that authorship makes a contribution to self-governance via the construction of self-narratives. The attitudes that can be 'authored' (deliberated about or justified on the basis of reasons) are likely to play a significant role in people's narratives. As a result, breakdowns of authorship can ensue in unsuccessful self-governance. In Section 5.5, we review some attempts to describe delusions and confabulations as unreliable self-narratives. In Section 5.6, we draw some general conclusions about the discussion of self-governance in people with delusions and confabulations, and we think about possible implications for policy.

In the paper we argue that, in most of the relevant cases, the best thing to say is that people with delusions and confabulations retain the basic capacity for self-governance but are unlikely to be successful at governing themselves due to their typical failures of rationality and self-knowledge. Failures of rationality and self-knowledge are also present in people without delusions and confabulations and they interfere with the exercise of self-governance in these cases too. However, the failures of rationality and self-knowledge that occur in delusions and confabulations may have more serious consequences, for instance by impairing social functioning.

5.2 **The epistemic faults of delusions and confabulations**

Usually, people distinguish between monothematic delusions which involve one central theme from polythematic delusions which are more pervasive. An example of a monothematic delusion is a person asserting sincerely and with conviction that she is dead (*Cotard delusion*). An example of a schizophrenic delusion is a person asserting sincerely and with conviction that he has just discovered a cure for all types of cancer and that the scientists keep ignoring it because they don't understand his genius (*grandiose delusion*). People confabulate when they report sincerely and with conviction false beliefs about the past or the present or false explanations about their current attitudes and behaviours. Confabulation can occur in the presence of dementia, amnesia, or delusions for instance, but is also common in normal cognition. One example of abnormal behaviour related to false beliefs about the present is that of SD, a 36-year-old man who began to confabulate following a bicycle accident (Metcalf et al. 2007). Upon his return home, SD acted upon his confabulations by searching for his swimsuit because he believed he was a schoolboy with a school swimming carnival to attend.

Delusions and confabulations are classified and diagnosed on the basis of their *surface* features, that is, on the basis of their manifestations. Moreover, these manifestations are normally described by reference to epistemic notions such as truth, rationality, justification, and belief.

Here are some definitions of delusions and confabulations where the two phenomena are presented as cases of false or ill-grounded beliefs or narratives:

> Delusion. A false belief based on incorrect inference about external reality that is firmly sustained despite what almost everyone else believes and despite what constitutes incontrovertible and obvious proof or evidence to the contrary. The belief is not one ordinarily accepted by other members of the person's culture or subculture (e.g., it is not an article of religious faith). When a false belief involves a value judgment, it is regarded as a delusion only when the judgment is so extreme as to defy credibility. (American Psychiatric Association (DSM-IV) 2000, p. 765)
>
> A person is deluded when they have come to hold a particular belief with a degree of firmness that is both utterly unwarranted by the evidence at hand, and that jeopardizes their day-to-day functioning. (McKay et al. 2005a, p. 315)
>
> Confabulations are typically understood to represent instances of false beliefs: opinions about the world that are manifestly incorrect and yet are held by the patient to be true in spite of clearly presented evidence to the contrary. (Turnbull et al. 2004, p. 6)
>
> In the broad sense confabulations are usually defined as false narratives or statements about world and/or self due to some pathological mechanisms or factors, but with no intention of lying. (Örulv and Hydén 2006, p. 648)

Epistemic features are highlighted not just in the definition of these conditions, but also in their further analysis and description (Bortolotti and Cox 2009). In particular, the epistemic features attributed to people with delusions and confabulations have been interpreted as infringements of norms of *rationality* for belief and as failures of *self-knowledge* (e.g. Bortolotti and Broome 2008, 2009; Gallagher 2003; Gerrans 2009).

In the literature, violations of rationality and failures of self-knowledge have been taken to explain why some delusions and confabulations are *un-understandable* (Jaspers 1963) or at the very least *puzzling* (Campbell 2001). Such epistemic faults have also been used as criteria of demarcation between pathological and non-pathological beliefs or narratives. Some of us have argued elsewhere (Bortolotti and Cox 2009; Bortolotti 2011) that people with delusions and confabulations typically violate norms of rationality and fail to acquire or preserve self-knowledge, but that these epistemic faults are also shared by other (non-pathological) beliefs or narratives. In addition, in some of the circumstances in which they occur, confabulations may also bring some epistemic benefits, as they may allow people with dementia or amnesia to 'reconstruct' autobiographical information that they can no longer access and, in this way, to maintain a sense of the self that is essential to some degree of social functioning (e.g. Fotopoulou 2008).

For these and other reasons, it is misleading and psychologically implausible to explain the pathological character of delusions and confabulations exclusively on the basis of their epistemic faults, because many non-pathological beliefs and narratives are irrational in similar ways, and can also contribute to unreliable autobiographies. For example, Wilson (2002) reminds us that we typically integrate in our self-narratives and remember more vividly, episodes in which we have been successful as opposed to episodes in which we have failed to achieve our objectives. As a result, we may form a skewed, and excessively optimistic, conception of ourselves.

It is plausible though, that delusions and confabulations violate norms of rationality and compromise self-knowledge to a higher degree and across more dimensions than non-pathological beliefs and narratives, and that they sometimes represent more *statistically unusual* violations of rationality by having wildly implausible content (Bortolotti 2009a, chapter 6). This might be due to the aetiology of delusions and confabulations, which typically involves neurobiological deficits giving rise to abnormal experiences or impairing memory and cognition, as well as deficits in the evaluation of the hypotheses aimed at explaining those experiences (McKay et al. 2005).

The main epistemic faults of delusions and confabulations are as follows:

- People with delusions and confabulations can endorse mutually conflicting or even inconsistent attitudes (*failure of procedural rationality*).
- Delusions and confabulations are typically formed in the absence of sufficient evidential support, are extremely resistant to counterevidence, and are rejected by other members of the community to which the person belongs (*failure of epistemic rationality*).
- Although people with delusions and confabulations are often disposed to act on their reports, and to defend their reports with sensible

reasons, there are circumstances in which their actions do not match their reports, and in which they offer no reasons in defence of their beliefs (*failure of agential rationality*). This may in some cases signal a lack of commitment towards the content of the delusion or the confabulation (*double bookkeeping*).

- People with delusions sometimes have a distorted conception of their personal boundaries. For instance, they may claim that an external force is responsible for moving their limbs or that a third person is inserting thoughts into their minds (*distortion of personal boundaries*).

- People with confabulations are likely to make false reports about their past experiences and life events, which lead to delusional memories and impact on their understanding of their present circumstances and on the accuracy of their predictions about their future behaviour (*unreliable autobiographies*).

If people with delusions and confabulations cannot typically satisfy the conditions for rationality and self-knowledge, at least with respect to the content of their delusional or confabulatory reports, what are the implications for their autonomy?

5.3 **Authorship**

This Friday, Claire has been invited to Rita's birthday party. She is not sure whether she should go. She likes Rita, although Rita is not one of her closest friends. However, the party would require Claire to drive quite a long way, and thus Claire would not be able to drink or to stay late. Should she go? Claire forms that belief that she shouldn't go. She can provide reasons for her belief: she is tired after a long day at work, and she is not too confident about driving her new car to Rita's place. But Claire's boyfriend, Ron, thinks differently. Ron suspects that Claire is becoming lazy, a 'couch potato', and that she would not have gone to the party even if her day at work had been easier and the party had been just a few blocks away.

The notion of authorship introduced by Moran (2001) and further elaborated in Bortolotti (2009b) and Bortolotti and Broome (2008) suggests that there is something special about the fact that Claire can give reasons for her belief, reasons that she takes to be her best reasons. Claire's own endorsement of her belief creates an asymmetry between Claire and Ron. When she defends her belief on the basis of reasons she takes to be her best reasons, Claire takes an *agential perspective* on her belief. Instead, Ron cannot have the same perspective, because he is not the person responsible for forming the belief. He can only adopt the *perspective of an observer* or *an interpreter*, and make sense of Claire's behaviour on the basis of the evidence available to him.

We could say that Claire is 'authoritative' about her decision, but here authority does not imply that the reasons she takes to be her best reasons are actually the true or the best reasons behind her decision. Claire's authority consists in this: she knows what her belief is because she formed that belief on the basis of reasons. She *authored* her belief by giving reasons for it, to herself and to others (rather than by tossing a coin). This does not mean that Ron is mistaken about what motivated Claire's belief. Ron may be right about what is driving Claire's behaviour. We know that people's behaviour is often driven by attitudes that may not be known to them (e.g. Nisbett and Wilson 1977). The sense in which Claire is authoritative about her belief does not make her infallible in assessing how good her reasons are, and is not sufficient to make her an overall rational agent.

Moran's message is not that the asymmetry between Claire and Ron lies in Claire having better *epistemic* access to her attitudes or processes. Ron forms beliefs about Claire's attitudes on the basis of evidence (*theoretical stance*), similar to a scientist who examines a certain environment and makes inductive generalizations about the causes of certain phenomena. In order to know her attitudes, Claire needs to rely neither on behavioural evidence about herself nor on introspection. She decides what to believe by weighing up reasons (*deliberative* or *agential stance*). In other words, it is not the case that Ron has a more modest evidential basis for interpreting Claire's attitudes than Claire herself. Ron needs to interrogate evidence about Claire to know what Claire believes, whereas Claire just needs to *do* something, that is, form a belief on the basis of reasons that she regards to be her best reasons. Deliberating offers

people an additional route to knowing the content of the attitudes they
endorse.

> If it is possible for a person to answer a deliberative question about his belief at all,
> this involves assuming an authority over, and a responsibility for, what his belief
> actually is. Thus a person able to exercise this capacity is in a position to declare
> what his belief is by reflection on the reasons in favor of that belief, rather than by
> examination of the psychological evidence. In this way . . . avowal can be seen as
> an expression of genuine self-knowledge. (Moran 2004, p. 425)

Does authorship *require* rationality? Being the author of one's beliefs
(intentions, decisions, etc.) requires the capacity for giving reasons.
This capacity requires the use of reason, but it is not sufficient for
rationality in the sense that it does not necessarily involve giving *good*
reasons or endorsing *rational* beliefs (intentions, decisions, etc.). Does
authorship *enhance* rationality? Not necessarily. The agential perspective is a stance in which reasons are evaluated and evidence is weighed
up. If the person engaging in reason giving adopts rational criteria for
the evaluation of reasons and weighs up all the evidence relevant to her
act of deliberation or justification, then we can expect the ensuing mental state (belief, intention, decision, etc.) to be rational all things considered, and to add to the rationality of the agent's behaviour (Bortolotti
2009b).

Does authorship require or enhance self-knowledge? Again, not necessarily. Authorship provides an additional route to knowledge of some
attitudes (those that can be deliberated about or justified with reasons).
Thus, we can say that it *contributes to* self-knowledge. However, this is
not equivalent to claiming that agents who author their attitudes by
default have self-knowledge with respect to those attitudes. Claire may
be receiving conflicting messages about the belief that she shouldn't go
to Rita's party. On the one hand, the reasons she considered speak
against going to the party; on the other hand, she may experience a little
spark of excitement at the mere idea of the party. What Claire genuinely believes, in some circumstances, may not be transparent to her,
partly because she may not realize what her 'best reasons' are.

Moreover, we should distinguish between knowledge of the content
of a mental state and knowledge of the reasons why that mental state

was endorsed. For instance, imagine that Ron's suspicions are well-founded and that the real reason why Claire believes that she shouldn't go to the party is that she is not attracted at all to the idea of going out and prefers to sit on the couch and watch TV instead (independent of how busy her day at work has been and how far the party venue is). Claire may identify correctly her belief that she should not go to the party, but identify incorrectly the reasons for her belief: that she is tired because she had a busy day at work, and because the party venue is not easy to reach by car. Claire thinks that she formed her belief on the basis of what she takes to be her true reasons, but she is mistaken about what her true reasons are. Although her 'error' has implications for the claim that Claire is an overall knowledgeable and rational agent, it does not compromise the claim that Claire is the *author* of her belief. As long as she adopts an agential stance towards her belief, she is the author.

Authorship contributes to self-knowledge: by giving reasons in support of their attitudes, people come to know that they have those attitudes in a way that differs from mere introspection or inference from behaviour. Moreover, they feel entitled to the beliefs (intentions, preferences, decisions) they author and recognize themselves as people who endorse beliefs (intentions, preferences, decisions) with those contents.

5.4 Self-narratives

The notion of self-narrative has been used in recent philosophical investigation to account for the notion of autonomy. The basic idea we shall explore here is that developing self-narratives contributes to people acquiring a sense of self and is necessary for self-governance. People tell stories about themselves which help them recollect memories about past experiences, identify certain patterns and a sense of direction in their life events, and have some concept of what kind of person they are, what they have achieved or failed to achieve, and what their future objectives are.

> Generation of explanations about our perceptions, memories, and actions, and the relationships between them, leads to the construction of a personal narrative that ties together elements of our conscious experience into a coherent whole. (Roser and Gazzaniga 2004, p. 58)

Authoring an attitude can be seen as a means to integrate an isolated preference or an apparently insignificant belief into a coherent whole that delivers a conception of the self. Suppose that Claire honestly believes that she is skipping Rita's birthday party because she is tired and not confident about her driving. On the basis of her belief, she will make further decisions, predictions about her future behaviour and commitments. People around her, instead, find that she is becoming increasingly lazy and less likely to go out, independent of whether the event is nearby or whether she is tired. Claire's self-narrative may be false, but the fact that she can offer plausible reasons for her belief, and recognize herself in that belief, might contribute to changing the truth about what kind of person she is. And at some time in the future, she might become a person who is not confident about her driving and will go to parties only when she is not too tired, as a result of (a) genuinely believing that those were the reasons why she skipped Rita's party and (b) trying to impose consistency on her own thoughts and actions.

In a different scenario, Claire may be convinced by Ron that she is becoming increasingly lazy and realize that the real motivation behind her belief that she shouldn't go to the party had very little to do with how hard her day at work had been and with the distance between her place and Rita's. As a result of this 'self revelation' (see Wilson 2002, chapter 10), Claire will change her own self-narrative and may attempt to change her future behaviour so as to beat the lazy disposition that her friends recently observed in her. Claire may think: 'I don't want to become a couch potato. From now on every weekend I will endeavour to do something special, something that requires energy and initiative on my part'. As a result of her resolution, Claire will become more active and more sociable. This change is brought about by (a) recognizing the real reasons for her previous behaviour and (b) attempting to make her life correspond with her own conception of herself as an active and lively person.

Contemporary philosophers have drawn attention to self-narrative in describing the nature of the self and the mechanisms underlying autonomous thought and action. For instance, Dennett (1992) argues that the self is a *centre of narrative gravity*: it is the fictional character the self-narrative talks about, a fiction by means of which we can impose some order on complicated autobiographical events. He argues that the narrative in which the self is the leading character is produced by the brain. This builds upon Gazzaniga's (1985) work where he describes what he calls an 'interpreter module' which provides a running commentary and forms hypotheses to explain the agent's actions. In the narrative, there is one single entity to which attitudes and actions are ascribed, a unified self, a locus of agency. But, according to Dennett, this is not necessarily how things are outside the fiction, where there is no self over and beyond the 'I' in the running commentary.

Velleman (2005) partially agrees with Dennett that the self is the character of a narrative, but argues that the narrative is not necessarily false, and thus the self may actually exist. The narrative is true in so far as it accurately describes past events that happened to the agent, and it is true in so far as it affects the future behaviour of the agent and 'makes itself true'. Velleman's main objective is to square the insight that the self is a fiction with the acknowledgement of a capacity that most humans have, that of self-constitution. This is the capacity to invent or create oneself.

> In Dennett's metaphor, the self is the non-existent author of a merely fictional autobiography composed by the human organism, which neither is nor embodies a real self. (Velleman 2005, p. 204)
> My only disagreement with Dennett will be that, whereas he regards an autobiography as fictive and consequently false in characterizing its protagonist, I regard it as both fictive and true. We invent ourselves, I shall argue, but we really are the characters whom we invent. (Velleman 2005, p. 206)

The key to Velleman's view is that the narrative can be produced by a module in the agent's brain, but the narrative ultimately reflects the behaviour of the agent and is also able to produce changes in such behaviour. As he puts it, an autobiography and the behaviour that it narrates are mutually determining. We produce a narrative in order to interpret the events in our lives, but then we also behave in such a way as to be faithful to the story we have been telling. This mutual determination is what explains the phenomenon of self-constitution, creating the self by making commitments about the future:

> As your hand hovers indecisively over the candy dish, you say, 'No, I won't', not because you weren't about to take a candy, but because saying so may stop you from taking one. (Velleman 2005, p. 214)

According to Velleman, an autonomous agent is precisely an individual with the power of self-constitution. An attitude that is authored and integrated in an agent's narrative is more likely to affect the decisions made and the actions performed by that agent. Arguably, the self intimations of the type 'No, I won't' are expressions of the agential stance we talked about in the previous section.

Motivated reconstruction and interpretation shape memories and contribute to the creation of the self as a narrative character—but this character exists outside the fiction, it is (to an extent at least) *created by* the narrative. This does not mean though that the narrative is always true and accurate. The narrative strives for coherence, and because of the very many factors that affect a person's behaviour, coherence can sometimes be achieved only at the cost of distorting the facts. This does not necessarily lead to pathological confabulation or delusional memories, but is a feature of normal cognition.

> [T]his value attached to narrativity in the representation of real events arises out of a desire to have real events display the coherence, integrity, fullness, and closure of an image of life that is and can only be imaginary. (White 1987, p. 24)

There are everyday examples of unreliable self-narratives that are not pathological: in general, people go a long way to preserve a positive conception of themselves and their perception of their own successes and failures (e.g. self-serving biases) is often different from a third-person's perception. However, when distortions are more severe, not even perceptual information or general principles of plausibility may serve as constraints on the narrative. For instance, patients with anosognosia (denial of illness) for arm paralysis may claim that their arm can and does move, even if they have no perceptual deficits and should be perfectly able to see that their arm lies motionless at their side. Such patients have not updated their narratives to include the presence of a serious impairment such as paralysis of their limbs, among their significant life events.

> Patients with severe cognitive deficits often confabulate wildly in order to produce an explanation of the world that is consistent with their conscious experience. These confabulations include completely denying the existence of a deficit and probably result from interpretations of incomplete information [. . .]. Wild confabulations that seem untenable to most people, because of conscious access

to information that contradicts them, probably seem completely normal to patients to whom only a subset of the elements of consciousness are available for integration. (Roser and Gazzaniga 2004, p. 57)

Self-narratives can be partial accounts of life events that are interpreted in a biased way and do not necessarily take into account all relevant unconscious or preconscious behavioural dispositions. In pathological cases, conditions involving memory impairment, motivational factors and limited access to personal information prevent the narrative from updating, and the narration is so insulated from the reality checks available to the narrator that it appears to others as blatantly false (as in Alzheimer's disease). But what is really interesting about narrations of this type is that they can start as being false and then become true, because in some circumstances they have the power to influence or determine behaviour.

5.5 **Unreliable autobiographies**

The literature on delusions has recently explored possible connections between delusions as a breakdown of rationality and delusions as failures of self-knowledge. Gerrans (2009) criticizes the inferential approach to the explanation of delusions, because it usually ignores the limitations of the capacity for accurate autobiographical narration in people with delusions.

> The inferential conception of delusion treats the delusional subject as a scientist in the grip of an intractable confirmation bias. She recalls and attends selectively to evidence consistent with her biased hypothesis with the result that the delusions become ever more firmly woven into her Quinean web of beliefs [. . .]. I propose instead that processes of selective attention and recall exert their effects, not on a process of hypothesis confirmation but of autobiographical narrative. Someone with a delusion is not a mad scientist but an unreliable narrator. (Gerrans 2009, p. 152)

Gerrans proposes that people with delusions attribute excessive significance to some of their experiences. According to Gerrans, it is relevant to the explanation of hypersalience in delusions (Kapur 2003) that retrieved experiences (which are either the object of memory or the basis for imagination) come with an 'emotional tone' attached to them. Kapur's idea is that without an emotional tone a person's experiences wouldn't come to their attention and wouldn't be regarded as meaningful. With Gerrans we can suppose that, when experiences are accompanied by salience, they become integrated in an autobiographical story that partially determines what comes next in the story by guiding deliberation. If only experiences attached to negative emotions are retrieved (as in depression), or if abnormal experiences are attributed excessive significance and weaved into the story as a dominant event (as in some delusions), thoughts and behaviours acquire pathological characteristics.

This approach vindicates the apparent success of some form of medication (D2 antagonists) and of cognitive behavioural therapy. Kapur argues that such medication can stop the generation of inappropriate salience and hence the emotional valence of relevant experiences is lessened. As a result, people become less preoccupied and more 'open' to psychological techniques and in particular to the cognitive probing of their pathological beliefs. Gerrans notices that in cognitive behavioural therapy people with delusions are encouraged to refocus attention on a different set of experiences from the ones that contribute to the delusional narrative, or to stop weaving the delusional experiences in their autobiographies by constructing scenarios in which such experiences would make sense even if the delusional state were false.

In one paper discussing the effects of certain forms of psychopathology on autonomy and moral responsibility, Kennett and Matthews (2009) argue that one condition that is necessary for a person to be autonomous is the capacity to make choices and decisions that commit one's future self to certain courses of action (p. 329). Summarizing a report from Levine and colleagues (1998), Kennett and Matthews make a case for the necessity of episodic memory for forward planning:

> M.L. suffered a severe brain injury and was in the immediate post-injury period amnesic both for events and persons as well as suffering impairments in semantic knowledge. He made a good recovery from his semantic deficits and he re-learned significant facts about his own past. However, his recall of events from his personal past remained fragmentary. Moreover and significantly, M.L. was unable to episodically re-experience post-injury events to the same extent as control subjects, although he could use familiarity or other non-episodic processes to distinguish events he had experienced from those he had not experienced. He continued to report a feeling of subjective distance from recall of events occurring after his recovery. He displayed errors of judgement and failures to understand

his responsibilities as a parent that required supervision of his behaviour and structured routines. He was unable to secure paid employment [. . .]. Cases such as M.L. bring out the importance of the kind of access we have to past episodes for the purposes of planning and deliberation. An effective agent is the true author of the project, fully invested in its completion, and above all she has a knowledge of it that is part and parcel of her self-knowledge. (Kennett and Matthews 2009, p. 340)

In conditions similar to that of ML, where access to previous thoughts, commitments and experiences is lost due to memory impairments, the agent can find herself thinking or doing things without being able to provide reasons for them because she has no access to relevant biographical data and cannot construct a coherent narrative. As ML cannot have episodic memories of events that occurred after his accident, his capacity for deliberation and his capacity to assume moral responsibility for his actions are both compromised. Similarly, the person with dissociative identity disorder who acts in one of her alter states cannot rely on the thoughts, commitments, and past experiences of her 'host' personality, as these are not available to her. There are good reasons to believe that seriously impaired access to autobiographical information of this type and lack of narrative integration result in the loss of the capacity for self-governance.

The case of people with delusions and confabulations is not typically a case in which self-narratives cannot be constructed at all, but in which they are constructed *unreliably*. Most delusions and confabulations are integrated in a person's narrative, at least to some extent, but they may be paid excessive attention, or may remain compartmentalized with respect to other beliefs. In general, integrating a belief into a self-narrative is beneficial. But when the belief is delusional or confabulatory, and thus likely to be false, integration might have disadvantages: by integrating delusional and confabulatory beliefs in a narrative, a person becomes less prone to revise her delusions or confabulations in the presence of external challenges. Delusions that are rationalized become ingrained and may lead to further false beliefs and to avoiding considering evidence that would lead to the revision of the delusions and confabulations.

The positive and negative aspects of confabulating and rationalizing have been observed in other contexts. Finding reasons for a false and irrational belief in general gives rise to more false and irrational beliefs, and thus is *epistemically* bad. But confabulations and rationalizations can have an adaptive function:

> The real reason for the evolution of these defense mechanisms (confabulations, rationalization), I suggest is to create a coherent system in order to impose stability in one's behaviour. [. . .] When something doesn't quite fit the script however, you very rarely tear up the entire story and start from scratch. What you do, instead, is to deny or confabulate in order to make the information fit the big picture. (Ramachandran 1996, p. 351)

Confabulation is sometimes the only means by which people can maintain a unified and coherent sense of self. Fotopoulou (2008) observes that after brain damage or memory loss, personal narratives can be disrupted, undermining people's sense of coherence and making the future less predictable. This is often associated with increased anxiety and depression.

> Despite their poor correspondence with reality, confabulations represent attempts to define one's self in time and in relation to the world. Thus, they are subject to motivational influences and they serve important identity formation functions. (Fotopoulou 2008, p. 542)

In the context of serious memory disorders, Fotopoulou argues that confabulators construct distorted or false selves. They may claim that they live in a different place, that they have a different profession, or a different family. The personal narrative confabulators construct is not 'anchored and constrained by reality' (2008, p. 548). These distortions are exaggerated by brain damage or memory loss, but are not different types of distortions from those present in normal subjects attempting to remember past events and making errors (see Burgess and Shallice 1996).

> Confabulators' narratives might also exhibit an exaggerated self-serving bias but the majority of people reconstruct memories that are consistent with their desired self-image. To some degree, and for the sake of creating a coherency to life, it is normal to confabulate and to enhance one's story. Self-deception is not unusual; false memories are frequent. (Gallagher 2003, p. 348)

It is what Fotopoulou calls the 'identity formation' of confabulation that interests us here. In dementia or amnesia, patients revisit their past and attempt to build a bridge with their premorbid self in order to make sense of their present experiences and feelings. Confabulations are instrumental for people to establish continuity between the image of themselves before the accident, the illness, or the memory loss, and the image of themselves afterwards. Confabulations are also an attempt to preserve a positive self-image. These two functions of confabulation can also be observed in normal subjects who tend to present their current selves in a way that is both coherent and largely favourable.

This reflection on the potential effects of confabulation suggests a tension between the aim of preserving coherence and the aim of being constrained by reality (Conway et al. 2004; Conway 2005). Consider confabulators with dementia or brain damage. They act out a script that is roughly known to them, and that links their current experiences with common experiences lived by their previous selves and remembered in a superficial, fragmented and possibly even biased way. Coherence trumps correspondence, as the 'reality' to which their stories should make reference (their past lives and their connection to their present lives) is poorly (if at all) remembered, and poorly understood. Now consider subjects with delusions. They find themselves with a certain belief, or experience, and they support it with secondary confabulations or delusional systematization that allows them to present a (largely) coherent and intelligible position, rather than crumble under the pressure of contradictions and challenges. Yet again coherence trumps correspondence, as the 'reality' they describe is coloured by beliefs whose process of acquisition is not necessarily introspectively available to them, or by experiences that are the result of a neurobiological deficit.

The obvious disadvantage of the preference for coherence over correspondence is that losing touch with reality can create a gulf between the person with delusions and confabulations and her interlocutors. Given that confabulations consist in ill-grounded statements about the present or the past, they do little to remedy the 'ignorance' (i.e. inaccessibility of information) that caused them in the first place, and they are not likely to be believed by others. Fotopoulou (2008, p. 560) remarks that in the most serious amnesic conditions there is often a lack of 'shared reality' between confabulators and the people who were once closest to them, which can be very distressing for patients and their families. Moreover, in the case of delusions, as previously suggested, rationalization can contribute to increasing the elaboration and the rigidity of delusions—this is likely to result in delusions becoming less sensitive to counterevidence or counterargument.

However, confabulating can also have some pragmatic benefits: it allows people to keep constructing self-narratives in situations where personal information is no longer available. As a result, it secures some psychological continuity with the confabulators' previous selves in the absence of reliable recollective capacities, and it contributes to the preservation of psychological integration in absence of introspective access to the reasons for conscious attitudes such as beliefs, desires, and preferences. It also allows people to include new facts into previously developed narratives that have become fragmented. When a delusion becomes integrated in a personal narrative and part of the self-concept, giving up the delusion can generate lack of self-esteem and confusion about one's identity.

Suppose Jimmy has mistakenly believed for some time that he is an Oscar-winning actor. As a consequence of this delusion, he tells people in the pub about his life in the spotlight, his friends in Hollywood, his excellent salary, and his exotic holidays. But in real life Jimmy lives on benefits, and has no real friends. What will happen if he is 'cured of' his delusion? He will start doubting that he is a famous actor, but he will also appreciate that many of the things he believed to be true about himself were false. Jimmy will start seeing his life as it really is—empty. The effects of making one's self-narrative correspond to reality can be devastating, and many people experience serious depression when they recover or acquire insight into their illness. From clinical experience we note that rates of suicide are highest in the first few years of a psychotic illness when people try to come to terms with their loss of social networks and their fear of chronic mental illness (Drake and Cotton 1986; Clarke et al. 2006).

5.6 **Implications and conclusions**

In this paper, we have explained the effects of the epistemic faults of delusions and confabulation on autonomy (intended as self-governance) by introducing the notions of authorship and self-narrative. Through authorship, attitudes can be integrated into self-narratives, and by constructing self-narratives, agents can make sense of their previous behaviour and exercise control over their future behaviour. When we justify our previous attitudes or form new ones on the basis of reasons, we also create meaningful connections between these attitudes and other attitudes we have. This leads to the construction of a largely coherent story. In this story about ourselves, our sense of self guides the formation of future attitudes, and shapes future behaviour.

The narrative module doesn't just describe and explain past behaviour, but causally determines future behaviour, attempting to give a certain direction to the story. A reformed Claire may be thinking something like this: 'I don't want to become a couch potato. I have to be more active, and get out more'. At other times, the behaviour causally determines the narration. Beliefs, actions, or decisions that haven't necessarily been authored need to be made consistent with previous beliefs, actions and decisions post hoc, often at the expense of correspondence. The patient with anosognosia who is denying arm paralysis may be thinking something along these lines: 'My arm can move, but it's slower than usual. I must be suffering from arthritis'.

Failures of rationality and self-knowledge do not necessarily compromise the capacity to construct self-narratives, and thus the capacity for self-governance, but can result in *unsuccessful* self-ruling. Although (trivially) you don't need to be a successful self-ruler in order to be a self-ruler, self-knowledge and rationality help you become a successful self-ruler, while lack of self-knowledge and irrationality may interfere with the exercise of self-governance (Broome et al. 2010).

When correspondence and coherence go hand in hand rather than clash, psychological well-being is expected to ensue. When coherence wins out, and delusions and confabulations are woven in, this might also result in well-being, but only temporarily, until the pressure of fitting the story with reality becomes too much to bear (this is especially true of far-fetched delusions and confabulations which are integrated in the story at the cost of creating a gulf between story and reality). When correspondence is irremediably compromised by neurobiological deficits afflicting cognition, experience, or memory, then maintaining coherence at the expense of correspondence might be desirable. Some sense of self (even if inaccurate) is better than no sense of self. When correspondence is not irremediably compromised, and can be restored at the cost of crossing out a bit of the story and rewriting it (as in a circumscribed delusion), cognitive behavioural therapy alongside appropriate medication can serve this purpose.

In conclusion, delusions and confabulations do not necessarily signal a lack of *capacity* for autonomy as self-governance, but are a reason for alarm since they often interfere with the *exercise* of self-governance. On this account, what are the implications for policy? It would be a mistake to assume that people have lost their capacity for self-governance just because they report delusional beliefs and engage in confabulation. Failures of rationality and self-knowledge do not necessarily compromise the capacity to make decisions about one's own future. But such failures make it likely that decisions about one's own future are based on unreliable information about oneself and about the surrounding social and physical environment. That is why it would also be a mistake to assume that people with delusions and confabulations can govern themselves *successfully*.

Depending on the nature of their delusions and confabulations, and on the extent to which their attitudes depart from rationality, people with delusions and confabulations can make decisions that may not lead to the satisfaction of their own preferences and interests. As a result, such decisions may not be conducive to promoting their own well-being. As we have argued in this chapter, failures of rationality and self-knowledge turn people with delusions and confabulations into unreliable autobiographers, compromising the coherence of their attitudes and interfering with the accuracy of the information they have about themselves. Minor inaccuracies in a self-narrative can be beneficial, e.g. when an overly optimistic reconstruction of one's own past performance contributes to one's self-esteem and social confidence in everyday situations. However, accounts of shared experiences that depart radically from other people's cause a breakdown of communication, possibly leading to social withdrawal and isolation, and conflicting 'evidence' about oneself can create fragmented narratives that cannot shape future action in a consistent and meaningful way.

References

Allport, G. (1937). The functional autonomy of motives. *American Journal of Psychology* 50: 141–56.

American Psychiatric Association (2000). *Diagnostic Statistical Manual of Mental Disorders. Fourth edition, Text Revision (DSM-IV-TR)*. Washington, DC: American Psychiatric Association.

Anderson, J. and Lux, W. (2004). Knowing your own strength: accurate self-assessment as a requirement for personal autonomy. *Philosophy, Psychiatry, & Psychology* 11(4): 279–94.

Bortolotti, L. (2009a). *Delusions and Other Irrational Beliefs*. Oxford: Oxford University Press.

Bortolotti, L. (2009b). Epistemic benefits of reason giving. *Theory & Psychology* 19(5): 624–45.

Bortolotti, L. (2011). Psychiatric classification and diagnosis. Delusions and confabulations. *Paradigmi* XXXIX(1): 99–112.

Bortolotti, L. and Broome, M.R. (2008). Delusional beliefs and reason giving. *Philosophical Psychology* 21(3): 1–21.

Bortolotti, L. and Broome, M.R. (2009). A role for ownership and authorship in the analysis of thought insertion. *Phenomenology and the Cognitive Sciences* 8(2): 205–24.

Bortolotti, L. and Cox, R.E. (2009). 'Faultless' ignorance: Strengths and limitations of epistemic definitions of confabulation. *Consciousness and Cognition*, 952–65.

Broome, M.R., Mameli, M., and Bortolotti, L. (2010). Moral responsibility and mental illness. *Cambridge Quarterly of Healthcare Ethics* 19: 179–87.

Burgess, P.W. and Shallice, T. (1996). Confabulation and the control of recollection. *Memory* 4(4): 359–41.

Campbell, J. (2001) Rationality, meaning and the analysis of delusion. *Philosophy, Psychiatry, & Psychology* 8(2–3): 89–100.

Clarke, M., Whitty, P., Browne, S., Mc Tigue, O., Kinsella, A., Waddington, J., *et al.* (2006). Suicidality in first episode psychosis. *Schizophrenia Research* 86(1): 221–25.

Conway, M.A. (2005). Memory and the self. *Journal of Memory and Language* 53(4): 594–628.

Conway, M.A., Singer, J.A., and Tagini, A. (2004). The self and autobiographical memory: Correspondence and coherence. *Social Cognition* 22(5): 495–537.

Dennett, D.C. (1992). The self as a center of narrative gravity. In F. Kessel, P. Cole and D. Johnson (eds.) *Self and Consciousness: Multiple Perspectives*. Hillsdale, NJ: Lawrence Erlbaum, pp. 103–15.

Drake, R.E. and Cotton, P.G. (1986). Depression, hopelessness and suicide in chronic schizophrenia. *British Journal of Psychiatry* 148(5): 554–59.

Fotopoulou, A. (2008) False-selves in neuropsychological rehabilitation: The challenge of confabulation. *Neuropsychological Rehabilitation* 18(5/6): 541–65.

Gallagher, S. (2003). Self-narrative in schizophrenia. In A.S. David and T. Kircher (eds.) *The Self in Neuroscience and Psychiatry*. Cambridge: Cambridge University Press, pp. 336–57.

Gazzaniga, M. (1985). *The Social Brain: Discovering the Networks of the Mind*. New York: Basic Books.

Gerrans, P. (2000). Refining the explanation of Cotard's delusion. *Mind and Language* 15(1): 111–22.

Gerrans, P. (2009). Mad scientists or unreliable autobiographers? Dopamine dysregulation and delusion. In M.R. Broome and L. Bortolotti (eds.) *Psychiatry as Cognitive Neuroscience: Philosophical Perspectives*. Oxford: Oxford University Press, pp. 151–72.

Jaspers, K. (1963). *General Psychopathology*, J. Hoenig and M. Hamilton (trans.). Manchester: Manchester University Press.

Kapur, S. (2003) Psychosis as a state of aberrant salience: a framework linking biology, phenomenology, and pharmacology in schizophrenia. *American Journal of Psychiatry* 160(1): 13–23.

Kennett, J. and Matthews, S. (2002). Identity, control and responsibility: the case of dissociative identity disorder. *Philosophical Psychology* 15: 509–26.

Kennett, J. and Matthews, S. (2009). Mental time travel, agency and responsibility. In M.R. Broome and L. Bortolotti (eds.) *Psychiatry as Cognitive Neuroscience: Philosophical Perspectives*. Oxford: Oxford University Press, pp. 327–50.

Levine, B., Black, S.E., Cabeza, R., Sinden, M., Mcintosh, A.R., Toth, J.P., *et al.* (1998). Episodic memory and the self in a case of isolated retrograde amnesia. *Brain* 121(10): 1951–73.

McKay, R. and Cipolotti, L. (2007). Attributional style in a case of Cotard delusion. *Consciousness and Cognition* 16 (22): 349–53.

McKay, R., Langdon, R., and Coltheart, M. (2005a). 'Sleights of mind': Delusions, defences, and self deception. *Cognitive Neuropsychology* 10: 305–26.

Metcalf, K., Langdon, R., and Coltheart, M. (2007). Models of confabulation: a critical review and a new framework. *Cognitive Neuropsychology* 24(1): 23–47.

Moran, R. (2001). *Authority and Estrangement*. Princeton, NJ: Princeton University Press.

Moran, R. (2004). Précis of authority and estrangement. *Philosophy and Phenomenological Research* LXIX: 423–6.

Nisbett, R. and Wilson, T. (1977). Telling more than we can know: Verbal reports on mental processes. *Psychological Review* 84(3): 231–59.

Örulv, L. and Hydén, L.-C. (2006). Confabulation: sense-making, self-making and world-making in dementia. *Discourse Studies* 8: 647–73.

Ramachandran, V.S. (1996). The evolutionary biology of self deception, laughter, dreaming and depression: some clues from anosognosia. *Medical Hypotheses* 47(5): 347–62.

Roser, M. and Gazzaniga, M. (2004). Automatic brains- interpretive minds. *Current Directions in Psychological Science* 13(2): 56–59.

Turnbull, O., Jenkins, S., and Rowley, M. (2004). The pleasantness of false beliefs: an emotion-based account of confabulation. *Neuro-Psychoanalysis* 6(1): 5–45 (including commentaries).

Velleman, D. (2006). *Self to Self*. Cambridge: Cambridge University Press.

Wegner, D. (2002). *The illusion of conscious will*. Cambridge, MA: MIT Press.

White, H. (1987). *The Content of the Form*. Baltimore, MD: John Hopkins University Press.

Wilson, T.D. (2002). *Strangers to ourselves*. Cambridge, MA: Belknap Press.

Chapter 6

Privacy and patient autonomy in mental healthcare

Jennifer Radden

6.1 Introduction

Autonomy is a category whose attribution is associated with a number of ideas pertinent to biomedical ethics.[1] These include ideas about the capabilities required for the exercise of informed consent, and ideas about the conditions for freedom or liberty. The individual with autonomy possesses the agency required for self-rule, and is free of any external constraints that might prevent her from exercising it. In the context of mental healthcare, issues of information privacy and confidentiality intersect with both aspects of autonomy. Agency is often compromised during episodes of severe disorder, and the recovered patient's subsequent freedom to exercise autonomy is reduced when confidentiality has been breached. Because autonomy is so importantly contingent on the preservation of privacy in these settings, respecting autonomy requires unsurpassed attention to patient privacy.

The several inter-related elements here include both the patient's own ability to ensure privacy of information (henceforth 'privacy'), and the duties of caregivers to maintain confidentiality. The nature of mental disorder, its distinctive treatment, and the social role of caregivers all combine to leave patient privacy in considerable jeopardy. Thus, in the throes of severe disorder, patients are often unable to ensure (and indifferent about), the protection of their privacy, and the

---

[1] The range of ways autonomy is appealed to suggest there are alternative, context-specific *conceptions* rather than a single concept of autonomy, it has been recognized (Arpaly 2004). For a review of these different conceptions see Buss (2008).

treatment they receive almost always expects heedless candour. By maintaining confidentiality, caregivers can protect patient privacy, and they have a prima facie duty to do so. Yet caregivers are required to break patient confidentiality when, because of the risk of harm to others and to the patient herself, they do so for purposes of public safety and social welfare, respectively.

What can be called the *privacy stakes* for the patient comprise: (1) the likelihood that confidentiality will be breached, and (2) the degree of subsequent harm resulting from that breach. And both are particularly high, I want to emphasize here. Even before the approaching digitization of medical records that will further jeopardize patient privacy, this mix of a high risk of disclosure combined with the highly negative consequences of such disclosure brings places the recipient of psychiatric care for severe disorder in a situation of extreme and continuing vulnerability.

Following the contrast between (1) and (2), the present discussion falls into two parts that correspond loosely to the two aspects of autonomy noted earlier. Laying out the ways patient privacy and confidentiality rights are in jeopardy, Section 6.2 ('Part one') emphasizes agency, that is, the aspect of autonomy embodied in the principle of informed consent. Section 6.3 ('Part two') notes how protecting patient privacy and confidentiality during episodes of severe disorder while the agency required for autonomy may be compromised, affects the subsequent freedom of the one-time patient when she has recovered.

6.2 Part one

6.2.1 The usual protections may be insufficient

One of the most obvious safeguards against a violation of privacy and breaches of confidentiality across all healthcare settings is the principle of informed consent. When any case material leaves the doctor's office, or information about any aspect of the treatment is exposed to others (such as when trainees are present to observe hospital rounds), the patient's consent must first be sought. The aspect of autonomy that involves the decisional capacities associated with *agency*, is employed here.

And preserving one's privacy has always been regarded as emblematic of exercising such autonomy (Allen 2009). This emphasis on consent is found in standard analyses of privacy and confidentiality, such as the following one:

> If a patient or research subject *authorizes* release of ... information to others, then no violation of rights of confidentiality occurs, although a loss of both confidentiality and privacy may occur.
>
> An infringement of person's right to confidentiality occurs only if the person (or institution) to whom the information was disclosed in confidence fails to protect the information or deliberately discloses it to someone without *first-party consent* (Beauchamp and Childress 2001, pp. 306, 304, emphasis added)

The right to privacy and duty of confidentiality are enshrined in several legal traditions. In tort law, privacy has traditionally been protected as an interest in having control over information about oneself (De Cew 1997). Echoing such notions of privacy are the above emphasis on the control we exercise over certain private information about ourselves, and the importance of consent in all matters to do with it. Thus, a right to privacy becomes 'valid claims against unauthorized access that have their basis in the right to authorize or decline access' (Beauchamp and Childress 2001, p. 296). Consent reflects not a waiving of the right, on this analysis, but an exercise of it (Beauchamp and Childress 2001, p. 297).

The principle of informed consent reflects our hallowed liberal conceptions of the person as an autonomous agent, possessed of the capacity to decide what is in her best interests, able to understand the risks and costs of proposed courses of action, and sufficiently stable in her guiding values and well-considered, planful judgments to abide by them.[2] This is a somewhat idealized depiction of the capacities making up the agency called for here. Indeed, research suggests that few subjects or patients of any kind actually achieve the level of rational agency as so depicted (Cassileth et al. 1980; Appelbaum et al. 2004; Flory and Emanuel 2004). Nonetheless, the patient in the throes of an episode of severe psychiatric disorder will not even be close. Episodes of this kind

---

[2] See Berg and Appelbaum (2001).

regularly compromise people's judgement over their immediate and long-term self-interests, as well as some or all of their: reasoning ability; insight into their own condition; self-control; steady allegiance to long-term goals and values; capacity to communicate their concerns and needs to others; and perceptions of other people's responses.[3]

At one time or another, these obstacles to autonomous functioning are an aspect of the experience of most psychiatric patients enduring episodes of severe disorder. This is not an accidental correlation. In the absence of other, biologically measurable markers, this is part of how such disorder is identified and its severity defined.

Informed consent to treatment and consent to research (as subjects) can be achieved, it has been shown, in spite of these obstacles, when time can be taken to coach the patient about the issues involved (Carpenter et al. 2000). And my claim here is not that psychiatric patients always lack the capabilities required for autonomous agency, nor that patient permission to disclose details (of diagnosis, prognosis, treatment, etc.) should not be sought—of course it should. Nonetheless, particularly when the condition is severe, during the turmoil of extreme psychosis for example, the protection provided by informed consent (to disclosure of information) will not get us far enough.

Many patients are fiercely concerned to protect their privacy, even irrationally so, it is true. But consider the following case examples, told in the words of a clinician, and also reportedly not untypical.

Case 1

The patient came in very manic and requested I give him a note for work explaining to his boss not only that he was out sick but that he is taking a few days off to solve the problem of global warming, using some chemical apparatus he's set up in his garage. 'Are you sure you want me to tell him all that, Mr M?' I asked. Of course, he answered: 'Tell him everything: I want him to know!' Again, I protested: 'I'd have to tell him why you were seeing me—this might not be wise'. But he was adamant: 'I don't care what you tell him! I authorize you—no, I insist—you tell him what's going on. He'll give me a bonus!'.

---

[3] For discussions of these kinds of disability when the psychiatric patient is a recipient of treatment and or a research subject, see Dresser (1996) and Roberts (2000).

Case 2

My patient was hospitalized in a locked ward and far from home, and it fell to me to talk to her family. She had come to believe that marks on the windshield of her car were messages from God, directing her to preach the Gospel to those around her. Explaining this directive to me, she urged me to share her revelation with her elderly mother and her school-age daughters. I explained that I was reluctant to do so, and that whatever the truth of these messages, her loved ones would be bothered by them. She was distressed over my decision, seeing me as an agent of the devil for my failure to tell the world of her revelation—this was a message from God, she stressed, and not to be kept secret.

Case 3

The patient (Mr J) was refused continuing treatment by his medical insurer. In attempting to intervene, I explained to him that the company's case manager would need information about the severity of his depressive illness, including details he had shared about suicidal thoughts. Mr J was indifferent and uncaring, entirely unable to respond to the issue presented to him: 'What does it matter? Tell them whatever you want— I don't care'.

Mr M, Ms S, and Mr J has each been informed and given consent to disclosure of information about their condition. But whether any can be said to offer informed consent seems debatable. The evident distortions and grandiosity in Mr M's reply, the apparently delusional aspects of Ms S's ideas, and the depressive indifference of Mr J's response each indicate autonomy-affecting capabilities that are temporarily disabled. Only on a very minimalist interpretation limited to basic comprehension—and such a standard has been explored—could any of these three patients be said to possess decisional capacity.[4]

On less minimal interpretations, the sort of decisional capacity required for informed consent has been seen to comprise at least four parts: comprehension, appreciation, reasoning, and choice (Charland 2010).[5] While he may understand and have articulated a choice, it seems

[4] The minimal interpretation is discussed in Grisso and Appelbaum (1998, pp. 37–42). See also Wirshing et.al (1998) and Sreenivasan (2003, 2005).

[5] These aspects of decisional capacity have also been depicted in terms of the more legal notion of voluntarism (Roberts 2002).

Mr M fails to appreciate of the nature and significance of releasing this information; and his optimistic predictions appear distorted, and unrealistic. Similarly, Ms S 's sense of its real world, as distinct to spiritual, implications suggests a failure of appreciation, and her account of why the marks on the windshield were messages from God rather than of some more prosaic origin, hints at flawed reasoning. Mr J's indifference presents the most puzzling case: his unconcern seems apt, given his apathetic attitude—the problem lies with the attitude. But perhaps we could invoke another criterion of decisional capacity, having a minimally consistent and stable set of values (Buchanan and Brock 1989, p. 24). Mr J's uncaring attitude exhibits a deficit with respect to valuing and values.

Fine-grained interpretations of decisional capacity based on criteria such as these will determine whether the case examples illustrate the success of the principle of informed consent in excluding Mr M's, Ms S's, and Mr J's avowels from the status of informed or consenting, or its failure (in including them).[6]

To successfully protect the patient's privacy, these cases seem to indicate, minimal standards of informed consent will need to be avoided. But a further reason to avoid minimal standards lies with the magnitude of the subsequent harm risked when privacy is not protected, discussed in 'Part two' (Section 6.3). Within research ethics a principle has been articulated that aligns that magnitude (of harm to the patient) with higher standards for attributing decisional capacity—or, as it is sometimes put, consent that is appropriately informed and voluntary (Dresser 1996).[7] Given the privacy stakes for the patient in the psychiatric setting, and applying that principle, such standards must be very high indeed. Moreover, to the extent that patients cannot protect themselves using informed consent procedures, the duties of caregivers will expand and become more weighty.

....

[6] For a review of the disparate interpretations of each of the four capacities noted here, on which Mr M's, Ms S's, and Mr J's status would seem to rest, see Charland (2010). See also Holroyd, Chapter 7, this volume.

[7] 'A higher level of decisional ability should be required when research participation presents significant risk and little or no chance of benefit to subjects than when the risk-benefit ratio is more favorable for subjects' (Dresser 1996, p. 69).

Legal structures take us some way in solving this problem of the patient temporarily incapable of protecting her own privacy though an exercise of autonomy, viz. advance care directives (also called 'Ulysses Contracts' within psychiatry), and the assigning of power of attorney or some other form of substituted judgement. The person who anticipates a return of a disabling condition can plan ahead, explaining the measure of confidentiality she will want at that future time. Or she can designate someone else to make those decisions for her. Both arrangements at times prove helpful, although they have limitations, and prompt additional, controversial questions. (Issues of personal identity are raised by advance care directives of this kind, for example; in particular, why—and when—should an earlier self be permitted to dictate what happens to a later self, including what degree of privacy it enjoys? (Radden 1996; DeGrazia 2005); and, again, at what level of competence or decisional capacity should the patient's present wishes be substituted by the earlier directive or substituted judgement (Buchanan and Brock 1989; Shiffrin 2004).) A more obvious limitation is perhaps the most easily solved: these arrangements have thus far been restricted to the recurrence of episodes of mental disorder. To help those suffering the first episode they would need to be more widely employed. (Just as the general living will has sufficient generality to anticipate hypothetical end of life healthcare situations, so the psychiatric advance care directive might be formulated, and administered, to anticipate hypothetical first episodes.)

Despite the potential of such advance planning, however, protecting patient privacy remains a joint effort: patients cannot protect their privacy rights alone, and a duty of confidentiality is incumbent on caregivers around them.

Employing the definitions and conceptions introduced thus far, we can sum up here by saying that when autonomy-affecting capabilities are compromised during episodes of severe mental disorder, informational privacy, and what Beauchamp and Childress call the right to decline or authorize access, will be under considerable strain. For this reason, the caregiver's obligations of confidentiality are profoundly important. Moreover, the privacy stakes are enormously high here in terms of future harm, affecting the standard of decisional capacity employed when consent (to disclose) is sought.

6.2.2 Psychiatric disorders and their treatment both place privacy at risk

Arguably, confidentiality around every aspect of mental health treatment, including record-keeping and research, must be guarded with greater attention and vigilance than is true in many other healthcare settings. This is so for several reasons, some concerning the nature of mental disorder and its treatment, and others the consequences of disclosure on the subsequent life of the recovered patient.

The subject matter that makes up symptoms, treatment goals, and focus, as well as other aspects of the therapeutic exchange when episodes of severe disorder are treated, is regularly *personal, delicate, intimate,* and/or *revealing*.[8] The content of the therapeutic exchange, for example, is rarely anything short of private in this sense because of the nature of severe mental illness. Intense and potentially embarrassing feelings, 'crazy' ideas and experiences, delusional and incomprehensible thoughts, often focused on sexuality, spiritual and metaphysical matters, fantasy life and dreams, are regularly present. Treatment for severe disorder involves aspects of ourselves that are (in varying degrees) usually: 1) concealed from public view, 2) often considered inappropriate for public presentation, and/or 3) involve material over which we exercise our right to 'decline or authorize access' with the utmost attention and discretion. At least presumptively, they are private. (This is not to suggest risks are only imposed by the content of the therapeutic exchange; exposure of information about anything that occurs in, and any aspect of, the therapeutic context has the potential to prove a damaging violation of privacy. But the delicate and presumptively private subject matter is nonetheless a distinctive aspect of psychiatric disorder and treatment.)

Psychiatrist Leston Havens speaks of the psychiatric interview as another secret place (Havens 1989, p. 133). In part he means what is

---

[8]   These terms are all inexact, of course. (So are legal attempts to capture the kinds of information over which privacy rights have been thought to apply—see Parent (1983).) Such vagueness is unsurprising, however. These matters are tied to cultural norms, and the scope of informational privacy rights is contested. There are unclear cases at the margins, undeniably; but core cases also exist.

discussed behind that closed door, the nature of the subject matter. But the customs governing the therapeutic 'frame', customs suited to the peculiar intensity of the therapeutic relationship, also in part explain the secrecy to which Havens alludes. Some of these customs, if we accept psychodynamic ideas, are attributable to the transferential nature of that relationship. Feelings and attitudes with unique intensity and significance are involved. Some sense of this quality emerges from discussions about the importance of maintaining therapeutic 'boundaries', that have been described as the 'structural characteristics of the relationship that allow the therapist to interact with warmth, empathy, and spontaneity within certain conditions that create a climate of safety' (Gabbard 1999, p. 143). Protected by these boundaries, the patient is encouraged to disclose, uninhibitedly, her innermost thoughts, feelings, and impulses.

This last is particularly critical. The stress on candour in describing symptoms varies widely across other medical conditions; in some it is essential to effective treatment, in others irrelevant. But within psychiatry, such disclosure forms an almost unfailing aspect of treatment. The strong presumption is that any failure on the patient's part to disclose her inner states in this way will detract from, or even sabotage, the therapeutic effort. Because so much depends on first-person, phenomenological description in efforts to identify and treat psychiatric conditions, patient candour is a fundamental ground rule of all practice.

Privacy and confidentiality are valued in every medical setting, it is true. In practising medical privacy, as Anita Allen puts it, institutions try to 'limit access to health information, respect medical autonomy, and honor expectations of modesty, intimacy, bodily integrity, and self-ownership' (Allen 2009).[9] There are undoubtedly some more straightforwardly medical conditions that, because of their embarrassing nature (bowel cancer), association with gender traits (breast cancer), or with behaviour that is frowned on (AIDS, obesity), for example, are viewed—rightly or wrongly—in something the same way as mental disorder with regard to the characterization of content privacy offered

[9] See also Allen (2003) and Humber and Almeder (2001).

in (1)–(3) earlier. Their strong link to self-identity may distinguish mental disorders even here: a diagnosis of mental illness, it has been pointed out 'more sweepingly and persuasively' than other medical diagnoses, affects how a person's whole identity is viewed, so that 'all the person's behaviors may come to be interpreted through the lens or label of the illness' (Mills 2009, p. 21). That link, the fact that severe mental disorder involves aspects of ourselves that are often concealed and closely guarded, added to the fact that mental disorder is still often seen as frighteningly inexplicable, combine to leave all or almost all mental disorders notably 'private' in these respects.

When they are recovered, these patients will be able to choose what to disclose and what to reveal, at least to the extent that other autonomous agents customarily do—although shame, embarrassment, and self stigmatizing attitudes have been observed as the sequel to such episodes, suggesting disclosure may be a freighted choice (Byrne 2000; Link et al. 2001.) In addition to these research observations, we can discern something about these privacy attitudes from the burgeoning literary genre of mental illness memoirs. (Other aspects of the social networking and interest group sites on the Internet are similarly revealing, but their anonymity alters and complicates them in relation to privacy matters, so I will restrict my attention to those memoirs in the present discussion.) At first observation, that writing suggests recovered patients will often choose the course of disclosure, rather than concealment. (Some evidence from recovery research even indicates that such disclosure may itself be healing (Young et al. 2008).) Nonetheless, these memoirs attest to attitudes towards the episodes of disturbance described that confirm how 'private' this material remains. Even when disclosure is chosen over concealment, the way these memoirs are framed suggests these matters are private, personal and potentially discomforting.[10]

---

[10] After such episodes, these states are often disowned, for example. In past, more religious times, recovered patients claimed their symptoms were the result of possession, or some other, external interfering agency ('the devil made me do it'; 'that was not me but my illness'); in earlier times and also today, those who suffered such episodes employ the language of earlier and later selves, to describe the changes that occurred ('I'm a different person now', 'That was not m'). See Radden (2008).

Thus far, we have spoken of privacy and confidentiality as *rights*, whose violation is intrinsically unacceptable, and this is the language within which much legal and bioethical discussion of privacy and confidentiality is conducted. But when we look at the privacy of the severely disordered mental patient, it is consequences that become inescapably important. The stakes are very high here because real world effects of breaches of confidentiality are incalculably severe. Telling, as it has been pointed out, is risky business (Wahl 1999).

Much stigma and consequent discrimination about mental disorder exist in the outside world: in housing, educational, and work opportunities, on the street, the shop, the underground. These harmful and far-reaching consequences also occur more personally, affecting relationships, opportunities for love and friendship, and access to many of the pleasures of human companionship and informal association.[11] Information about any aspect of the person's encounter with the psychiatrist, including the fact that he sees her at all, the nature of the diagnosis, the type of treatment, the prognosis, and the matters discussed in the therapeutic setting, all put the patient at risk of negative sequelae of these kinds.

Medical conditions involving private facts disclosure of which are comparably personal and delicate include not only those noted already (embarrassing, associated with gender traits, or behaviour that is frowned on), but sexually transmitted diseases, and genetic information. Within biomedical ethics, discussions of the harmful consequences that could result from the revelation of such facts have often focused on cases like these.[12] But so much is at risk in lapses of confidentiality for the psychiatric patient, that we can wonder whether the cases noted in bioethics discussions offer helpful analogies. The privacy stakes in the mental healthcare setting seem higher—or at least different. In the broader culture, if not within professional opinion, uncertainties and scepticism surround the aetiology, boundaries, diagnosis,

---

[11] See Fink and Tasman (1992), Hayward and Bright (1997), Wahl (1999), Bryne (2000), and Mental Health Foundation (2000).

[12] See, e.g. Beauchamp and Childress (2001).

and prognosis of mental disorders, for example, and no definitive test confirms their presence as it does with infectious diseases or genetic information. Moreover, even today mental disorders are widely regarded with dread, as well as distaste, discomfort, scepticism, and, sometimes, moral condemnation.

The set of reasons offered here included some that stem from the nature of severe mental disorder, its diagnosis and treatment, and others from cultural attitudes. Together, they impose strain on privacy and show why the demands on discretion are magnified in the psychiatry setting. But rather than supporting this injunction, public safety and social welfare obligations on caregivers sometimes work against it.

6.2.3 Other societal obligations jeopardize confidentiality

Considerations of privacy are over-ridden and patient confidentiality set aside for certain social goals and goods in a number of spheres—they are for purposes of public health in the case of infectious diseases, for example. Psychiatrists (and other mental healthcare workers) are often required—both legally and morally—to expose, report, and notify others about matters relating to their patients also, though for reasons not of public health, but public safety. Indeed, our system extends an extraordinary power to the mental health practitioner, who may seclude and treat innocent individuals against their wishes when there is reason to suppose they pose a wide range of threats to the safely or well-being of other people, and even to themselves.[13] Since Tarasoff, in the USA, for example, there is a positive legal duty to violate patient confidentiality by warning police and potential victims of harm when there is reason to believe a patient intends harm to others (*Tarasoff*

---

[13] The wording of the various civil commitment statutes varies, and some go further in permitting such involuntary treatment merely because the patient is in need of care. I note that these are very different standards; from the point of view of a Millian liberal the difference between preventing a mentally ill person from harming *others*, and preventing him from harming or even just neglecting, himself, is profound. However, ours are paternalistic times, the world over (see Appelbaum 1997). And that is the nature of our current medico-legal structures.

vs Regents of the University of California 1976).[14] A patient's suicidality or voiced intention to harm himself similarly trigger breaches of confidentiality in a range of cases. When the threat is judged to be real and to present a danger, for example, enforced hospitalization is often regarded as the ethically and legally accepted response and police powers are regularly employed to manage potential suicides (Potter 1996; Martin 2011). (Clinicians also report situations where such action would be regarded as inappropriate, it should be added—if the threat is judged rational, or improbable, or merely provocative, for example.)

Arguably, this social arrangement poses an unacceptable professional role dilemma, and should be changed.[15] It constitutes an irresoluble ethical tension for practitioners, certainly, the more so as the patient trust secured by confidentiality is a sine qua non of an effective therapeutic alliance. What is important here, however, is that present policy further jeopardizes patient privacy. The final source of vulnerability then, from the perspective of patient privacy, lies with the risk that the caregiver's role in the service of other social goals will require confidentiality to be overridden.

6.3 **Part two**

Breaches of confidentiality leave the patient disadvantaged when, the episode of disorder over, her personal agency has been restored. The real world sequelae affecting every aspect of everyday life, noted earlier, limit personal choices and opportunities.

A person is unfree when external conditions that are not outcomes of his or her own autonomous decisions and actions prevent the achievement of self-rule and self-determination. If I cannot get work in a day-care centre because my medical record is alluded to by a referee; or my girlfriend breaks off the engagement when her mother finds out I have

---

[14] Tarasoff is not a very popular ruling, it must be added. Certainly clinicians find it oppressive in that it leaves no room for their clinical judgment—to discern the difference between realistic threats, voiced fantasies, and mere sounding off, for example.

[15] The extent to which the professional goals of healing and forensic concerns conflict is a source of considerable controversy. See, for example, Strasburger et al. (1997); also Radden and Sadler (2010).

a history of mental illness; or I am dropped from the bowling team when it's rumoured I take antipsychotic medicine—options are closed to me. When these outcomes are the result not of my voluntary disclosures, but of breaches of confidentiality, the scope of my freedom is decreased. In this respect then, privacy is a form of social power, like money.[16] There is philosophical disagreement over how to express this relationship. Some would say privacy is a *means* to freedom, some that it affects the *worth* of freedom, others that it confers freedom. [17,18,19] Following Cohen, I will adopt the latter formulation.

These impediments are public, and actual. Yet breaches of confidentiality also result in many that are neither, and these too seem to jeopardize elements we associate with autonomous choice. To be marked as 'mentally ill' it has been said, carries consequences both *external*, in social exclusion, prejudice and discrimination, and '*internal* (secrecy, lower self-esteem and shame)' (Byrne 2001, p. 281). A residue of discomforting shame and embarrassment are an almost universal aftermath of severe disorder, research indicates, and these feelings can be expected to be magnified, in many cases at least, when details of psychiatric history are known by others. They would also be magnified with the knowledge that such details *are at risk of becoming*, or *may be* known to others. My freedom is diminished not only if I am prevented from doing what I want, but if my fear of being prevented stops me from trying. And this situation is described in research on the effects of stigma. Not only exposure, but fear of it, and of consequent stigma, are barriers to using health services, it has been shown, as well as to other ways of re-entering the everyday world of health, work, and relationships (Wahl 1999; Corrigan 2004; Rusch et al. 2005; Hinshaw 2007). There will be

---

[16] See Cohen (2008).

[17] For a discussion of these alternative positions, see Cohen (2008).

[18] In this respect it is what Cohen calls an inus condition (of freedom/unfreedom)—viz. a condition that prevents one from overcoming interference. Inus conditions include not only lack of money, but ignorance, stupidity, or ugliness, he explains: 'they constitute lack of freedom, they are inus conditions of unfreedom, in particular circumstances' (Cohen 2008:14).

[19] Impediments to freedom such as lack of money, or in our case, of privacy, would on Rawls account be deemed to affect the *worth* of liberty. (See Rawls 1971).

normative constraints here, obviously. Only a reasonable and warranted fear of exposure can be laid at the feet of breaches of confidentiality;
and a similar qualification will apply to cases where the fear of stigma
originates in voluntary disclosure of information by the one-time
patient.

Arguably, the recovered patient's actual autonomy, and not merely
her freedom to exercise it, are implicated here. If on recovery the person fears her history is insecure, or is unsure whether or not it is known
to others, it would seem that she lacks information important to making decisions about her life—where to go, what to do, what to say, how
to present herself, and so on. This suggests something closer to an aspect
of agency noted earlier in this chapter, or to conceptions of autonomy
that emphasize the relationship between a person's motives and enduring values and goals.[20] Lacking information so profoundly material
to how she lives her life, the fear of stigma may prevent the recovered
patient from pursuing goals in ways compatible with her defining
values.

The internalized negative assessments that mirror surrounding societal attitudes, known as *self-stigma*, appear to stand in the way of the
person's agency in somewhat the same way: they deprive the person of
knowledge (more accurate assessments of her worth) that in turn can
be expected to impede her efforts to proceed planfully and freely in
light of her own values. These observations are apparently supported by
a small body of research concluding that internalized stigma ('self-
stigma') weakens 'self-mastery' (Wright et al. 2000; Link et al. 2001);
and diminished 'empowerment' in recovered patients has been tied
to both fear of stigma and to self stigma (Rusch et al. 2005). (This is
not to attribute the effects of self-stigma to breaches of confidentiality,
but to point to ways social attitudes can also affect autonomy, it should
be stressed.)

Whether patient privacy is breached through failure to set the right
standard of decisional capacity for informed consent, or failure to

---

[20] This view is focused on authenticity conditions rather than competency conditions of
autonomy (Christman 2009), and associated with philosophers such as Harry Frankfurt.

adhere to duties of confidentiality, the recovered patient's subsequent freedom, and arguably even her autonomy itself, are diminished.

6.4 **Conclusion**

The most urgent recommendations stemming from the preceding discussion are two. First, the dangers to information privacy in this setting and the magnitude of the stakes for recovered patients must both be recognized. Adhering to the principle that the greater the harm risked, the higher should be the standard by which decisional capacity is assessed, we need also to acknowledge that the bulwark provided by the informed consent model in this setting will be effective only when interpreted stringently, and in such a way as to increase the legal and ethical burden on caregivers to preserve confidentiality. (Respect for personal autonomy does not *reduce to* informed consent, nonetheless informed consent is emblematic of personal autonomy.) Additional, more practical steps also suggest themselves, both within and outside the clinic. A routine use of advance care directives that would include instructions about privacy has already been noted; special safeguards might also be applied to confidential material, governing the 'need to know' guidelines on which medical records are generally shared—a proposal made the more pressing by the added risks incumbent in digitalized records. Another suggestion concerns the fate of patients' records upon their recovery. Just as the records of felons who have completed their sentences are in some courts permanently sealed, so when patients have demonstrated their past disorder was behind them, perhaps they alone should be permitted to access their medical records.[21] (As policy, this would have some untoward results in particular cases, where knowledge of past psychiatric history might have permitted more effective prediction and handling of later episodes. Viewed in aggregative terms, however, the harms associated with privacy violations arguably outweigh those risks.)[22]

---

[21] This policy over felon records occurs in Germany, for example.

[22] This will at best be so only while some therapeutic interventions remain less than consistently effective, and the exact prediction of dangerousness from past information continues to elude experts.

In a societal context where autonomy and privacy are highly valued, several of these recommendations seem very obvious. Yet their benefits may not be entirely beyond criticism, and deserve a final word of explanation. The baleful effects of ignorance, alarm, abhorrence, stigma, and discrimination about mental illness are widely documented, and efforts to eradicate this legacy repeatedly support disclosure over secrecy, and point to the societal advantages of awareness rather than ignorance about mental disorder (Byrne 2000; Rusch et al. 2005; Mills 2009). However, the relationship between patient privacy, autonomy, and freedom outlined in the preceding pages suggests that individuals cannot shoulder the burden of furthering the public interest this way. Governments, policies, and education programs should do so.[23,24] But one-time patients may have too much to lose.

Acknowledgements

For help with this chapter I wish to acknowledge Dr Lubomira Radoilska and fellow participants at the Autonomy and Mental Health conference supported by the Centre for Research in the Arts, Social Sciences and Humanities at the University of Cambridge, held in January 2010; I also thank Amelie Rorty, Alec Bodkin, and members of PHAEDRA Jane Roland Martin, Susan Douglas Franzosa, Ann Diller, Beatrice Kipp Nelson, and Barbara Houston.

References

Allen, A. (2003). *Why privacy isn't everything: Feminist reflections on personal accountability*. New York: Rowman and Littlefield.

Allen, A. (2009). Privacy and medicine. In E.N. Zalta (ed.) *Stanford Encyclopedia of Philosophy* [Online] http://plato.stanford.edu/archives/entries/privacy-medicine/

Appelbaum, P. (1997). Almost a revolution: An international perspective on the law of involuntary commitment. *Journal of the American Academy of Psychiatry and Law* 25: 135–47.

Appelbaum, P.S., Lidz, C.W., and Grisso, T. (2004). Therapeutic misconceptions in clinical research: Frequency and risk factors. *Irb* 2: 1–8.

---

[23] See, for example, the Royal College of Psychiatrists' 'Changing Minds' campaign to counter stigma (White 1998; Crisp 2000). http://www.stigma.org. See also Rusch et al. (2005).

[24] Peter Byrne urges that it is institutional psychiatry itself, not service users, that must take the lead in acknowledging and countering stigma (Byrne 2000).

Arpaly, N. (2004). Which autonomy? In J.K. Campbell, M. O'Rourke, and D. Shier (eds.) *Freedom and determinism*. Cambridge: MIT Press, pp. 173–88.

Beauchamp, T.L. and Childress, J.F. (2001). *Principles of biomedical ethics* (5th edn.). New York: Oxford University Press.

Berg, J.W. and Appelbaum, P.S. (2001). *Informed consent: Legal theory and clinical practice* (2nd edn). New York: Oxford University Press.

Buchanan, A.E. and Brock, D.W. (1989). *Deciding for others: The ethics of surrogate decision-making*. Cambridge: Cambridge University Press.

Buss, S. (2008). Personal autonomy. In E.N. Zalta (ed.) *The Stanford Encyclopedia of Philosophy* [Online] http://plato.stanford.edu/archives/win2003/entries/personal autonomy/

Byrne, P. (2000). Stigma of mental illness and ways of diminishing it. *Advances in Psychiatric Treatment* 6: 65–72.

Carpenter, W.T., Gold, J.M., Lahti, A.C., Queern, C.A., Conley, R.R., Bartko, J.J., *et al.* (2000). Decisional capacity for informed consent in schizophrenia. *Archives of General Psychiatry* 57: 533–38.

Cassileth, B.R., Zupkis, R.V., Sutton-Smith, K., and March, V. (1980). Informed consent—Why are its goals imperfectly realized? *New England Journal of Medicine* 302: 896–900.

Charland, L. (2010). Decisional capacity. In E.N. Zalta (ed.) *The Stanford Encyclopedia of Philosophy (Fall 2010 Edition)* [Online] http://plato.stanford.edu/archives/win2003/entries/decisional capacity/

Christman, J. (2009). Autonomy. In E.N. Zalta (ed) *The Stanford Encyclopedia of Philosophy (Fall 2010 Edition)* [Online] http://plato.stanford.edu/archives/win2003/entries/autonomy/

Cohen, G.A. (2008). Freedom and money. In L. Thomas (ed.) *Contemporary Debates in Social Philosophy*. London: Blackwell, pp. 19–42.

Corrigan, P. (2004). How stigma interferes with mental health care. *American Psychologist* 59: 614–25.

Crisp, A.H. (2000). Changing Minds: every family in the land. *An update of the College's campaign. Psychiatric Bulletin* 24: 267–68.

DeCew, J. (1997). *In pursuit of privacy: Law, ethics and the rise of technology*. Ithaca, NY: Cornell.

DeGrazia, D. (2005). *Human identity and bioethics*. Cambridge: Cambridge University Press.

Dresser, R. (1996). Mentally disabled research subjects: The enduring policy issues. *Journal of the American Medical Association* 276: 67–72.

Fink, P.J. and Tasman, A. (1992). *Stigma and mental illness*. Washington DC: American Psychiatric Press.

Flory, J. and Emanual, E. (2004). Interventions to improve research participants' understanding in informed consent for research: a systematic review. *Journal of the American Medical Association* 292: 1593–601.

Gabbard, G. (1999). Boundary violations. In S. Bloch, P. Chodoff, and S. Green (eds.) *Psychiatric Ethics* (3rd edn.) New York: Oxford University Press, pp. 141–60.

Grisso, T. and Appelbaum, P.S. (1998). *Assessing competence to consent to treatment.* New York: Oxford University Press.

Havens, L. (1989). *A safe place: Laying the groundwork for psychotherapy.* New York: Harcourt Brace.

Hayward, P. and Bright, J. (1997). Stigma and mental illness: a review and critique. *Journal of Mental Health* 6: 345–54.

Hinshaw, S. (2007). *The mark of shame: Stigma of mental illness and an agenda for change.* Oxford: Oxford University Press.

Humber, J.M. and Almeder, R.F. (2001). *Privacy and health care.* New York: Humana Press.

Link, B.G., Struening, E.L., Neese-Todd, S., Asmussen, S., and Phelan, J.C. (2001). Stigma as a barrier to recovery: The consequences of stigma for the self-esteem of people with mental illnesses. *Psychiatric Services* 52: 1621–26.

Martin, N. (2011). Preserving trust, maintaining care, and saving lives; Competing feminist values in suicide prevention. *Journal of Feminist Bioethics* 4: 164–87.

Mental Health Foundation. (2000). *Pull yourself together: a survey of the stigma and discrimination faced by people who experience mental disorders.* London: Mental Health Foundation.

Mills, C. (2009). Stigma and openness. *Philosophy & Public Policy Quarterly* 29: 19–23.

Parent, W.A. (1983). Privacy, morality and the law. *Philosophy and Public Affairs* 12: 269–88.

Potter, N. (1996). Discretionary power, lies, and broken trust: Justification and discomfort. *Theoretical Medicine* 17: 329–52.

Radden, J. (1996). *Divided minds and successive selves: Ethical issues in disorders of identity and personality.* Cambridge, MA: MIT Press.

Radden, J. (2008). My symptoms, myself: Reading mental illness memoirs for identity assumptions. In H. Clark (ed.) *Depression and narrative: Telling the dark.* New York: SUNY Press, pp. 15–28.

Radden, J. and Sadler, J. (2010). *The virtuous psychiatrist: Character ethics in psychiatric practice.* New York: Oxford University Press.

Rawls, J. (1971). *A Theory of Justice.* Oxford: Oxford University Press.

Roberts L. (2000). Evidence-based ethics and informed consent in mental illness research. *Archives of General Psychiatry* 57: 540–42.

Roberts, L. (2002). Informed consent and the capacity for voluntarism. *American Journal of Psychiatry* 159: 705–12.

Rusch, N., Angermeyer, M.C., and Corrigan, P.W. (2005). Mental illness stigma: Concepts, consequences and initiatives to reduce stigma. *Journal of European Psychiatry* 20: 529–39.

Shiffrin, S.V. (2004). Advance directives, beneficence, and the permanently demented. In J. Burley (ed.) *Dworkin and His Critics with Replies by Dworkin*. Oxford: Blackwell, pp. 195–217.

Sreenivasan, G. (2003). Does informed consent to research require comprehension? *Lancet* 362: 2016–8.

Sreenivasan, G. (2005). Informed consent and the therapeutic misconception: clarifying the challenge. *Journal of Clinical Ethics* 16: 369–71.

Strasburger, L., Gutheil, T., and Brodsky, A. (1997). On wearing two hats: Role conflict in serving as both psychotherapist and expert witness. *American Journal of Psychiatry* 154: 448–56.

Wahl, O.F. (1999). *Telling is risky business—Mental health consumers confront stigma.* New Brunswick, NJ: Rutgers University Press.

White, P. (1998). Changing minds: Banishing the stigma of mental illness. *Journal of the Royal Society of Medicine* 91: 509–10.

Wirshing, D.A., Wirshing, W.C., Marder, S.R., Liberman, R.P., and Mintz, J. (1998). Informed consent: Assessment of comprehension. *American Journal of Psychiatry* 155: 1508–11.

Wright, E.R., Gronfein, W.P., and Owens, T.J. (2000). Deinstitutionalization, social jejection, and the self-esteem of former mental patients. *Journal of Health and Social Behavior* 41: 68–90.

Young, A.T., Green, C.A., and Estroff, S.E. (2008). New endeavors, risk taking and personal growth in the recovery process: Findings from the STARS study. *Psychiatric Services* 59: 1430–36.

Part III

Rethinking capacity and respect for autonomy

Chapter 7

Clarifying capacity: value and reasons

Jules Holroyd

7.1 Introduction

The aim of this paper is to clarify what is involved in the notion of capacity as used in the Mental Capacity Act of 2005. This act (hereafter MCA) sets out the conditions for ascertaining whether an individual lacks the mental capacity to make a decision. Where there is evidence for an individual lacking capacity, and further inquiry confirms this to be the case, then another individual is assigned to decide in the individual's best interests. Because judgements about whether someone has or lacks capacity can have significant consequences, in particular in the context of healthcare, it is crucial to come to a full and accurate understanding of what it is to have—or lack—capacity. Considered in the context of mental healthcare, we will see that ascertaining whether an individual has capacity is not only an ethical matter concerning the avoidance of harms, but also has political implications concerning what choices or conceptions of value the state should, via the health service, permit.

I will be asking whether meeting the conditions set out in the MCA requires certain evaluative commitments. This question is particularly testing in the context of issues that arise concerning mental health, where what is believed relevant or given weight in making a decision appears to be bound up with the mental health problems about which decisions are being made. In this paper I will first clarify and elaborate on the claim that the conditions for capacity as set out in the MCA are value-laden (cf. Owens et al. 2009; Sections 7.2–7.4). Then I will show that whilst the conditions are indeed value-laden, and presuppose that certain evaluative commitments are held by capacitous individuals, significant difficulties arise in attempts to rationalize value-laden judgements about capacity, and much work still remains in this regard.

How is capacity relevant to the various understandings of autonomy? One might view capacity (with respect to a particular decision) as coextensive with being autonomous (with respect to that decision)—if so, then given the role that the notion of capacity is playing, it is clear that the particular target concept of autonomy at work is concerned with the boundaries of interference and paternalism. If one does not take capacity to be coextensive with autonomy, then individuals might be autonomous whilst lacking capacity, or vice versa (depending on the notion of autonomy adopted). Discussion of which strategy one might adopt is deferred for another time.[1]

7.2 **Mental capacity**

Whilst it is usually appropriate for adults to make decisions about what kinds of medical treatments they undergo, sometimes impairments are suffered—either temporary or permanent—which render an individual unable to make such decisions. The Mental Capacity Act 2005 sets out the conditions under which it is appropriate to regard an individual as lacking the capacity to make a particular decision about treatment. It is important to note that the MCA is different from the Mental Health Act (2007), which sets out the conditions under which patients with mental illnesses may be detained for their own health or safety, or that of others, for the provision of treatment for the mental disorder. The two acts serve quite different purposes; individuals who have not been diagnosed with a mental illness may fail to meet the conditions for capacity—if they are in a state of temporary confusion or debilitation or are in a coma, say. Likewise, individuals who have been diagnosed with mental health problems may still meet the conditions for capacity. However, as we will see, suffering from certain mental health problems or illnesses can make meeting these conditions difficult; patients who

[1] See also the contributions to this volume by Jane Heal (Chapter 1) and Hallvard Lillehammer (Chapter 9).

suffer from dementia may be unable to retain information in the way required; patients suffering from delusions may be unable to understand the relevant information, for example. I will focus in later sections on sufferers of anorexia nervosa, and what we might say about the ability to weigh the relevant information in coming to a decision.

As stated, the MCA specifies that an individual lacks the capacity to make a decision if:

> At the time he is unable to make a decision for himself in relation to the matter because of an impairment of, or a disturbance in, the functioning of the mind or brain. (MCA, 2.(1))

An individual is in turn judged unable to make a decision about such a matter, if he is unable

(a) to understand the information relevant to the decision
(b) to retain that information [for sufficiently long to make the decision, at least]
(c) to use or weigh that information as part of the process of making the decision, or
(d) to communicate his decision (whether by talking, using sign language or any other means). (MCA 3(1))

One of the striking principles stated in the MCA is that: 'a person is not to be treated as unable to make a decision merely because he makes an unwise decision' (1(4)). In so claiming we are encouraged to consider these conditions as content-neutral, or procedural—whether an individual has capacity should not depend upon the content of her decisions, or commitments.

However, in a recent discussion of the MCA, the authors conclude that 'if psychiatry aims at a completely value-neutral or even value-free conception of mental capacity it will come unstuck' (Owens et al. 2009, p. 100). If these authors are right, then it is important to work out precisely at what point values play a role in the conditions for capacity. Ascertaining this is important for three reasons: first, to clarify what considerations are relevant to judging capacity, especially in difficult cases—for some such cases seem to hinge upon whether the individual endorses certain values; second, understanding the relationship between autonomy and capacity requires first being clear on what the conditions for capacity demand; third, clarity on the evaluative content of the conditions may have implications more broadly for public health ethics.

I will be primarily concerned with the first of these considerations, leaving the other two for detailed discussion elsewhere. It is clear that it is of crucial importance that the conditions for identifying when an individual lacks capacity are properly understood and applied; misapplication of those principles will lead to medical paternalism, infliction of moral harm, and imposition of the (risk of) physical harm attendant upon most medical procedures. Whether or not the conditions are value-laden also intersects with concerns in public health ethics. When it comes to which choices to respect, many have argued that the state should not make such decisions based on whether those choices cohere with certain state-sanctioned values; that individuals should be free to pursue whatever conception of the good they choose, so long as it does not harm or wrong others.[2] It will be important, then, to ascertain whether the conditions for capacity are value-laden, and in what way: might being judged to have capacity ultimately turn on whether one accepts certain values?

7.3 **Evaluative components of MCA**

An agent is deemed to lack capacity insofar as she is unable to do any one of the four things set out in the MCA. Precisely what is involved in meeting these conditions needs considerable unpacking. I aim to focus on the extent to which being able to understand information relevant to the decision, and to weigh that information in making the decision, are value-laden. Do judgements about when an individual is able to understand or weigh information in deliberation depend upon which values she endorses? This focus coheres with some aspects of Owens et al.'s treatment of the MCA. The authors identify four dimensions in

---

[2] For a discussion of when and whether it is appropriate to override individuals' choices, see Dworkin (1983, 1972), Christman (2004), and Oshana (1998). The target of autonomy in much of this writing is that which sets the boundaries for paternalism. See Arpaly (2003) for a taxonomy of the different notions of autonomy.

For discussion of whether the state should be in the business of promoting certain values in healthcare, see Radoilska (2009).

which the conditions for capacity rely on value-laden, rather than purely descriptive criteria. These include (2009, pp. 92, 95–100):

The patient having 'insight into illness'.

The patient's evaluations and the role these play in their reasoning.

The emotional states of the patient and the role these play in practical reasoning and decision-making.

The gravity of the decision, and the risk of falsely judging capacity when the potential harms are great.

The first two of these dimensions, the patient's insight into illness and her evaluative commitments, correspond to the two aspects of the MCA I have picked out as warranting further scrutiny; the understanding and weighing requirements. I will focus on the first two aspects, and set aside the other two, although these also deserve further scrutiny.[3]

---

[3] A few notes on the latter two conditions are in order: first, the authors focus on the impact of 'altered emotional states' upon the individual's decision-making process. Such emotional states may influence 'in a detectable and identifiable way, the meaning, value and weight given to treatment risks and benefits, such that the patient may be unable to appreciate the benefits side of the equation, or may become unduly concerned about the risks' (2009, p. 98). The question of what are appropriate emotional responses to certain benefits or risks, and what amounts to undue concern, becomes salient. Whilst some of these issues will be peripherally addressed in the discussion of the patient's evaluations, the matter of the appropriateness of certain (strengths of) emotional responses and their relevance to capacity will not be tackled head on here. The question of whether any the agent must hold certain evaluative commitments (believe certain things to be valuable) in order to have capacity can be addressed without settling this matter, and insofar as emotional responses are attached to certain evaluative dispositions (and perhaps are constitutive of them) we will touch upon this matter indirectly. Moreover, ascertaining whether capacity requires certain evaluative commitments may then help with later assessments of the rationality of certain emotional responses to the objects of those commitments.

The fourth dimension picked out by Owens et al. focuses on the evaluations of the assessors—the weight assigned to the risks and benefits of the decision undertaken, and how this may affect where the bar for capacity is set. They write:

> To judge incapacity falsely results in treatment in the patient's best interests, whereas to judge capacity falsely may result in serious harm or death which may have been preventable and which the patient did not autonomously choose. It is more valuable, by implication, for risky decisions which are incapable to be blocked than risky decisions which are capable to be permitted. This makes it imperative, so the argument goes, for assessors of capacity to be surer about capacity in the context of a risky decision. (2009, pp. 99–100)

7.3.1 **Understanding relevant information**

The text of the MCA adds that the information relevant to the decision includes (but as we shall see is not limited to):

> Information about the reasonably foreseeable consequences of a) deciding one way or another, or b) failing to make the decision. (MCA, 3(4))

What more is required for understanding the information relevant to a decision? In this section I will argue that the understanding condition requires that individuals subscribe to a certain range of values, and that this is most clearly the case in relation to the requirement for 'insight', namely, understanding that one is ill.

What is deemed to be relevant to the decision in hand will, in part, be determined by the evaluative commitments of the agent. For example, that one course of treatment violates a religious doctrine (to draw on an example to which we will return) might be considered relevant by a patient who is committed to that religious system and its doctrines, but not deemed (independently) important by some medical practitioners. The grounds for regarding such information as relevant (and the patient's attendant beliefs that receiving certain treatment would be sinful, say) is not independent of the evaluative weight that the patient gives to different considerations; the considerations to which an individual accords significant weight will presumably correlate with what she regards as relevant. I return to the issue of weighing the information in Section 7.4. The considerations that arise in this regard will not only be relevant to decisions made in medical contexts, but will pertain to judgements about capacity in relation to decisions in other domains also. In the context of healthcare—particularly mental healthcare—some specific propositions are regarded as relevant, and this section will focus on the extent to which these are value-laden.

Note that here, the claim is that despite the moral and physical harms that may ensue, when the stakes are high a false negative judgement of capacity is better ('more valuable') than a false positive. Once again, this issue is not wholly isolated from the matter of what evaluative commitments a patient must have in order to meet the conditions for capacity, for her evaluation of the risks may differ from that of the assessors. Our focus for now is not primarily upon the evaluations of those assessing capacity, but rather on what evaluative commitments an agent may be required to have if she is to meet the conditions for capacity.

7.3.2 **Insight into illness**

Owens et al. identify 'insight into illness' as a value-laden dimension of capacity (2009, p. 95). The notion of 'having insight into illness' pertains to whether or not the patient recognizes that she has an illness. Clearly, such a recognition is necessary in order to make sense of why certain treatment options (or their refusal) are on the table—that is, why any decision needs to be made at all. Unless one understands that one is unwell and that treatment may remedy this, the only sensible option will be to refuse treatment. Thus we see that having insight falls under the specification of the MCA which requires that one 'understand the information relevant to the decision'. What is required in having insight?

Owens et al. refer to 'a judgement about the patient's ability to recognise certain experiential states as pathological. And such judgements are value-laden' (2009, p. 95). The focus of their discussion is on the evaluative nature of the judgements (by practitioners) about whether an individual has insight. We should want to know a great deal more about the ways in which such a judgement is value-laden. I will focus on the question of whether an individual's having an awareness of their illness requires that they accept certain evaluative propositions or values more broadly (in particular, those which correspond to the practitioners judgement regarding what it is to be in good health, or ill). Whilst this is important for the cases that Owens et al. raise—cases in which a feature of the illness is that the symptoms are not recognized as such (2009, p. 95)—we will see that the evaluative requirements are necessary even in run of the mill acknowledgements of illness.

A first gloss on what 'insight' requires is as follows: a patient suffering from an illness with symptoms S ought, insofar as she has insight, to subscribe to the beliefs:

(a) I am experiencing (symptom) S, and

(b) S is indicative of a disease/illness

However, articulated in this way, it is not clear precisely what the evaluative element is: (a) and (b) may appear to be purely descriptive statements; one about the patient's experiential states, the other about the relationship between these states and disease. If this is so, then it is not clear that insight is an evaluative matter, but rather a matter of simply forming certain beliefs about one's own states and about what these states mean in terms of one's state as diseased or not.

However, in such judgements there are in fact (at least) two evaluative aspects. Fulford (1989) has argued for an understanding of the notions of health and disease as evaluative. Roughly put, on his view to 'be in good health' or 'to be well' is to meet certain standards of functioning designated as valuable states. To suffer from illness is to fall short of these evaluative standards (first evaluative component) in a way that is disvalued or regarded as undesirable (second evaluative component). If this is right, then having insight into illness will involve recognizing:

(a) I am experiencing (symptom) S, and

(b) S indicates a negative departure from the norms of good health, H.

If this is right, then having insight into illness (and understanding this bit of relevant information) requires accepting certain normative ideals of health.

7.3.3 The evaluative content of assessments of health

Does this mean that coming to an understanding of the relevant information is only possible insofar as one subscribes to certain ideals of health? If so, an individual's disagreement over a state being pathological would mean that she lacked insight, and thereby lacking the capacity to make the relevant decision. But Fulford's understanding of illness as evaluative acknowledges that there might be some variation in the relevant ideals and evaluations. Whilst there might be general agreement on the existence of a certain experiential state, whether that state gives cause for diagnosis of an illness or disease will sometimes depend upon the patient's evaluation of it, as Fulford and colleagues write:

> What is a problem for one person – having an ache or pain, being a certain weight, having a given level of energy or a particular sleep pattern – may not be a problem for another person . . . medical diagnosis is . . . a matter of negative evaluation. (Fulford et al. 2002, p. 6)

On this view, being ill will involve the patient taking a negative evaluation towards her experiential state. An agent might evaluate a state negatively because it departs from certain norms of health that she accepts (and that others do not). Alternatively, she might note that it departs from these norms, but not find that departure problematic. Thus two individuals with similar experiential states may differ with respect to whether they regard themselves (or are diagnosed as) suffering from some illness or defect of health. The differing conceptions of the norms of health might lead A and B to differ in their judgements about whether (e.g.) an erratic sleep pattern is a health problem. Or such disagreement might be characterized differently: even if A and B accept the same norms of health, B might not find the departure from the norms she accepts as problematic.

If there is sometimes room for divergent understandings of the norms of health, or of evaluations of departures from them, this is relevant to the evaluative nature of the condition of understanding 'insight into illness'. It may be that an individual does not accept a certain experiential state is symptomatic of an illness. This may be because that individual is unable to recognize that symptom as a departure from the norms of health she accepts, and so cannot understand that she is ill (hence cannot meet the 'understanding' condition of the MCA).

However, it might be that an individual's conception of the norms of health differs from those norms accepted by many others (it might also be that the importance she attributes to some state deemed by some pathological differs significantly—a point to which I return in Section 7.4). As Fulford et al. note, many norms are widely shared: a heart attack is generally accepted as bad for a person (2002, p. 8). Plausibly, there are some such states which are bad for a person irrespective of their evaluation of it. But it will not be the case that all norms of good functioning are shared, nor that all symptoms or experiential states will be bad for a person independently of their evaluation of it.[4]

---

[4] It is worth also noting the distinction, discussed by Fulford (2001), between dysfunction and illness; the textbooks may set out what scientists, with complex understanding of physiology, identify as good or bad functioning. Whether or not a divergence from this

There is scope for divergent conceptions of some norms, as well as divergent evaluations of departures from the set of norms that agents accept.[5] This value laden understanding is supported by Derek Bolton's claim that, in the context of mental healthcare:

> A primary task should be to define what the problem is and for whom, according to whose values, in an active collaboration with the individual or others concerned. (Bolton 2000, p. 151)

Thus understood, it appears that there are a range of ideals that might be accepted consistently with having mental capacity: people diverge in their ideas about what good health involves (even if there are some norms on which all (should) agree). Moreover, that individuals do diverge in their views of good health, and that having such preferences ignored can be upsetting and distressing (see Lillehammer Chapter 9, this volume), provides pragmatic reason in favour of operating with a more pluralist understanding of the norms of health.

Plausibly, then, for an individual to have insight, she must make evaluative judgements concerning the norms of health to which she subscribes; and concerning whether her experiential states are divergences from these.[6] Whilst value-laden, then, we haven't yet seen that making judgements about capacity would be determined by whether or not an individual accepts certain values or not; rather, it is a matter of looking for a coherent understanding of how an individual's experiences fit with her conception of health.

---

function is a divergence from the norms of health that an individual accepts, or evaluates negatively, will determine whether or not a medical diagnosis of illness is appropriate.

[5] Strictly speaking, we should understand the patient's evaluation as in accordance (or not) with the norms of health H that she would accept, were she to reflect upon them under optimal conditions. This is required so that the analysis is not hostage to the patient's current mental states (which may in fact be subject to distortion or mistake).

This understanding is different to, but (I believe) consistent with, the account of insight that Fulford develops—he understands lacking insight in terms of misconstrued attributions—for example, seeing some trait as done to oneself, rather than as done by oneself (or vice versa). See Fulford (2004, esp p.56). Such wrongful attributions would presumably not be recognized as departures from the endorsed norms of health.

[6] As Fulford (2004) notes, some failures of insight will be due to the failure to recognize an experiential state as a divergence from endorsed norms of health, but rather to attribute it to, e.g. one's environment (to which one's response is normal).

But can any conception of health be endorsed?[7] I've noted that there are strong intuitions that some norms of health are just wrong. Further intuitions can be found in various feminists' arguments for women's rights in relation to health: Chambers considers women who, having undergone female genital cutting rituals suffered significant health complications but did not regard their bodily functions (prolonged menstruation and urination, painful penetration, and childbirth) as abnormally difficult (2007, p. 213). The intuition is that it is simply mistaken to fail to regard such difficulties as a departure from good health (rather than a different but reasonable conception of health). Such an intuition is vindicated by the fact that, with more information, such women changed their views: 'once women do realise that they have been harmed by FGM, they are keen to put in place the village-wide declarations that are necessary to abandon the practice, as field-work demonstrates' (Chambers 2007, p. 214). Whilst on the one hand consideration of such cases appears to support the thought that there are limits to the norms of health that can be accepted, one might maintain that such a conclusion does not rely on assumptions about what is and what is not a norm or ideal of good health. (Doing so would yield a value-laden notion of capacity, as whether an individual has insight will depend upon whether she accepts certain ideals of health, and is able to recognize her symptoms as departures from these.) Rather, content-neutral conditions pertaining to the information an individual has available to her whilst formulating understandings of good health can be appealed to: the women's understanding was mistaken, in being formed without relevant information (rather than mistaken because it was substantively wrong).[8] Perhaps this kind of content-neutral condition can account for intuitions about which norms of health are

---

[7] Parallel concerns may arise in other domains in which considerations of capacity arise (in social care, or legal settings, say, where decisions are to be made about responsibility for welfare, or property): can any conception of the good life be consistent with capacity, or do some commitments indicate a lack of understanding of the relevant information? Thanks to Edward Harcourt for pressing this point.

[8] Compare some of Dworkin's (1988) necessary conditions for autonomy, requiring that endorsements are formed with relevant information, and under conditions of procedural independence.

mistaken or wrong. However, when we look to work in mental health-care, it appears that there are some cases in which, even when equipped with all the relevant information, seemingly problematic norms of health are subscribed to.[9]

Some sufferers of anorexia nervosa reject the ideal of a certain weight that affords good functioning (physically and mentally). Certain experiential states may be recognized (say, dizziness, weakness resulting from malnourishment), but not regarded as a departure from the individuals accepted norms of health (which do not feature adequate nutrition). Is this indicative of lack of capacity to decide about treatment? This brings us to the weighing condition.

7.4 **Weighing information**

In addition to understanding the relevant information—understanding, say, that one is ill, or that according to certain standards of wellness one's experiential states are divergent from these norms—one must also be able:

> (c) To use or weigh that information as part of the process of making the decision (MCA (1))

What might we look to in order to determine whether an individual is able to weigh information? The ability to weigh information as part of a deliberation process is in the first instance subject to certain formal constraints—such as consistency and transitivity. Inconsistent evaluations thwart stable processes of deliberation and weighing, as does the

---

[9] A further concern is that conditions pertaining to having the relevant information may also be practically difficult to implement. Consider a condition pertaining to whether or not one had the relevant information in forming a norm of health. Most individuals do not have reflective access to when they formed views on what good health consists in, less still what influenced them in doing so; nor is such information likely to be readily available from others. The point is not that this condition may not ultimately be able to identify circumstances that threaten the capacity to make decisions (perhaps undermining insight or the ability to weigh information). Rather, the worry is that the application of those conditions to ascertain whether an individual has capacity or not will not be practically possible: it will require information about processes according to which individuals formed desires or endorsed values—information that is not easily discerned, least of all in contexts where decisions may be required with some urgency.

inconsistent ranking of options in order of value. In the instance in which an agent violates these constraints, we may have reason to suppose that they are unable to weigh the information in a manner required for capacity (or perhaps may be unable to retain information long enough (as required by the second condition) in order to make consistent evaluative rankings). Certainly, failure to meet such constraints would lead to erratic patterns of valuing, which would be difficult to reconcile into a stable decision about treatment options.

Such constraints, however, do not require that any *particular* weights are assigned to certain options or experiential states: these formal constraints are consistent with assigning a low value to some physiological functions, and a high value to treatment avoidance (insofar as such commitments are consistent with other values held). Does weighing information require that certain specific evaluative commitments and rankings are held? For example, would refusing treatment because one cannot see any value in continuing what would be an otherwise physically healthy life indicate that one is not properly weighing the information, giving too little weight to the harms of leaving the condition untreated? Or would refusing treatment for severe malnourishment due to anorexia nervosa, in order to maintain a low weight and avoid food consumption, indicate that one is improperly valuing nourishment and giving too much weight to food avoidance and maintaining a low weight? Would refusing life-saving treatment on the basis of religious doctrine? I want to focus in this section on the case of anorexia nervosa as it locates our discussion in the context of mental health, and provides a particular challenge for content-neutral understandings of capacity.

Tan and Hope (2008)'s research implies that certain evaluative weightings are required for capacity, and that this can be seen in considering the competences and capacities of patients with anorexia nervosa. Such patients are described as (frequently) meeting the formal conditions for capacity, manifesting high standards of rationality. However, these individuals, it is argued, 'overvalue' maintaining a low weight, leading them to assign to it a greater evaluative weight than that assigned to participating in treatment programs that would ensure a healthier body weight. In an earlier piece (Tan et al. 2003) the formal competence of the patients is described; however, it is remarked that anorexic individuals experience difficulties in their substantive valuings:

> All the participants were already highly conversant with the facts of their disorder, the exercise of going through information about anorexia nervosa and its treatment [. . .] was experienced as onerous and patronising to the participants and awkward and painful to carry out for the interviewer. This suggests that the standard concept of capacity to consent to treatment, as being one of understanding and reasoning [. . .] may not be relevant to the difficulties that these participants may experience in their decision making.
>
> One important area, which emerged from the qualitative analysis, is attitudes to death and disability. Treatment refusal may occur, not because the patient wishes to die, but because of the relative unimportance of death and disability as compared to anorexia nervosa, or because of the particular meaning death and disability may acquire in the context of anorexia nervosa. (Tan et al. 2003 p. 704).[10]

In remarking on the 'relative unimportance' to these patients of death and disability, Tan et al. identify the patterns of valuing which diverge from those deemed normal. Many people endorse as a norm of health the maintenance of a body weight that permits daily activities and does not risk disability or death. But such a norm does not figure—or not significantly—in the norms accepted by the patients Tan describes. We tend to think that someone who weighs being thin or avoiding food over death or disability is not just endorsing a different set of values; rather, they are making an evaluative mistake. This seems to indicate, then, that our understanding of what it is to be able to weigh information in a way relevant to capacity concerns the assignment of *appropriate* weights to certain objects or options or norms, which determines how one should rank them: to value life over food avoidance; to value treatment over significant risk of death or disability. Similarly, it has

---

[10] Some anorexia sufferers may have false beliefs about their size or weight, or experience significant emotional resistance to eating or weight gain. In such cases, they may not meet the formal requirements; or it may be that conditions that make reference to emotional states (as recommended by Owens et al.) are relevant to capacity. My claims in this section, then, are of most relevance in the cases described by Tan et al., where formal conditions are met, and insofar as the conditions for capacity do not make explicit reference to emotional states. I thank Agnieska Jaworska and Lisa Bortolotti for raising these considerations.

been argued that depression involves undervaluing continued existence (Moorhead and Turkington 2002). And controversial cases in which individuals with religious commitments refuse potentially life-saving treatment centre on whether the weight given to considerations of faith and religious doctrine undermines ability to properly weigh other relevant information (cf. Martin, 2007). If this is so, then meeting the conditions for capacity seems to require not merely that the agent hold some evaluative commitments (as is required for understanding the information relevant to the decision); but also that the agent hold some specific and substantive evaluative commitments.

I take it there are two key thoughts underpinning these judgements: first, that an agent who makes such divergent evaluations is not merely engaging in different patterns of valuing, but rather in distorted patterns; she is not simply diverging from the (statistical) norm, but is somehow getting something wrong. Again, an evaluative conception of this condition for capacity, which rules out at least some value-commitments, must be endorsed if this thought can be accepted. The second thought is that it might be appropriate to make decisions on behalf of an individual, if her distorted understanding means she is unable to weigh information in making a decision (and where the consequences of that decision are grave).

7.4.1 Consequences of value-laden conditions for capacity

I haven't offered a watertight argument for the conclusion that meeting the weighing condition for capacity requires certain evaluative commitments; rather, I have shown that the structure of the understanding and weighing conditions presupposes that certain values are held, drawn out strong intuitions in favour of this conclusion, and appealed to empirical research findings. There are strong reasons for supposing that both the understanding and the weighing conditions require certain evaluative commitments: insight into illness requires that some values are endorsed; the weighing condition appears to require that this endorsement is of values, given appropriate relative weight, from a limited set. It is plausible that those values in play might be plural, leaving some room for individual divergences regarding what is of value. But certain beliefs or commitments, or rankings of them, will be ruled out.

This preliminary conclusion may be an uncomfortable one: it is certainly in tension with the stated principle that judgements of capacity should not be determined by the content of an individual's decision. The following consequences of a value-laden set of conditions stand out:

1 If over-valuing some option is taken as evidence that an individual cannot weigh the information in coming to a decision, some 'unwise' decisions will be relevant to ascertaining whether an individual meets the conditions for capacity. Such a conclusion implies that whether an individual's values are unorthodox may be relevant to her decisional capacity.

2 This also suggests that there may be an asymmetry in ascertaining capacity: individuals who make 'orthodox' weightings of value and relevant information may not be pressed to explain or justify their decisions in a way that an individual who is regarded as 'over-' or 'under-' valuing some considerations may be.

3 Further, this conclusion poses a challenge for those who defend a value-neutral understanding of the state's obligations in public healthcare; we will need to see how such a framework can be consistent with the MCA, which seems to rely on the conceptions of value an individual endorses in making assessments of decisional capacity.

4 Finally, if the MCA does contain value-laden criteria in this way, then further discussion will be required about which values are consistent with capacity and which are not. The alternative would be to re-formulate the MCA so as to avoid reliance on a 'weighing condition'.

However, as we will see in the following section, there is significant difficulty in systematizing intuitions about what undermines decisional capacity.

7.5 Systematizing intuitions

The preliminary conclusion is that, as Owens et al. argue, it is mistaken to maintain that the conditions for capacity are value-free. I have drawn out two ways in which the conditions for capacity require that individuals accept certain values, most notably the weighing condition. If it is right that assessing decisional capacity depends upon an individual's evaluative commitments in this way, then it is essential that some systematic way of ascertaining which value commitments are consistent with being able to weigh information, and which threaten to undermine this ability.

As it stands, intuitions seem to pull in different directions: it appears intuitively plausible that over-valuing food avoidance or under-valuing continued existence thwarts the ability to weigh information relevant to treatment decisions. On the other hand it is less intuitively compelling to think that under-valuing the risk of death or disability due to a commitment to religious doctrine undermines decisional capacity (although anecdotally, intuitions seem to vary significantly on this).

In a recent Hastings Center Report, Adrienne Martin (2007) has offered arguments which may account for such conflicting intuitions. In this section, I address these claims, arguing that they cannot explain our divergent intuitions. These arguments are also important in addressing which considerations, beyond decisional capacity, may speak in favour of respecting treatment choice.

If one does not share the intuition that religious believers lack decisional capacity, and rather should have their choices respected, this would speak against a value-laden understanding of the conditions for capacity: over-valuing other options relative to avoiding death or disability cannot be what undermines capacity. The treatment decisions of certain religious individuals involve certain weighting or assignments of value that may, to non-religious individuals, be as distorted and misguided as those evaluations of the anorexic patient. For example, in cases in which life is threatened unless a blood transfusion occurs, some followers of the Jehovah's Witness faith will assign a greater value to maintaining a pure soul (believing an interpretation of the bible according to which God prohibits the transference of blood) than to remaining alive.[11] For those who give no weight to the commands

---

[11] It is important to note that many do not so believe, and campaign for the legitimacy of their pro-transfusion views within the Jehovah's Witness faith. See the website of the Associated Jehovah's Witnesses for Reform on Blood.

of God or the purity of the soul, such evaluations are misguided and distorted.

However, the tendency to see these beliefs and evaluations as undermining of capacity is weaker than in the case of the anorexic patient; whilst one might disagree with the evaluative weighting, one might nonetheless maintain that, because of her religious commitments, it is appropriate to respect this divergent evaluation. Such cases might be appealed to in support of the claim, then, that evaluative commitments do not inform judgements of capacity—otherwise intuitions and decisions about some such religious believers would pull in the same direction as those regarding the anorexia sufferer.

Martin's arguments may provide a way of accounting for such divergent intuitions. She argues that even if individuals are lacking capacity, there may be other reasons for which it is important to respect their choices. These other considerations may be informing intuitions about the case of religious believers. If her arguments work, this would explain how a value-laden understanding of capacity can be consistent with divergent intuitions about which choices to respect. However I will argue that her arguments not successful, which leaves the situation somewhat vexed with respect to our intuitions about intervention and capacity, showing the need for more attention to which values are consistent with decisional capacity and why.

7.5.1 Respect for autonomy

In this paper, I have left open whether we should identify capacity with autonomy, or whether the two notions might come apart. The stance one takes on this will depend (in part) upon whether the conditions for capacity are value-laden (whether or not autonomy is value-laden or content-neutral is itself contentious). However, in order to base an argument for respecting the decision of an agent who lacks capacity in respect for autonomy, the notions of autonomy and capacity cannot be seen as coextensive. For if so, an agent who lacked capacity, would also lack autonomy; respect for her autonomy could not then provide an additional reason for respecting her choice.

Martin suggests that we consider the possibility that 'even a person lacking capacity qualifies as autonomous' (2007, p. 38), and that their status as autonomous might provide reason to respect a choice even if capacity is lacking (due to, say, 'distorted' evaluative judgements). Martin works with an understanding of autonomous agency as 'coherence or consistency across one's value hierarchy and how one acts in relation to that hierarchy' (2007, p. 38) such that autonomous persons are unified in their endorsement of and action upon certain values (cf. Frankfurt 1971). She suggests that certain evaluations based in false beliefs (about, e.g. valuing treatment refusal over acceptance, due to the belief that eternal damnation is a consequence of the latter) might nonetheless play an important unifying role for the agent. If this is so, then respect for that agent's autonomy (her capacity for coherent evaluative endorsements which guide action) might mean respecting a choice that would not meet the conditions for capacity:

> The requirement to respect autonomy may therefore require respecting some incapacitated decisions [. . .]. For some decisions, respect for autonomy might require that we respect her treatment decision based in her [false] belief, even when she 'unreasonably' retains that belief [. . .] – even when the belief renders her incapacitated' (Martin 2007, p. 39).

Martin is here (with her reference to the unreasonable retention of belief rendering the agent incapacitated) supposing that some beliefs might get in the way of understanding the relevant information, or weighing it appropriately (she writes that the 'Jehovah's Witnesses religious beliefs prevent them from arriving at an even remotely accurate assessment of the risks of blood transfusion' (2007, p. 36)). But Martin claims that even if the agent does not meet the conditions for capacity—if her false belief prevents her from understanding or weighing the relevant information—it might nonetheless be appropriate to treat her as if she has capacity for the sake of respecting her autonomy.

Whilst this might be so, it will not help us in explaining any divergent intuitions about the anorexia sufferer and the religious believer; for we might suppose (plausibly, given what was said about the formal competence of many sufferers of anorexia) that the anorexic meets the relevant coherence and endorsement conditions in order to be considered autonomous, in this sense. An individual—particularly if she has suffered from anorexia over a prolonged period—might consider anorexia 'part of herself', identifying and endorsing the abstinent motives and evaluative commitments to thinness and food-avoidance, much in the same way that individuals regard other evaluative commitments as constituting their identity.

That anorexic individuals could meet these conditions on the structure of the will may place in doubt their sufficiency for self-governance or autonomy. Indeed, that anorexic patients might endorse at a higher order their desires for abstinence is precisely what leads Marilyn Friedman (1986) to express concern about such accounts: the first order desires for food from which the sufferer is alienated, she maintains, are ones we might be inclined to regard as her 'true' desires: authentic and constitutive of her 'true self'.

But on an account that privileges higher order endorsements, respect for autonomy might require respect for the anorexic's refusal of life-saving treatment, for the sake of her 'overvaluing' thinness or food avoidance. Insofar as this is counter-intuitive, it cannot be that these structures of endorsement (understood as autonomy) provide sufficient reason for respecting choice. For these structures of the will could be found in religious believers and anorexic individuals alike, and would provide reason for respecting the choice of both, even if both also lacked capacity.

7.5.2 **Respect for institutions**

An alternative argument Martin offers concerns whether an individual's 'distorted' evaluative commitments are located within established practices or institutions. She writes that:

> It may be appropriate, even important, to evince attitudes of tolerance, admiration, or even respect for some of the communal practices people participate in, regardless of whether those practices or participation in them are connected to individuals' autonomy. Religion can be a deep source of meaning in individual and community lives. (Martin 2007, p. 39).

The thought here seems to be that respect for certain valuable practices requires respecting choices based on values embedded in those practices, even if the commitment to those values undermines the agent's ability to meet the conditions for capacity, or her autonomy. So supposing the believer's faith prevents her from meeting the conditions for capacity, there might nonetheless be reason to respect her choice for the sake of respecting or sustaining those practices that have informed her evaluations. This is because those practices perform other important functions, even if they also serve to undermine the capacity to make important decisions of those who partake in them.

This argument is problematic on a number of grounds. First, it expresses a worryingly instrumental attitude towards the individual whose decisional capacity is at issue; recall (as mentioned in Section 7.2) that the decisions at issue in the medical realm may frequently be ones which involve significant risks and burdensome costs. To allow an individual who is not equipped to make such significant decisions to do so for the sake of preserving some traditions or practices is to use that individual as a mere means. This seems to be a significant failure of respect for that individual, and fails to demonstrate adequate concern for their welfare.

Second, the argument has strongly conservative tendencies; consider the practices described in Section 7.3 of female genital cutting, which detrimentally impacted upon the health of those women who partook in those practices. Suppose (as is not implausible, but does not, of course, leave those practices impervious to critique) that these practices of female genital cutting serve some role in securing social cohesion, and have significance and meaning for those who participate in them: the practice is an initiation rite which secures for young women the status of eligibility for marriage, and confers some esteem upon them as well as those who perform the rituals.[12] In the example we considered, many of the women had insufficient information to understand the impact of these practices upon their urinary and sexual functioning. With the relevant information, they revised their assessment of their experiential states in relation to a likewise revised conception of the norms of good health. It seems deeply troubling to maintain that, whilst lacking the understanding of the relevant facts to enable informed

[12] Indeed, in her discussion of practices of genital cutting in Senegal, Anne Phillips notes that the difficulties ending rituals of female genital cutting are essentially coordination problems: whilst no individuals were strongly attached to the practice, no community wanted their daughters to miss out on the social benefits accessible to those who underwent FGC. Hence the success of projects that signed communities up to a collective pledge to end FGC. See Phillips (2007, esp. pp. 46-47).

decisions, the value of those practices in maintaining social cohesion and individual meaning provides reason to respect a decision which supports that institution. The mere fact that there is a social practice, and that this social practice serves some useful function, cannot provide sufficient reason to respect choices that cohere with and reinforce those practices. This would be especially so when (as in Martin's example, and unlike the Sudanese women in Chambers' example) we have reason to believe that those choices are made by individuals who do not meet the conditions for capacity.

Finally, we can see the inadequacy of this argument by considering what might be said with regards the choices of anorexic patients. If the value provided by certain practices legitimizes respecting choices irrespective of whether they are made with capacity, then if it were the case that the valuing of thinness were embedded in certain practices that gave significance and meaning to a community, then there would be reason to respect those choices. Indeed, one might argue that such communities and practices exist: perhaps with the existence of 'pro-ana' communities (where anorexic individuals provide support and motivation for each other in online forums, engaging in projects which have become known as 'thinspiration'), or in the increasingly prevalent social norms of thinness, reinforced daily on catwalks and billboards, and in the myriad women's magazines that provide normative frameworks in which many women find meaning. But to cite such practices as providing reason to respect choices that value thinness over life is as unappealing as citing practices of genital cutting as providing reason to respect choices that lead to damaging health consequences (although of course there are many significant differences between the cases).

In short, considerations that might be marshalled in favour of respecting choices based on divergent religious values do not seem able to provide sufficient reason for respecting those choices. This leaves things in a bit of a muddle: one explanation for the intuition that treatment which is in the best interests of the individual may be imposed on an anorexia sufferer who faces death or disability, it seemed, was that according to a value-laden conception of capacity, such an individual lacked decisional capacity, being unable to properly weigh information in coming to a decision. But nor, on such a value-laden conception, do religious believers, who privilege their commitments over life-saving treatment. But we (tend to) have different intuitions about whether such religious believers have capacity. These different intuitions cannot be explained away by appealing to the value of respecting autonomy or institutions, as I have just argued. This is relevant to the MCA, because intuitions about the evaluative capacities of anorexic patients pushed us towards a value-laden conception of capacity, whilst intuitions about the religious believers seem to pull in the other direction. If it is accepted that the conditions of the MCA are value-laden, in the ways I have set out, then significant work remains in systematizing intuitions about which value commitments or rankings undermine decisional capacity, and which do not.

7.6 **Conclusions**

The considerations I have raised indicate that the conditions for capacity presuppose that individuals endorse certain evaluative commitments, both in regard to what information is relevant to the decision (in particular, relevant to insight into illness), and in regard to the ability to weigh information in deliberation. If this is right, then it is a mistake to suppose that whether or not one meets the conditions for capacity can be determined purely formally, without reference to the content of an individual's choice or commitments. I have drawn out certain consequences of this conclusion, regarding the different requirements that face individuals with conventional or unconventional value commitments; the consequences for value-neutral conceptions of public health; and the need to consider further which values are deemed to be inconsistent with decisional capacity. If such value-judgements do play a role in assessments of capacity, it is then important to open discussion of which values are to be respected and when, rather than to suppose that any choice is permitted, no matter how unwise or irrational. This is especially so as intuitions about which evaluative commitments hinder decisional capacity appear to conflict, and a value-laden notion of capacity seems to require that some of our intuitive judgements are revised or rejected.

Acknowledgements

This paper has benefited greatly from discussions with Lubomira Radoilska and with the members of the reading group on Autonomy and Mental Health at the University of Cambridge, to whom I am grateful for their generous feedback. I am also grateful for feedback from Agnieszka Jaworska, Elizabeth Fistein, Fabian Freyenhagen, and Lisa Bortolotti, and from the audiences at the conference on Autonomy and Mental Health at The University of Cambridge.

References

Arpaly, N. (2003). Varieties of autonomy. In *Unprincipled Virtue*. Oxford, Oxford University Press, pp. 117–49.

Associated Jehovah's Witnesses for Reform on Blood website. http://www.ajwrb.org/about.shtml

Bolton, D. (2000). Continuing commentary: Alternatives to disorder. *Philosophy, Psychiatry, & Psychology* 7(2): 141–53.

Chambers, C. (2007). *Sex, Culture, and Justice: The Limits of Choice*. Pennsylvania, PA: Pennsylvania State University Press.

Christman, J. (1991). Autonomy and personal history. *Canadian Journal of Philosophy* 21: 1–24.

Christman, J. (2004). Relational autonomy, liberal individualism, and the social constitution of selves. *Philosophical Studies* 117: 143–64.

Dworkin, G. (1972). Paternalism. *Monist* 56: 64–8.

Dworkin, G. (1983). Paternalism: Some second thoughts. In R. Sartorius (ed.) *Paternalism*. Minneapolis, MN: University of Minnesota Press, pp. 105–12.

Dworkin, G. (1988). *The Theory and Practice of Autonomy*. Cambridge: Cambridge University Press.

Frankfurt, H. (1971). Freedom of the will and the concept of a person. *The Journal of Philosophy* 68(1): 5–20.

Friedman, M. (1986). Autonomy and the split-level self. *Journal of Social Philosophy* 24: 19–35.

Fulford, K.W.M. (1989). *Moral Theory and Medical Practice*. Cambridge: Cambridge University Press.

Fulford, K.W.M. (2001). 'What is (mental) disease?': an open letter to Christopher Boorse. *Journal of Medical Ethics* 27: 80–85.

Fulford, K.W.M. (2004). Completing Kraeplin's psychopathology: Insight, delusion and the phenomenology of illness. In X. Amador, and A. David (eds.) *Insight and Psychosis*. Oxford: Oxford University Press, pp. 47–66.

Fulford, K.W.M., Dickenson, D., and Murray, T.H. (2002). Introduction: Many voices, human values in healthcare ethics. In K.W.M. Fulford, D. Dickenson and

T.H. Murray (eds.) *Healthcare Ethics and Human Values*. Oxford: Blackwell Publishers Ltd., pp. 1–21.

Martin, A.M. (2007). Tales publicly allowed: Competence, capacity, and religious belief. *Hastings Center Report* 37(1): 33–40.

Moorhead, S. and Turkington, D. (2002). Letter: Role of emotional capacity in consent should be clarified. *British Medical Journal* 325: 1039.

Oshana, M. (1998). Personal autonomy and society. *The Journal of Social Philosophy* 29(1): 81–102.

Owens, G.S., Freyenhagen, F., Richardson, G., and Hotopf, M. (2009). Mental capacity and decisional autonomy: An interdisciplinary challenge. *Inquiry* 52(1) 79–107.

Phillips, A. (2007). *Multiculturalism without Culture*. Princeton, NJ: Princeton University Press.

Radoilska, L. (2009). Public health ethics and liberalism. *Public Health Ethics* 2(2): 135–45.

Tan, J., Hope, T., and Stewart, A. (2003). Competence to refuse treatment in anorexia nervosa. *International Journal of Law and Psychiatry* 26(6): 697–707.

Tan, J. and Hope, T. (2008). Treatment refusal in anorexia nervosa: A challenge to current concepts of capacity. In G. Widdershoven (ed.) *Empirical Ethics in Psychiatry*. Oxford: Oxford University Press, pp. 187–210.

The Mental Capacity Act. (2005). *Office of Public Sector Information*. http://www.opsi.gov.uk/acts/acts2005/ukpga_20050009_en_1

The Mental Health Act, Department of Health. *The National Archives*. http://www.dh.gov.uk/en/Healthcare/Mentalhealth/Policy/InformationontheMentalHealthActs/index.htm

The Mental Health Act. (2007). *Office of Public Sector Information*. http://www.opsi.gov.uk/acts/acts2007/ukpga_20070012_en_1

Chapter 8

The Mental Capacity Act and conceptions of the good

Elizabeth Fistein

8.1 Introduction

Respect for personal autonomy is widely accepted as an important ethical principle in medical practice. Generally, the principle is enacted by seeking informed consent for acts connected with medical care and treatment, and by respecting refusals of the care and treatment on offer. However, a problem arises when a patient is thought to lack the mental capacities necessary for participation in the consent process. Paternalism has been defined as 'the interference of a state or an individual with another person, against their will, and defended or motivated by a claim that the person interfered with will be better off or protected from harm' (Dworkin 2009). Whilst 'soft' paternalism, or interference with actions that are not the products of an autonomous will, is often considered justifiable, 'hard' paternalism, interference with autonomous individuals, has fewer defenders (McMillan 2007).

In some circumstances (e.g. unconsciousness, infancy) the lack of capacity is uncontroversial, as is the imperative to intervene in treatable cases rather than letting the patient die simply for wont of consent. Such cases are generally considered to be examples of justified paternalism. However, in medicine circumstances are rarely as clear-cut as these. Different forms of mental disorder may, to a greater or lesser extent, interfere with a person's ability to participate in informed decision-making (Okai et al. 2007) and it may, in practice, be difficult to determine whether choices are sufficiently autonomous to demand respect. Moreover, even if decision-making ability is impaired to the extent that a person is deemed unable to give legally valid consent, he may remain capable of expressing preferences. In addition to the expression of preferences, patients with progressive or relapsing and remitting conditions may in the past have expressed deeply held values that are pertinent to the decision to be made on their behalf in the present. To what extent should practitioners take such preferences and values into account when providing care or treatment for people who are currently unable to give legally valid consent?

In England and Wales, the Mental Capacity Act 2005 (MCA), has been developed to regulate this difficult area of practice. The Act defines the circumstances under which a person's decision will be deemed insufficiently autonomous to carry legal weight. If someone is found to lack the legal capacity to make a particular decision, that decision will be made on his behalf. The Act also provides guidance on the factors to be considered when making a decision on behalf of somebody else. However, despite the implementation of this comprehensive regulatory framework, it can be difficult to decide how to treat a person who has a degree of cognitive impairment but nonetheless retains strong views about care and treatment which appear to stem from longstanding values.

In this chapter, I reflect upon this difficulty from the perspective of a psychiatrist considering the real case of a woman with dementia who does not want to be placed in a residential care home. Drawing on the idea of reflective equilibrium as a method for resolving ethical problems (Rawls 1971; Beauchamp and Childress 2001), theoretical accounts of the boundaries of personal autonomy and justifications for paternalism are considered alongside the discussion of the clinical case which took place at a multi-disciplinary team meeting. The moral intuitions apparent in the deliberations of the clinicians are explicated and used to reconsider theory, while theory is used to inform a critique of practice.

Case 1: Mrs Day

Mrs Day, a widow in her 70s, had lived alone for 23 years. She was admitted to hospital for assessment when she was discovered by the busy road outside her flat in a confused state, unable to find her way home from the shops. She was diagnosed with moderately severe dementia and found to have impaired decision-making abilities as a result. A decision had to be made concerning where she should live when she left hospital.

The discussion which follows is based upon an anonymized transcript of the meeting during which health and social care practitioners discussed the case with Mrs Day's representatives i.e. her sons and an independent mental capacity advocate.

Mrs Day was able to convey her current wishes and feelings to her advocate, who described their conversation in the following terms: 'She told me that she wants to go home ... She couldn't actually remember her home where she lived, because I asked her to tell me a little bit about it and she can't remember it at all. But she did say she wants to go somewhere nice where she's on her own. She doesn't want to live with other people, wants to be on her own but to have other people that can pop in and see her'.

Mrs Day's sons were able to infer values that would be likely to influence any decision she was able to make, describing them in the following terms: 'Mum's always lived on her own. She's always been independent'.

Nonetheless, the clinical team struggled to come to a decision. They did not seem comfortable with the option of discharging Mrs Day home to her flat, expressing concerns about her physical safety. They hoped to discharge her to a specialist residential care home for people with dementia, where she could be monitored at all times. The Day family contested this plan, which they characterized as unnecessarily restrictive to their mother's independence and contrary to her overall well-being. They asked the clinical team to delay discharging Mrs Day until her social worker could arrange a new, warden-controlled, flat in a sheltered complex for elderly residents well away from busy roads. The social worker, who was responsible for making the final decision on behalf of Mrs Day, was required to apply the framework laid down in the Mental Capacity Act 2005. She was faced with the task of reviewing all the relevant information and selecting the best option. Some of the difficulties she encountered can be attributed to a lack of consensus over the meaning of one of the central doctrines of the Act: best interests.

8.2 The Mental Capacity Act 2005 and the concept of best interests

In England and Wales, the MCA regulates the process of decision-making on behalf of people who are found legally incompetent to make a particular decision. The Act sets out a two-stage process for determining whether or not a person has the capacity to make a specific decision. Stage one is establishing whether the person has an: 'impairment of, or a disturbance in the functioning of, their mind or brain' (s.2). This is a necessary, but not sufficient condition. A person is deemed to lack capacity only if, as a result of this impairment, he cannot (i) understand information relevant to the decision, (ii) retain that information in his mind, (iii) use or weigh that information as part of the decision-making process, and (iv) communicate his decision (s.3). Only when all practical and appropriate support has failed can it be said that the person lacks the capacity to make a decision.

This approach to the determination of capacity is sometimes termed a test of ability to understand (Gunn 1994) or functional ability. It is based on a procedural account of personal autonomy which protects decisions made by people with the cognitive ability to work out what would be best for them (even if they then choose something else) and has the advantage of relative clarity and ease of application. It is not too difficult, in practice, to determine whether somebody has the cognitive capacity to handle relevant information about a particular healthcare intervention and therefore whether any refusal of that intervention must, in law, be respected. A potential weakness of the functional ability approach, however, arises from its failure to include consideration of the deeply held feelings and values that may persist even when mental ill health has significantly impaired functional cognitive ability.

In the case of Mrs Day, professionals and family carers alike appeared reluctant to override her longstanding preference for independence and living alone, either arguing that it should be respected or, at the very least, holding themselves under a duty to provide adequate justification for making decisions that conflicted with this preference. This intuition that long-standing values or even preferences are morally significant relates to an argument that the capacity for autonomous action is retained as long as long-standing preferences or values persist (Jaworska 1999). It would follow that enacting respect for autonomy entails acting in accordance with those values, including undertaking decision-making on behalf of a person who no longer has the intellectual capacity to make the choices that will best serve her own values. However, it does not necessarily follow from the fact that we tend to treat the values and preferences of others as worthy of a degree of respect that people should be considered capable of autonomous agency simply because they are capable of valuing or preferring particular states of affairs (Kittay 2007). Indeed, the prominence of the 'respect for autonomy' principle in applied bioethics may even be creating something of a distortion, with other intuitively significant principles such as 'respect for values' or 'respect for persons' becoming conflated with the notion of 'respect for autonomy', which then becomes a placeholder for respect in general (Lysaught 2004). There is a risk that by extending the margins of autonomy to promote respect for values, we could inadvertently undermine other elements of respect for persons such as care (Mol 2008) and trust (O'Neill 2002). The MCA uses the notion of *best interests* as a means of incorporating respect for values into medical care, without necessarily extending the margins of what is to be treated as autonomous agency.

Once it has been established that: 1) a person lacks the capacity to make a specific decision, and 2) there is no valid advance refusal of treatment (which must be respected) then, according to the MCA, that decision must be made on her behalf, acting in her 'best interests'. The MCA does not, therefore, appear to go as far as incorporating the capacity to value into its test of decisional capacity, perhaps because, in comparison with functional decision-making ability, this would be more difficult to test reliably. It does, however, treat past and present wishes and feelings, and longstanding beliefs and values, as significant and requires that they are taken into account by decision-makers, during the determination of 'best interests'. The concept of 'best interests' lacks a clear definition, and this lack of conceptual clarity creates a series of potential problems for clinicians which are illustrated by the case of Mrs Day. Various attempts at clarification have been made by both ethicists and judges. Three examples are outlined as follows, for the purpose of comparison with the conception of 'best interests' that emerges from the MCA.

8.2.1 An alternative to substituted judgement

Buchanan and Brock's normative analysis of the ethics of decision-making on behalf of others identifies two alternative principles to be used to guide surrogate decision-making: substituted judgement and best interests (Buchanan and Brock 1990). Loss of the capacities considered necessary for decision-making competence is not, in itself, treated as sufficient reason for reliance on the notion of best interests as the guiding principle. Wherever possible, decision-makers are advised to respect self-determination, for both its intrinsic value and its instrumental value in highlighting the course of action that would be most in keeping with the patient's overall well-being. Therefore, decision-makers are advised to take account of clear expressions of preference, *made before capacity was lost,* which could be used to help them to 'don the mantle of the incompetent patient' and attempt to make the decision he would have made, had he retained capacity (assuming that the competent patient, in possession of a set of values and conception of the good, is usually the person best placed to understand what will be most in keeping with her own values and long-term projects). This process is referred to as substituted judgement. It extends the scope of autonomous agency beyond loss of the cognitive capacities needed to make decisions, by providing external assistance with the cognitive aspects of decision-making without substituting the values of the decision-maker for the values of the patient.

However, this may be difficult to achieve, particularly for those clinicians who hold themselves accountable to a strong professional duty to care for the health of their patients (Mol 2008). Indeed, in the case of Mrs Day, healthcare professionals appeared particularly reluctant to endorse any plan that would leave their patient unsupervised and therefore at risk of coming to harm. An illustrative example is a nurse's comment that 'But if there's issues of safety in her home, maybe there may be issues of safety in a warden controlled flat. Like, if you were concerned that she's likely to turn the taps on . . . I mean, she hasn't done that here, but . . .'. There appears to be a widespread intuition amongst the clinical staff that their primary duty is to safeguard the physical well-being of their patients, particularly those with impaired decision-making capacity.

Possibly less difficult for clinicians to adhere to, then, is the alternative guidance principle: best interests. When there is no expression of preference on which to base substituted judgement, decision-makers are advised to select the treatment or care option that carries the greatest net benefit for the patient. This raises the question of how to define 'benefit'. Approaches to the definition of what is good for persons can be grouped into three categories: first, *hedonist theories* hold that it is good for people to have positive conscious experiences e.g. pleasure or the satisfaction of aims or desires. Second, *corrected preference satisfaction theories* hold that it is good for people when what they want to happen actually does happen, to the maximum extent possible over their lifetimes, allowing for correction of desires based upon mistakes or lack of relevant knowledge. Third, *objective list or ideal theories* hold that it is good for people to have experiences that are defined externally as 'good', regardless of whether they produce positive conscious experiences and even if these are not always what the person would prefer. Nonetheless, an externally defined list of 'good things' is likely to include pleasure and having one's preferences satisfied where possible. This is important because, as we will see in the case of Mrs Day, the conception of the good used by a decision-maker will influence the scope of justifiable paternalism. A version of the objective list approach which prioritizes good health will justify more paternalistic actions than a corrected preference satisfaction approach, which accepts that people may value other goods, such as pleasure or liberty, above their own health.

8.2.2 A response to health needs

Buchanan and Brock's framework makes a clear distinction between substituted judgement and best interests approaches. In English law, however, the distinction is less clear, as the following description of the development of the doctrine of necessity demonstrates. This doctrine was developed by the courts to legitimize treatment without consent when the need was urgent and the patient was unconscious (*Marshall v Curry* [1933]). In the early cases, treatment was deemed to be justified when immediately necessary to preserve the life or health of the patient. In *Re F (mental patient: sterilisation)* [1990], the doctrine of necessity was extended beyond the provision of emergency life-saving treatment, to cover treatment necessary in the best interests of any patient who lacked the mental capacity to give valid consent. Lord Goff identified best interests as being for the 'life, health or well-being' of the patient, while Lord Brandon stated that: 'The operation or other treatment will be in their best interests if, but only if, it is carried out in order either to save their lives, or to ensure improvement or prevent deterioration in their physical or mental health'. This development broadened the conception of best interests, basing it upon welfare interests rather than immediate physical safety.

8.2.3 Broader considerations

The doctrine of necessity was developed to deal with a potential problem for doctors treating people unable to give consent: in failing to provide treatment at all, they may be failing in their legal duty of care and potentially negligent; but treatment without valid consent, would, in the absence of a legal defence, be classed as assault. Clearly, the surrogate decision-maker was treated as responsible for the consequences of the decision and blame-worthy if harm arose. Initially, the determination of best interests was treated as identical to the legal definition of the doctor's duty of care, from the law of negligence. A doctor did not breach his duty of care, and therefore acted in the patient's best interests, if he provided treatment or otherwise acted 'in accordance with a practice accepted as proper by a responsible body of medical men skilled in that particular art' (*Bolam v Friern Hospital Management Committee* [1957]). However, using the *Bolam* test to determine the patient's best interests created a conceptual difficulty: potentially, numerous treatment options could be accepted as proper by a responsible body of doctors, who may differ in their opinions as to what is actually best for the patient. The Court of Appeal addressed this problem in 2000: If several options are available that are all in the interests of the patient's health, the option in the *best* interests must be chosen. Butler-Sloss P identified that such a decision 'will incorporate broader ethical, social, moral and welfare considerations' (*Re S (adult: sterilisation)*). Thus, the conception of 'best interests' used in law began as vital interests, grew to incorporate other health interests, and then developed scope to incorporate other considerations including an interest in the satisfaction of preferences.

The MCA does not define what a person's best interests might be, rather it sets out what must be done and considered when making a best interests decision. The following clauses are of particular significance here:

> He must, so far as reasonably practicable, permit and encourage the person to participate, or to improve his ability to participate, as fully as possible in any act done for him and any decision affecting him.

He must consider, so far as is reasonably ascertainable the person's past and present wishes and feelings (and, in particular, any relevant written statement made by him when he had capacity), the beliefs and values that would be likely to influence his decision if he had capacity, and the other factors that he would be likely to consider if he were able to do so.

He must take into account, if it is practicable and appropriate to consult them, the views of anyone named by the person as someone to be consulted on the matter in question or on matters of that kind, anyone engaged in caring for the person or interested in his welfare, any donee of a lasting power of attorney granted by the person, and any deputy appointed for the person by the court, as to what would be in the person's best interests and, in particular, as to the matters mentioned [above].

The Code of Practice that accompanies the MCA adds that:

[t]his checklist is only the starting point: in many cases, extra factors will need to be considered. When working out what is in the best interests of the person who lacks capacity to make a decision or act for themselves, decision-makers must take into account all relevant factors that it would be reasonable to consider, not just those that they think are important. They must not act or make a decision based on what they would want to do if they were the person who lacked capacity.

The MCA explicitly includes the wishes, feelings, beliefs, and values of the person who lacks capacity among the 'broader ethical, social, moral and welfare considerations' to be considered when determining best interests. This could be interpreted as a form of paternalism based upon an objective list theory of good that included (but did not necessarily prioritize) satisfaction of preferences. This interpretation would be in line with the approach of the case law that the MCA was enacted to codify. Equally, it could be viewed as paternalism based upon a preference satisfaction theory of the good for persons, particularly as wishes, feelings, beliefs and values are the only factors explicitly named. It is also open to interpretation as an attempt to limit the need for and scope of paternalistic intervention by facilitating a form of self-determination via substituted judgement. The reference to written statements made when the patient had capacity and the requirement to consult with people who know the patient or were named by him as someone he wished to be consulted both suggest that the intention was to enable substituted judgement.

8.3 **Three conceptions of best interests**

In the case of Mrs Day, the interpretation placed on the notion of best interests had direct implications for the planning of her care. The difficulties that arose appear, at least in part, to be due to the fact that those involved adopted different approaches to the determination of her best interests and arrived at different conclusions.

8.3.1 **Paternalism based on an ideal theory of good**

Mrs Day's condition was progressive and her healthcare needs were complex and contested, leading to a protracted argument between the in-patient team who characterized her as very impaired and in need of constant supervision, and her family, social worker, and advocate who all questioned whether she might be less impaired than the confusing hospital environment made her appear. Nonetheless, in the discussion of what would be in Mrs Day's overall best interests, consideration of how best to protect her health and safety was clearly given priority. In particular, the hospital staff appeared extremely reluctant to take any action that might leave her at risk of harm, to the extent that they constructed risks when there was no evidence that they were likely to occur, in order to justify a recommendation for constant supervision, as the following exchange illustrates:

> Nurse: There may be issues of safety in a warden controlled flat, like if you were concerned that she's likely to turn the taps on—I mean she hasn't done here, but . . .
> Occupational therapist: Would there be someone there all the time?
> Nurse: Yes, this is what concerns me really.

However, they refused to seek evidence to support their characterization of Mrs Day as impaired and at risk, implying that even doing this represented an unjustifiable risk, for example:

> Social worker: . . . . I know you did the assessment in the house, did you do anything outside of the house, around the roads and where the . . . shop is and see whether she could get back. Did you do anything like that on the assessment?
> Occupational therapist: No, no.
> Social worker: Would you be prepared to do it?
> Occupational therapist: Would it show anything up, sorry?

The social worker summed up her problem with this situation:

> It's always been the road hasn't it. This is why I asked for community safety tests
> so that we could find out once and for all whether this lady is going to be at high
> risk of crossing the road, but that's never materialized so we still don't know.

Thus, the determination of best interests by hospital staff appeared to be based upon a conception of the good derived from an objective list, with maximal health and physical safety at the top. This in turn led them to propose a paternalistic solution to the problem: Mrs Day should be discharged to a specialist residential home where she could be supervised at all times, despite her clearly expressed preference for living alone.

8.3.2 Paternalism based on satisfaction of corrected preferences

Mrs Day's sons also considered her safety, but this was limited to concern about the specific problem with wandering on the busy road outside her flat which had led to her hospitalization. Their response to the hypothetical concerns of the hospital staff was to refute their existence and to focus upon road safety: 'Well I'm more worried about the main road where she is at the moment; that's my biggest worry'. They demonstrated a concern for Mrs Day's overall well-being that honoured her preference for independence, repeatedly challenging the idea that it would be best for her to move to a residential home. For example, when the doctor stated that 'Personally, I think she'll benefit from having more people around; once she's in a stable environment with people around, I think she'd be . . . she'd flourish in something like a residential home', the sons, in response, placed a preference for independence at the heart of what well-being means for Mrs Day: 'I disagree'; 'Yes, I disagree as well. Mum's always lived on her own. She's always been independent'.

Their determination of best interests appeared to be based upon a satisfaction of corrected preferences theory. The stable preference for independence lay at the core, but they considered how best this might be achieved: not by returning home to a flat where the risk of an accident on the road might lead to a swift return to hospital, but by an alternative approach that took into account Mrs Day's reduced cognitive abilities while keeping restrictions on her independence to a minimum. They suggested a flat with an on-site warden, in a quiet area away from busy roads.

8.3.3 Respect for autonomy based on substituted judgement

For the advocate, Mrs Day's preferences were both clear and deserving of serious consideration: 'She doesn't want to live with other people, wants to be on her own, but to have other people that can pop in and see her . . . And I made sure that I would make sure that everyone here heard that, that that's what she wants'. However, she did imply that risks should be taken into account, provided that these were things Mrs Day would have taken into account if she was able to: 'I'm not allowed to have an opinion on what I think is right for Mrs Day. I'm just raising questions . . . that she might ask if she was in here and was able to ask them'.

The advocate's conception of best interests appeared to be based upon a substituted judgement approach. She voiced Mrs Day's views, as she understood them, to the team and stressed the importance of listening to them. She acknowledged the need to consider the risks associated with a return to the old flat, but implied that the task for the team was to consider how Mrs Day would evaluate those risks, if she were still able to understand what they were, in relation to her desire for independence. Like the social worker, she wanted clear evidence of a significant risk to vital interests before she would condone a care plan that did not honour Mrs Day's expressed preference for her own home. The question was not what was good or best for Mrs Day, but what would Mrs Day have chosen for herself if she had retained the ability to take in relevant information and weigh it up?

These three different conceptions of best interests led to three quite different care plans. As two plans had to be eliminated, the clinicians had to find some way of resolving the conflict.

In all three models, the fact that Mrs Day had wandered onto a busy road outside her old flat made it an unsuitable choice. The documented risk of injury conflicted: 1) with her health and safety interests, as prioritized in the hospital staff's model based upon an objective list; 2) with her interest in the satisfaction of her preference for independence, as returning to a situation where she could be seriously injured would reduce the likelihood of her maintaining her independence in the long run; and 3) with her personal autonomy, assuming that she would not knowingly choose to risk serious injury (a reasonable assumption in the absence of clear evidence to the contrary).

The option of a warden-controlled flat appeared compatible with both preference satisfaction paternalism and with substituted judgement. However, in practice, this option was successfully resisted by the hospital staff, initially on the grounds that it was incompatible with their conception of her best interests. This was unproductive, because their conception was not accepted by the others involved in the decision.

Finally, the doctor raised an excuse rather than a justification for over-riding Mrs Day's preference. There was a waiting list for warden-controlled flats, whereas a residential home place could be arranged relatively quickly. Economic reality prevented him from respecting Mrs Day's preference: 'In an ideal world I would agree that it would be nice for you to just have that one move and all settled. But realistically, this is an acute medical ward and we are desperate for beds. I know that sounds horrible, but . . .'.

This excuse was immediately accepted by the Day family, who told the doctor that they were 'just being selfish' and that his plan to discharge Mrs Day to a residential care home was 'fair enough'. Everyone appears to have considered it reasonable to take into consideration not only the interests of Mrs Day, but also the wider interests of society and the need to distribute healthcare resources equitably, something which is not acknowledged in the MCA. Having accepted the necessity of a move to a residential home rather than the (currently unavailable) warden-controlled accommodation, the Day family revised their account of what would be best: 'Yes, if she's settled and that, happy and making friends, that'll be fine'.

By the end of this exchange, consideration of Mrs Day's *happiness* has been made relevant to the determination of what is best for her.

The one thing everyone seems to agree upon is that they must avoid making Mrs Day unhappy. Thus, the conflict was resolved by resorting to a hedonistic conception of the good, whereby best interests are served when the patient is happy and provided with pleasurable experiences to compensate for disappointments. However, the compensation appears inconsistent with what is known about the patient; why did the decision-makers suppose that living with others would result in Mrs Day making friends and feeling happy, when she had always preferred her own company? The possibility is raised that the decision-makers were offering to provide experiences that they themselves find pleasurable, in contravention of the Code of Practice which states that decision-makers 'must not act or make a decision based on what they would want to do if they were the person who lacked capacity'.

8.4 **Discussion**

In the MCA, decision-makers are warned of the danger of inappropriately imposing their own values. However, the case of Mrs Day illustrates how this may nonetheless occur, in response to difficulty agreeing on what is meant by the term 'best interests' in general, and the significance of patient preference in particular. This moulding of the meaning of 'best interests' illustrates a potential problem with any normative framework for surrogate decision-making: 'a theory that makes unrealistic moral demands on people by ignoring human psychology and the financial and institutional incentives under which individuals operate is of little practical significance' (Buchanan and Brock 1990, p. 89).

In the MCA, decision-makers are instructed to consider 'the person's past and present wishes and feelings'. Expressions of preference are treated as relevant, *even if made when the patient lacked capacity*. It is open to interpretation whether this conception of best interests is based upon a satisfaction of corrected preferences theory; an objective list theory that treats the satisfaction of preferences as one of the things that is good for persons, or even an attempt to broaden the scope of self-determination through substituted judgement. Whilst this may have the advantage of leaving scope for flexibility, the lack of conceptual clarity does appear to create difficulties for clinicians.

Theorists have noted that 'There is a long tradition in medicine that the physician's first and most important commitment should be to serve the well-being of the patient' and argued that this tendency needs to be accounted for in a normative framework for surrogate decision-making, by adopting a preference satisfaction approach to the determination of what is good for people, to avoid the risks of unwarranted paternalism or even abuse associated with an objective list developed from a limited perspective (Buchanan and Brock 1990). However, the case of Mrs Day illustrates a more complex process of meaning-making amongst clinicians than simply equating best interests with health and safety and therefore judging that best interests are served by the option than most rigorously safeguards the patient. There is evidence of an intuition that it is wrong to enforce a state of affairs that makes a person unhappy. Mrs Day's doctor and family all agreed that a move to a residential home may be morally justifiable, provided she turned out to be content to stay there, 'flourish[ing]', 'happy and making friends'. Health interests were not their only concern; they were also concerned with not causing negative or unpleasant conscious mental experiences and promoting opportunities for positive ones. However, in the heat of the moment it appeared to be difficult to make the imaginative leap necessary to determine the sort of things that might make Mrs Day happy and persuade her to accept the proposed move. Perhaps only careful observation and a process of trial and error would reveal this.

Besides the lack of conceptual clarity around the notion of 'best interests' used in the MCA, a second problem illustrated by the case of Mrs Day was the difficulty in determining the degree of significance to be accorded to requests for a particular form of care or treatment. The concept of informed consent carries with it a right to refuse treatment, but no right to demand treatment that a healthcare practitioner believes to be unsuitable. People are generally able to take into account their own aims and values and to judge whether to accept or refuse offers of treatment accordingly. Preferences play an important role in deciding when to *refuse* treatment. When a patient lacks capacity, however, she is not in a position to weigh up these considerations and accept or refuse the assistance being offered. Instead, healthcare practitioners must take them into consideration on behalf of the patient and use them to decide what treatment to *provide*. In Mrs Day's case, this process appeared to generate a 'fantasy option' that may well have been in her overall best interests, but the resources were never available to make the fantasy a reality. Moreover, making the necessary resources available would have impacted negatively on the interests of other patients. In practice, the clinicians treated her preferences not as reasons for providing a particular type of care, analogous to requests, but as reasons for not imposing care that she would, in all likelihood, have refused if she had the legal capacity to do so, because it would make her unhappy or distressed.

Taking these two issues (the meaning of 'best interests' and the significance of requests) together, the shared insights of the people involved in Mrs Day's case begin to illuminate the boundaries of autonomy and paternalism, as they are drawn in practice. Their actions were based upon a presumption that Mrs Day was unable to understand, retain or weigh up information relevant to the decision, and appeared to be directed towards the avoidance of three wrongs: 1) failure to protect Mrs Day from unknowingly risking serious injury; 2) the imposition of a state of affairs which made Mrs Day unhappy; and 3) the inequitable distribution of limited resources. Moreover, they appeared to hold themselves accountable for the outcomes making them, not Mrs Day, responsible for any harm arising as a result of their surrogate decision-making.

How does this relate to the core meanings of autonomy or paternalism? It is instructive to re-visit autonomy's roots in political philosophy, where self-rule acts as a protection against tyranny. In most cases, people will choose to minimize their risk of serious injury (although they may tolerate a degree of risk in order to obtain some other benefit such as excitement, a sense of freedom or the defence of a cause they care deeply about) and to avoid states of affairs which will make them unhappy (although they may tolerate a degree of unhappiness in order to obtain more happiness or some other benefit in the long term). Procedural accounts of personal autonomy call for a society in which this is made possible through a duty of non-interference with most choices, leaving people free to pursue their own projects as they see fit (to the extent that this leaves other people equally free to do the same). Thus, people are protected from tyranny from outside. However, people with impaired capacity for autonomous agency would be unable to flourish in an environment where all their wishes were respected: they may be unable to work out how to go about achieving the states of affairs that they value or care about, or they may be unaware of dangers associated with pursuing their goals and, moreover, incapable of becoming aware of them thereby unwittingly risking serious harm. This could be interpreted as a form of unwitting tyranny from inside which paternalism could prevent, by enabling people to pursue the things they care about through the provision of a surrogate to undertake the necessary cognitive tasks on their behalf.

However, once such assistance becomes necessary, account must be taken of the rights and responsibilities of the surrogate. If, prior to loss of capacity, Mrs Day had made an Advance Decision to refuse residential care, even if this put her at risk of serious injury, the clinicians could honour her preference for her own home confident that they were not enforcing a serious risk she had unwittingly imposed upon herself through ignorance. If it were clearly her choice to run that risk, in order to maintain the independence she so valued, then responsibility for the consequences might rightly be accorded to her. In reality, the clinicians had to decide whether her apparent desire to return home should be honoured as an authentic expression of her independence or overruled in order to protect her from serious harm. By facilitating a return home, the decision-makers would have effectively collaborated with Mrs Day in enacting plan that put her at risk, without being sure that this was what she would have chosen had she been able to use all the relevant information. If the risk was not of her choosing, then it would be unreasonable to hold her fully responsible for the consequences and the clinicians would have to accept a share of the responsibility.

Conversely, whilst decision-makers appeared to treat as unjustifiable any attempt to collaborate with a plan that would put her at significant risk of harm, they were also unwilling to enforce plans that seemed likely to make her unhappy, even if they would maximize her safety.

It seems that they *were* mindful of the possibility that Mrs Day might value her independence over her health or even safety, and that they treated this as something they ought to take into account, to the extent that they would not impose their own values at the cost of her happiness, thereby avoiding tyranny through the enforcement of the values of others. Instead, they attempted to plot a course between misery under tyranny from outside and injury under unwitting tyranny from inside.

Finally, they were faced with the task of doing whatever was in the best interests of Mrs Day. On the face of it, this would appear to be finding her a new placement in warden-controlled accommodation, thereby respecting her preference for independence whilst keeping her safe from harm. However, the clinicians appeared unwilling to enact a plan that compromised their ability to respond to the health needs of other patients without providing any immediate health benefit for Mrs Day, even if this meant enacting a less-than-ideal plan for her. The doctor acknowledged that warden-controlled accommodation would have been best 'in an ideal world', and the family appeared to accept that it would be 'selfish' to insist upon Mrs Day remaining in a hospital bed that might be needed by somebody else for health reasons until accommodation that met her preference for independence without risking her safety could be arranged. Faced with a choice between doing what appeared *best* for Mrs Day, but at the cost of the health of others, and what appeared to be *good enough*, because it achieved the twin goals of avoiding tyranny from inside and outside, the good enough option was selected. The final twist, however, is the way the decision-makers decided what was good enough to make Mrs Day feel 'settled', 'content', and 'happy'. Rather than asking her, they assumed that the opportunity to make friends would be adequate compensation for the loss of a home of her own, raising the possibility that the values of the majority had prevailed after all.

Can all of this be incorporated into a coherent approach to the treatment of people with impaired decision-making capacity? The justifications for any interference at all seem to be: 1) to assist those who are, as a result of a mental disorder, unable to develop the plans that would allow them to pursue the ends that they value and 2) in order to prevent harm risked unwittingly. The scope of justifiable paternalism would be, in condition (1), to do good by enabling the incapacitated person to maximize the satisfaction of her preferences and, in condition (2), to do good by preventing outcomes objectively considered bad or harmful but risked unknowingly (a limited form of ideal list theory of the good). The concept of best interests, therefore, needs to capture both of these conditions. Justification 1 is value-neutral, in that it requires the person to have a set of values, or at least things they appear to care about, but does not determine what those values should be. An explicit commitment to a satisfaction of corrected preferences theory within the Code of Practice would preserve this value neutrality. Justification 2, whilst apparently objective, may in fact be value-laden, as most healthcare interventions carry some risk of harm (complications, side effects, loss of liberty) and surrogate decision-makers must determine whether the likely harmful consequences of a decision outweigh the potential benefits, a task with an evaluative component. In the case of Mrs Day, the harmful effects of the proposed intervention were judged by their anticipated effect on mental state: an intervention to maximize safety would be doing more good than harm provided Mrs Day seemed happy or content. A threshold prohibition on the enforcement of ongoing care to which the patient appears to object could achieve this end.

Finally, consideration of the effects of decisions on the decision-makers and third parties appeared to be an important aspect of this case. Arguably, any putative right to assistance in the pursuit of one's own aims is limited by the freedom of others to refuse to assist in projects that conflict with their own values. A system which expects decision-makers to enact plans that conflict with their personal or professional ethics, even if they are consistent with the values of the patient, is unlikely to succeed in practice. A potential compromise is to use Advance Decisions to both promote personal autonomy and preserve the link between autonomous agency and responsibility. As these decisions are made before the loss of capacity, it seems reasonable to hold the patient who made the decision, not the clinicians who acts upon it, responsible for the consequences (assuming continuity of personal identity). In the absence of such a clear indication of objection, care and treatment in the interests of the patient's health, safety, and comfort would remain potentially justifiable.

The issue of resource allocation between the patient and third parties applies to people with and without decision-making capacity, but is highlighted by the problem of what to do when the best interests of one patient conflict with the vital interests of another or with the health interests of many others. Nobody involved in Mrs Day's case appeared to believe it would be reasonable to maintain her desire for independence at the cost of the health of other people who needed the hospital bed she would have to occupy while waiting for a new flat. On a broader scale, it would be illogical to require clinicians to devote all available resources to furthering the best interests of one patient at the cost of the interests of others. This leaves the question of how to balance the interests of different patients in practice. The concept of avoidance of tyranny provides a potential solution: wherever possible, the broad interests of people who lack capacity, based upon a corrected preference satisfaction theory of the good, should be promoted in the provision of health and social care. However, where resources are limited, promotion of best interests may be treated as an aspiration whilst the imposition of treatment plans that cause ongoing unhappiness would remain prohibited.

In summary, the case of Mrs Day illustrates some of the intellectual difficulties faced by clinicians applying the MCA. The lack of conceptual clarity around the notion of best interests leaves it open to interpretation as a requirement to promote personal autonomy through the exercise of substitute judgement or a justification for paternalism. Furthermore, different degrees of paternalism may be viewed as justifiable, depending on the conception of the good that decision-makers adopt, making the determination of best interests in practice contentious. Once best interests have been determined, other factors such as the responsibilities of decision-makers and the needs of others may place reasonable limits on the extent to which clinicians can be expected to pursue what is best for, or desired by, an individual patient, but the MCA does not acknowledge this, creating further difficulties.

Ideally, a form of best interests based upon substituted judgement (when relevant wishes prior to loss of capacity are known) or satisfaction of corrected preferences (when they are not) should be pursued. This encourages respect for the values of the patient which survive the loss of cognitive decision-making capacities without undermining trust and caring relationships by requiring clinicians to enact plans that risk significant harm to the patient (in the absence of a clear advance directive in which the patient assumes responsibility for any adverse consequences). When the best interests of the patient impact adversely on the interests of others, the interests of all concerned will have to be balanced. An explicit acknowledgement that best interests cannot always be served would be more straightforward and honest, in comparison with the practice of stretching the definition of best interests to match what is available which carries the risk of inappropriate imposition of the decision-maker's values. Nonetheless, a threshold test which focuses on the patient's current mental state and protects her from the imposition of care that causes ongoing unhappiness may be an appropriate safety net.

Acknowledgements .

The author wishes to acknowledge the following people who assisted in the writing of this paper: Dr Marcus Redley, of the Cambridge Intellectual and Developmental Disabilities Research Group, who supervised an ethnography of the process of surrogate decision-making in clinical meetings. Our discussions regarding the motivations of clinicians were the inspiration for undertaking the analysis presented in this paper. The Autonomy and Mental Health Group, convened by Dr Lubomira Radoilska in the University of Cambridge Faculty of Philosophy, for the stimulating and helpful discussion of an earlier version of this paper. The editor of this volume, Dr Lubomira Radoilska, for her constructive suggestions on the first draft of this paper.

References

Beauchamp, T. L., and Childress, J. F. (2001). *Principles of biomedical ethics* (5th edn.). Oxford: Oxford University Press.

Bolam v Friern Hospital Management Committee [1957] 2 All ER 118, [1957]1 WLR 582.

Buchanan, A. E. and Brock, D. W. (1990). *Deciding for others: The ethics of surrogate decision-making* (1st edn.). Cambridge: Cambridge University Press.

Dworkin, G. (2009). Paternalism. In E.N. Zalta (ed.) *The Stanford Encyclopedia of Philosophy.* [Online] http://plato.stanford.edu/entries/paternalism/

Gunn, M. (1994). The meaning of incapacity. *Medical Law Review* 2: 8–29.

Jaworska, A. (1999). Respecting the margins of agency: Alzheimer's patients and the capacity to value. *Philosophy and Public Affairs* 28(2): 105–38.

Kittay, E. (2007). Beyond autonomy and paternalism—the caring, transparent self. In T. Nys, Y. Denier, and T. Vandevelde (eds.) *Autonomy and paternalism: Reflections on the theory and practice of health care.* Leuven: Peeters Publishing, pp. 23–70.

Lysaught, M.T. (2004). Respect: Or, how respect for persons became respect for autonomy. *Journal of Medicine and Philosophy* 29(6): 665–80.

Marshall v Curry [1933] 3 DLR 260.

McMillan, J.R. (2007). Mental illness and compulsory treatment. In R.E. Ashcroft, A. Dawson, H. Draper, and J.R. McMillan (eds.) *Principles of health care ethics* (2nd edn.) Chichester: John Wiley and Sons, pp. 443–48.

Mental Capacity Act 2005. London: The Stationery Office.

Mol, A. (2008). *The logic of care: Health and the problem of patient choice.* Abingdon: Routledge.

O'Neill, O. (2002). *Autonomy and trust in bioethics.* Cambridge: Cambridge University Press.

Okai, D., Owen, G., McGuire, H., Singh, S., Churchill, R., and Hotopf, M. (2007). Mental capacity in psychiatric patients. *British Journal of Psychiatry* 191: 291–97.

Rawls, J. (2005 [1971]). *A theory of justice.* Cambridge, MA: Harvard University Press.

Re F (mental patient: sterilisation) [1990] 2 AC 1.

Re S (adult: sterilisation) (2000) *The Times* 26 May (CA).

Chapter 9

Autonomy, value, and the first person

Hallvard Lillehammer

9.1 **Autonomy and the first person**

Considerations of autonomy normally play a different role in ethical thought depending on whether we take a first-person or an other-person perspective (by which for present purposes I include both a second-person and a third-person perspective) on practical reasoning (cf. Darwall 2006). For many of us and for much of the time, at least when things go well, autonomy is what I call 'reflectively transparent' from the first-person point of view. What I mean by this is that considerations of autonomy very often play no substantial role in the content of our practical reasoning, which when things go well is directly targeted at the pursuit of what we see as desirable outcomes. Thus, the thought that my efforts to settle on ends and to take means to those ends had better not be coercively interfered with by others does not normally play a part in my practical reasoning when I wonder what product on the shelf I should go for at Boots while shopping for toothpaste. Instead I focus directly on getting the best toothpaste, given what I take my needs and preferences to be. In so doing, I implicitly take my autonomy thus understood for granted. Similarly, the thought that I might not be a very good judge of what is best for me all things considered does not prevent me from making an effective decision when I choose between Colgate and Boots' own brand. Perhaps I read the information provided. Perhaps I ask the pharmacist for advice. But in the end I will normally assume that the stage is set for me to make a final decision based on my own judgement. The thought that in buying some toothpaste I am exercising my autonomy as a self-governing agent does not enter my practical reasoning in this context. I simply aim to get some decent toothpaste. Indeed, the introduction of explicit thoughts about the ethical significance of my autonomy would as likely as not be counterproductive, and in the worst case would short-circuit my attempt to get some decent and affordable toothpaste by leaving me flustered and uncertain, unable to make what is a comparatively simple and trivial decision.

This presumption of reflective transparency often disappears when we move to an other-person perspective on agency. It is a well-known fact that we constantly disagree about which options are best to take, even on matters as simple and trivial as buying toothpaste. Suppose, for example, that I am about to buy the most expensive toothpaste in the shop. In your view, there is no relevant difference between this tooth-paste and Boots' own brand, the latter being much cheaper and tasting much the same. It is simply a matter of branding. If so, thoughts about autonomy may enter your practical reasoning from a second-person perspective to the extent that although you may fairly try to convince me that I am wasting my money in buying the more expensive label, you will normally stop short of coercing me into not doing so. In this way, considerations of autonomy sometimes figure in the foreground of practical reasoning from an other-person perspective in a way they do not from a first-person perspective. To respect someone's autonomy in this sense is in part to respect their freedom to make a mistaken (or at least a suboptimal) decision. That is what you are granting me by not coercively interfering, and the thought of doing so is in no way para-doxical from your other-person perspective. From my first-person perspective, on the other hand, the idea that you are respecting my autonomy to make a mistaken (or suboptimal) decision will not nor-mally play any direct role in my deliberation there and then without appearing paradoxical. Unless I have either conferred on you the authority to decide for me or am being deliberately perverse, I will sim-ply choose what I judge to be (in some relevant sense) the best option. The fact that I may also, from some abstract or theoretical point of view, value the freedom to make my own mistakes no more under-mines my claim to be making a sensible decision in this individual case than the fact that some scientific authors apologize in advance for mistakes in their works thereby undermines their claim to believe every individual sentence put forward in those works.

When considerations of autonomy enter practical reasoning from the first-person perspective, this is often because the agent's own capacity to choose well is in question. First, someone might try to take my freedom over some decision away from me or prevent me from having it in the first place. Legal constraints work that way, as do various forms of personal and social oppression. It is natural for us to protest at restrictions on our freedom when we judge them unjustified, and it is natural to appeal to some conception of autonomy in doing so. Second, there are some options about which we may know that we are not good, or even competent, judges. Thus, there are products that, in virtue of their nature and use, I do not consider myself well placed to judge the value of. If I need a drug to cure a serious intestinal infection I will normally be willing to grant authority over its selection to a relevant health professional and will normally judge that I ought to do so.[1] Third, there are situations in which I may doubt whether I am a good judge about an arbitrarily wide range of questions relating to my own best interest. If I am going through a period when I am beset by constant panic attacks I may consider having the power of decision about a range of issues taken away from me and handed to another person. In doing so, I may actually be placing a high value on autonomy in some sense even as I hand over control of some aspect of my life to someone else. If I present myself voluntarily for extended psychiatric treatment, for example, I might be placing myself in this category. A more difficult case is where my capacity to choose well is put into question and I either mistakenly refuse to admit that my ability to choose well is seriously compromised, or where I refuse to hand over control of some aspect of my own life in spite of having previously judged correctly that my

---

[1] I may still, of course, expect my autonomy to be respected by having the pros and cons of different drugs explained to me and by not having any drug forcibly administered against my will.

ability to choose well is seriously compromised.[2] In such cases, it may be tempting to describe the situation as one in which considerations of autonomy either might, or ought to, have figured centrally in practical reasoning from the first-person perspective, but did not (or not in the right way). It may also be tempting to think that in such cases the absence of considerations of autonomy from the first-person perspective combined with the absence of a capacity to judge well implies that the normal considerations associated with autonomy as an ethically significant value are not in play: the only (or main) duty held by others towards me is to act in what is my best interest. In other words, for persons incapable of exercising their autonomy the question of respecting their autonomy need (or should) not arise.

This kind of scenario gives rise to a puzzle about our ethical relationship to mentally ill or other psychologically challenged individuals who are capable of forming, expressing, and acting on judgements about what is in their best interest, but who systematically fail to either judge well about their own self-interest or to successfully translate such judgements (well-founded or otherwise) into prudentially coherent plans or actions. On the one hand, such patients are sometimes described as incapable of judging, choosing, or acting autonomously to the point that even their personhood is put into question (cf. McMahan 1996; Kittay 2005). So it might seem permissible to act towards them in the way we judge to be their own best interest from an other-personal perspective without giving any thought to considerations of autonomy. On the other hand, such patients are human beings towards whom it is natural to think we owe a kind of respect that extends beyond the care we extend to other beings with a bare capacity for agency or sentience (Kittay 2005; Nussbaum 2009). So it might seem impermissible to treat them in whichever way we reasonably judge is in their own best interest regardless of how the situation appears to them from their own first-person perspective on practical reasoning. The first thought may seem to be an inescapable implication of the facts of the case. The second

---

[2] The first case may capture an aspect of my personality if am prone to exhibit certain forms of manic behaviour. The second case may capture an aspect of my personality if am suffering from some form of mental incapacity, such as advancing dementia.

thought may seem to be an inescapable part of any ethics that is distinctively human (cf. Williams 2006; Singer 2009). When combined, these two thoughts may reasonably be thought to be in serious tension. One aim of this paper is to get clearer about what this tension amounts to. A second aim is to expose one source of danger embodied in the move towards an other-personal perspective on agency in cases where things are not going well, namely the danger of losing sight of the fact that even individuals who suffer from mental illness or incapacity have a first-personal perspective on agency that can matter from an ethical point of view.

9.2 Two kinds of autonomy

The term 'autonomy' is used in a wide variety of ways. This fact is a cause of much disagreement and confusion. In this paper I make use of two distinctive interpretations of 'autonomy', each of which has had some currency in the philosophical and medical literature. I do not claim that these two interpretations are the only coherent interpretations of the term 'autonomy' in these contexts, or that other interpretations of the term either can or ought to be analysed in terms of these two. I believe the appropriate attitude to take towards the many different interpretations of 'autonomy' in medical ethics and elsewhere is one of pluralism. I shall not, however, defend this claim here (cf. Christman 1988; Arpaly 2003; Beauchamp 2005).

On my first interpretation, 'being autonomous' means not being subject to coercive interference. Autonomy thus understood is a state of someone (or something) being (negatively) free, or independent, with respect to a certain range of options. Thus, I can be autonomous in this sense with respect to whether or not to take up residence for tax purposes in Spain, England, or Norway, even if I am not free in the relevant sense to either take up residence for tax purposes somewhere or not to take up such residence at all. I shall henceforth refer to autonomy so understood as 'choice autonomy'. The idea of choice autonomy has played a central role in contemporary debates in medical ethics (cf. O'Neill 2002). Respect for choice autonomy is embodied in the idea that health professionals normally have a duty to acquire informed consent for medical procedures and treatment plans, that patients normally have a right to refuse treatment (even after having given informed consent), and that the normal relationship between carer and patient is one in which everyday interactions, such as taking meals or going to the toilet, are constrained by the need to respect the patient's wishes where this is practical. There has been much discussion among philosophers about what does, and what does not, qualify as coercive interference and voluntary choice (cf. Nozick 1997; Olsaretti 2004). I shall have nothing new to say about this here. Instead, I stipulate that, for present purposes, an agent has choice autonomy with respect to a given option *only if* the agent is faced with a non-empty set of (in the relevant circumstances) reasonable options between which to choose (cf. Raz 1986). I take this to exclude from the domain of choice autonomy subjection to medical treatment as a result of physical force, psychological manipulation, serious and credible threats, and the like.

One central question in the ethics of mental health is whether, and if so when, it is ever reasonable to deny someone choice autonomy in the sense just defined. Thus, it is sometimes argued that it is justifiable to subject human beings who suffer from severe mental illness or disability to coercive medical treatment in order to reduce the risk of harm to themselves or others, even if incurring the risk of such harm is not taken to licence the coercion of other persons in a normal (but often less than perfect) state of mental health or intellectual ability (cf. Wikler 1979; Scoccia 1990). Given a prior ethical commitment to respect choice autonomy, such a distinction between when it is, and when it is not, justified to subject someone to coercive medical treatment stands in need of explanation.

On my second interpretation, 'being autonomous' means being a self-governing agent. Autonomy so understood is a state of realizing a set of higher-order capacities of rational thought and agency, whereby practical options are reflectively endorsed and plans of action formulated or brought to execution (with or without the assistance of others). There is a wide range of conflicting accounts of what does, and what does not, qualify as genuine self-governance (cf. Frankfurt 1987; Dworkin 1988; Korsgaard 2009). I shall make no attempt to choose between these accounts here. Instead, I stipulate that any plausible account of autonomy in this sense will include the following four conditions as necessary for genuine self-governance. First, self-governance requires the actual manifestation of a capacity of higher order reflection and endorsement of practical options (where under 'practical option' I include the option to have one set of motivations rather than another and 'some, non-trivial' is meant to exclude a purely latent potentiality but not to require anything like a 'maximal' realization of this capacity). Second, self-governance requires the actual manifestation of a capacity for planning and executing actions that accord with practical options endorsed (where this is taken to imply a non-trivial degree of practical consistency and the formulation and execution of plans over time). Third, self-governance requires that an agent's reflection, endorsement, and execution of practical options are each responsive to minimally intelligible standards of rational argument (where this is taken to exclude extreme forms of irrationality but to include the scope for substantial disagreement about what does, or does not, count as good or bad reasons for and against a practical option). Fourth, self-governance requires reflection, endorsement, and execution of practical options that involve a conception of oneself as a single person living a certain kind of life (i.e. having a substantial self-conception), although the conception in question need not include in its scope one's entire life as a whole or be in any sense maximally unified (cf. Dworkin 1994). I shall henceforth refer to autonomy so understood as 'agent autonomy'.

One central question in the ethics of mental health is whether, and if so when, it is reasonable to appeal to agent autonomy when deciding how to respond to someone's expressed or assumed preferences. Thus, it might be asked whether the informed consent of a mentally ill, but legally competent, patient is ever sufficient to establish the ethical permissibility of treating them in the way consented to, given that the informed consent of a mentally ill patient may well conflict with the judgement they would make if they were (in some suitable sense) genuinely self-governing, and therefore agent autonomous.[3] Given a prior

---

[3] The current legal understanding of competence in the United Kingdom classifies a patient as having capacity or competence if they 1) can understand and retain information

commitment to respect agent autonomy, any decision to either include or exclude appeals to agent autonomy in treatment decisions where the patient is thought to not meet the conditions of agent autonomy stands in need of explanation.

The idea of agent autonomy is a core component of the liberal individualism defended in much contemporary moral and political philosophy. In particular, the idea of agent autonomy plays a central role in some very influential accounts of the individual as a potential duty holder, and thereby also a potential holder of the rights that correspond with such duties (cf. O'Neill 2000).[4] First, a genuinely self-governing individual is a paradigm candidate for being someone who has the capacity to make, be held to, or hold others to, ethically or legally binding promises or contracts the ethical significance of which they can themselves understand. Second, the self-governing individual is someone who has the capacity to form and execute their own reflectively endorsed life-plans, and to whom reasons are sometimes said to be 'owed' by others (whether individuals or institutions) to justify actions that interfere with or otherwise undermine those life-plans (cf. Scanlon 1998). Third, the self-governing individual is someone who has the capacity to make ethically significant requests or decisions about what should happen to them in conditions of extreme vulnerability, such as a demented state of life beyond reason (cf. Dworkin 1994). Fourth, the self-governing individual is the standard model of the liberal citizen, whose capacity for autonomous agency is often said to stand as a normative limit on the collective promotion of impartial and other social goods (cf. Rawls 1970). On this view, the self-governing individual is someone who has the capacity, and therefore the right, to participate in

---

relevant to the decision in question, 2) believes it, and can reflect on that information to arrive at a choice and use that information as part of the decision-making process, and 3) can express or otherwise communicate that choice (Alzheimer's Society 2010). It is widely agreed that many persons diagnosed with some form of mental illness can satisfy each of these criteria at the same time. For further discussion of the legal definition of mental incapacity, see Holroyd (Chapter 7, this volume).

[4] Some philosophers argue that the domain of right holders extends beyond the domain of duty holders, rights being identified with special justifications for imposing a certain duty (cf. Raz 1986). I return to the relevance of this debate below in my discussion of duties of care to non-autonomous agents.

an arbitrarily wide range of mutually beneficial but inherently risky cooperative practices, such as market exchanges or the democratic process. In these and other ways, some idea of autonomy as self-governance has played a central role in liberal explanations of the idea that there is a distinctive kind of respect that we owe to each other as persons, and that the rationale for this respect is intimately connected to our capacity for self conscious reflection and endorsement of ethically significant goals.

Choice autonomy is possible in the absence of agent autonomy. Some agents are incapable of agent autonomy but still make choices that may, or may not, be threatened by coercion. These include young children and some persons with severe mental health conditions, such as patients in a state of advanced dementia. Some non-human animals also arguably experience choice autonomy without agent autonomy, as when my dog decides to go for my carelessly placed lunch as opposed to some processed food from a tin (cf. McMahan 1996; Kittay 2005).

The complete absence of choice autonomy is incompatible with agent autonomy. An agent subjected to coercion in every imaginable respect would be unable to genuinely exercise any capacity for self-governance. Yet some degree of agent autonomy is compatible with absence of choice autonomy in a wide range of respects, at least some of which are beyond ethical criticism. Thus, coercive interference in attempts to cause serious harm to others may restrict your choice autonomy but are not normally thought to undermine your capacity for self-governance. To the extent that it does, we are prone to accept it, or even question whether such actions should really be counted as autonomous at all (cf. O'Neill 2002). To value agent autonomy does not mean to value it absolutely, or as a uniquely supreme value. Coercive interference with your choice of such various goods as hairstyle, hobbies, friends, career, or life-plan on the other hand, not only restrict your choice autonomy but are widely thought to undermine your capacity for self-governance. To the extent that it does, contemporary liberals are prone to condemn it. Failure to respect agent autonomy therefore stands in need of special justification. In the absence of such justification, any subversive interference with agent autonomy is expressive of an ethically undesirable form of disrespect towards the other as an independent locus of self-governance, authority and value.

It is natural to think that the notions of agent autonomy and choice autonomy stand in an asymmetrical justificatory relationship. One reason (perhaps the most important reason) one might think we should respect choice autonomy is that we should respect agent autonomy. This thought is clearly visible in contemporary justifications of advance directives for end-of-life medical treatment and in the controversial debate over how to respond to the wishes of severely demented persons (cf. Dworkin 1994). In each case, the underlying thought is that whether or not we are required to respect choice autonomy depends on whether or not in doing so we will also respect agent autonomy, where agent autonomy is understood in terms of some prior exercise of genuine self-governance, such as publicly expressing one's reflective, or critical, endorsement of a life-plan. It is therefore unsurprising that much theoretical attention has been paid, first, to the philosophical task of specifying the necessary and sufficient conditions for agent autonomy, and second, to the empirical task of establishing whether patients in some given medical condition (e.g. advanced dementia, severe personality disorder, etc.) in fact meet these conditions. If they do, there is a deep ethical justification in favour of respecting choice autonomy where this is at all practical. And if they do not, there is no such justification, in which case paternalistic intervention or other forms of coercion might in principle be justified, either by appeal to the patient's own interest or to the interests of others.

I do not wish to suggest that this is a worthless project. It is, however, a project that has the potential to create both ethical and conceptual confusion, and arguably continues to do so. I have two reasons for making this claim. The first is that some of the most controversial debates concerning our ethical relations to people with serious mental health conditions are premised, either implicitly or explicitly, on the assumption that these people do *not* meet all the standard conditions for agent autonomy. Thus, contemporary disagreements about the ethics of advanced dementia and severe personality disorder, for example, are not always focused on whether or not patients who suffer from these conditions are capable of genuine self-governance. On the contrary, it is often assumed that they are not; one question being how to then evaluate their choice autonomy, and whether we should think of choice autonomy as generating substantial constraints on the treatment of such patients in the absence of some appeal to a prior, future or potential capacity for, or exercise of, self-governance. No real progress is made on this question by giving an account of the conditions for agent autonomy and then showing that the patients in question fail to meet them.

Second, the claim that the notions of agent autonomy and choice autonomy stand in an asymmetrical justificatory relationship does not entail that the value of respecting agent autonomy is the only justification there could be for why we should respect choice autonomy. There is a plurality of reasons why we might want to respect the choice autonomy of someone who is not agent autonomous, some of which essentially involve the idea of agent autonomy and some of which do not (cf. Kittay 2005; Nussbaum 2009). Here I shall mention eight (the list is not exhaustive). First, you might want to respect the choice autonomy of someone because you believe that by doing so you will help them to become agent autonomous. Some people may adopt this attitude toward their children or people with curable mental health conditions. Second, you might want to respect the choice autonomy of someone because you believe that by doing so you will arrest or delay their progressive loss of agent autonomy. Some people may adopt this attitude toward people with advancing dementia. Third, you may want to respect the choice autonomy of someone because you believe that doing so is expressive of respect for the person they once were (and to a decreasing, but not negligible, extent still are). This is a potentially more problematic example, but any satisfactory account of our ethical relationship to ageing and death needs to have something to say about it. Fourth, you might want to respect the choice autonomy of someone because you believe that not doing so would be unpleasant or frustrating for them. This thought is arguably independent of ideas about agent autonomy. Yet it can be shown to play a central part in discussions of mental health where the values of agent autonomy and choice autonomy are believed to conflict, including cases of patients with reduced mental capacities who express preferences that conflict with prior agent autonomous requests, such as an advanced directive.[5] Fifth, you may want to respect the choice autonomy of someone because you believe that it is in their best interest to be given the freedom to choose, either in this case or in general. This is perhaps the most obvious and uncontroversial way in which respect for choice autonomy can be justified without appealing to agent autonomy. Sixth, you may want to respect the choice autonomy of someone because you believe that doing so is in the general interest, where this includes the interests of anyone else likely to be affected by the decision in question. Thus, it might be thought that drawing a sharp line around agent autonomy as a source of constraints against coercive interference with individual choice may have detrimental effects on respect for persons in general, leading to unacceptable forms of stigmatization, repression or violations of basic legal rights.[6] Seventh, you may want to respect the choice autonomy of someone because they manifest a number, but not all, of the standard features associated with agent autonomy. Some of these features will be intrinsic to the person so respected, such as having or expressing a recognizable outlook on their existence, however unstable or fragmentary. Other features will be extrinsic to the person so respected, such as being someone with whom one stands in an intimate, or otherwise special, relationship of familiarity or dependence. Eighth, you may want to respect someone's choice autonomy because he or she is another human being. Once more, this may come down to the possession of intrinsic characteristics by the person in question, such as

---

[5] The conditions for enforcing an advanced directive in the UK include the qualifications that no advance directive can be used to 1) refuse basic nursing care essential to keep a person comfortable, such as washing, bathing and mouth care; 2) refuse the offer of food or drink by mouth; 3) refuse the use of measures solely designed to maintain comfort, such as painkillers, 4) demand treatment that a healthcare team considers inappropriate, 5) ask for anything that is against the law, such as euthanasia or assisted suicide (Alzheimer's Society 2010).

[6] In this context it is worth mentioning that at some times and places (including some places in the present) the standard treatment of people with serious mental health conditions has been worse than the treatment of many animals (cf. Foucault 1989).

human sentience or human form. Yet it may also be a question of extrinsic characteristics, including the relations in which they either stand or have stood to other human beings. Such forms of respect should not necessarily be thought of as respect for a second-rate form of agent autonomy. We may have deep reasons to value the relevant features of the agency of another human being that do not boil down to our valuing them as potential or second-rate manifestations of self-governance in the standard sense invoked in liberal moral and political philosophy. A human being whose mental capacities does not fully meet all the criteria of genuine self-governance need not be thought of as a second-rate person any more than a traffic warden need be thought of as a second-rate policeman or a European Union citizen claiming residential rights in the UK need be thought of as a second-rate Brit. The categories of agency we value as giving rise to ethically significant limitations on our treatment of others come in a cluster, not in a pair. They involve both intrinsic and extrinsic features of the agents in question. Their presence or otherwise are hardly, if ever, an all-or-nothing thing. They are also highly context sensitive. Thus, the virtues involved in caring for a friend or a family member are unlikely to be exactly the same as the virtues involved in creating and operating public institutions designed to care for any patient meeting a certain diagnostic description. To think that the only feature of a human being that could justify respect for their choice autonomy is that of their agent autonomy is therefore both an overly simplistic and a potentially dangerous idea.

Agent autonomy and choice autonomy are two related, but separable, factors of ethical significance for our treatment of other human beings. One of the most important reasons for respecting choice autonomy is that in doing so we will often also be respecting agent autonomy. Yet respect for agent autonomy is not the only justification for respecting choice autonomy. It follows that we can have good reasons for respecting someone's choice autonomy even if they do not meet the conditions of genuine self-governance that are necessary for agent autonomy. This conclusion has potentially significant consequences for the ethics of mental health, including our attitudes towards people with mental disabilities and patients who suffer from advancing stages of dementia.

9.3 **Autonomy as a value**

Considerations of autonomy are sometimes thought to be in potential conflict with considerations relating to what is in someone's best interest. This conflict is sometimes phrased in terms of how autonomy relates to value or the promotion of desirable outcomes, whether the desirable outcomes in question are conceived of as broadly ethical or more narrowly prudential. In fact, there is a plurality of ways in which considerations of autonomy can be coherently related to considerations of value or the promotion of desirable outcomes. Here I shall mention three.

First, autonomy is sometimes thought of as a conducive to the promotion of value or desirable outcomes (cf. Keown 2002). There are at least two ways in which autonomy can be thought of as valuable in this way (the two are not mutually exclusive (cf. Dworkin 1994)). First, it is sometimes argued that agents themselves are generally better placed to know what it is valuable for them to pursue, especially regarding what is in their own best interest. Preventing an agent's unconstrained pursuit of what they regard as being in their own best interest is therefore likely to be epistemologically counterproductive. Second, it is sometimes argued that agents themselves are generally better placed to successfully promote desirable outcomes, especially regarding what is in their own best interest. Preventing an agent's unconstrained pursuit of what they regard as being in their own best interest is therefore likely to be pragmatically counterproductive. In each case autonomy is valued as a means to the promotion of some desirable outcome, such as the agent's well-being. The issue of whether to respect someone's autonomy so valued then comes down to such questions as whether or not the agent in question is, in fact, better placed to know what is in his or her own best interest and/or whether or not the agent is, in fact, better placed to act in his or her own best interest. These claims are highly sensitive to context. Thus, it might be argued that with respect to some agents, such as patients suffering from severe mental disorders, paternalistic intervention is a more reliable mechanism for the promotion of the relevant desirable outcomes. If so, in these cases appeals to the value of autonomy do not gain support from appeals to the conduciveness of autonomy to the promotion of desirable outcomes.

The claim that autonomy is conducive to the promotion of desirable outcomes can be understood as invoking both agent and choice autonomy. An agent's exercise of self-governance can be thought of as conducive to the promotion of desirable outcomes for at least three reasons. First, an agent's reflective endorsement of a practical option is often evidential of that option being valuable, such as when someone decides upon reflection that participating in a dangerous sport either is, or is not, for them. Second, reflective endorsement sometimes implies that the option so endorsed is valuable. Arguably, some things in life are good for you at least in part because you reflectively endorse them. Third, being substantially self-governing entails a capacity for carrying one's reflectively endorsed plans out in practice, thereby enhancing the probability of realizing the desirable outcomes in question. When autonomy is valued as conducive to value in any of these three ways, it is therefore often the idea of agent autonomy that is the focal point of evaluation, choice autonomy being valued as a necessary condition for agent autonomy. The basic ability to act without coercive interference is at best contingently related to the promotion of desirable outcomes, being equally compatible with actions that frustrate the promotion of valuable states of affairs as with actions that realize them. It does not follow, however, that the only way for choice autonomy to be valuable as conducive to the promotion of desirable outcomes is as a necessary condition for agent autonomy. As I argued in the previous section, respect for choice autonomy can be valuable for reasons unrelated to agent autonomy, such as avoidance of pain and frustration that would reduce the agent's overall well-being. It might be tempting to think that autonomy being conducive to the promotion of desirable outcomes is inevitably a matter of agent autonomy being so conducive if we focus exclusively on the epistemological aspect of autonomy being conducive to desirable outcomes. This temptation ought to disappear once we remember that something can be conducive to the promotion of desirable outcomes without being epistemologically so conducive.

Second, autonomy is sometimes thought of as itself valuable as an end, and not merely as a means to the promotion of desirable outcomes.

Thus understood, it is natural to think that agent autonomy is valuable to a very high degree. On at least one influential conception of the self-governing individual as a primary holder of rights and duties, the failure to respect agent autonomy is the failure of treating someone with the basic respect they merit in virtue of being a locus of continuous and self-conscious rational agency (cf. Dworkin 1994). Thus understood, respect for agent autonomy is likely to be assigned a fundamental place in any broadly liberal conception of medical ethics. Yet choice autonomy can also be valued for its own sake. The fact of coercion is itself often a negative feature of action considered from the first-personal point of view. Thus, it is perfectly coherent to think that the basic ability to choose between available options is preferable to coercion, even for beings, such as some non-human animals, that have no capacity for agent autonomy. Yet the value of agent autonomy is often thought of as trumping the value of choice autonomy where the two conflict, as in the famous case of Ulysses and the Sirens (cf. Elster 1984). Faced with lethal temptation, Ulysses is willing to trade his choice autonomy for a limited period in order to protect his continued agent autonomy in the long run. More difficult cases arise where a capacity for choice autonomy is present but a capacity for agent autonomy is not. Such cases include the treatment of patients with severe mental incapacities, such as advanced dementia. In these cases, it is more controversial to what extent a prior exercise of agent autonomy (including the endorsement of practical options involving a future self who will not be agent autonomous) can reasonably be thought to trump a current exercise of choice autonomy (cf. Shiffrin 2004). We can only hope to get clear about such cases if we consider the fact, mentioned in the previous section, that the features associated with agent autonomy come in clusters, have both first-personal and third-personal aspects, and are not always present or absent as an all-or-nothing thing (cf. Heal Chapter 1, this volume). Thus, you may want to respect the choice autonomy of someone because they manifest some, but not all, the features associated with agent autonomy. Furthermore, in doing so you may not be interested in these features exclusively, or even primarily, to the extent that they serve as markers for an ideal, but imperfectly realized, condition of autonomous agency. In doing so, your aim can be to respect someone else as exactly the kind of agent they actually are.

To assign agent autonomy or choice autonomy intrinsic value as ends opens up the question of how to compare such autonomy with other values, including personal well-being or impartial goods. Choice autonomy certainly, and agent autonomy probably, is not guaranteed to be the most important value in every situation where it conflicts with other values of these kinds. Furthermore, if the ethical significance of autonomy in either sense were exhausted by its role as a value understood thus far, it should be legitimate to think of this value in broadly consequentialist terms. On broadly consequentialist terms, the value of autonomy belongs on a scale of goods to be valued along with other ethically significant goods. Thus, it must always be legitimate in principle to override autonomy in one case in order, for example, to respect more autonomy overall. Perhaps there is no principled obstacle to taking this consequentialist approach to choice autonomy. Yet for agent autonomy, considered as the primary locus of certain rights and duties, this consequentialist model arguably fails to do full justice to the idea that respect for an individual's capacity for self-governance ought to constrain our treatment of them in promotion of either their own or impartial goods (cf. Scheffler 1988). This fact suggests that thinking of autonomy as either an instrumental or an intrinsic value in the sense discussed so far fails to capture the full ethical significance of considerations of autonomy, not only in the context of mental health, but also in the context of ethical and political philosophy more generally.

Third, autonomy is sometimes thought of it as a (deontological) constraint on the promotion of desirable outcomes (cf. Nozick 1974). When thought of in this way, autonomy is not one further value to be weighed on a scale of goods, but instead an independent prohibition on, or obstacle to, taking certain means to promote otherwise desirable outcomes. As conceived by contemporary liberals, rights are paradigmatic candidates for the status of constraints in this sense. Thus, an individual's right to physical integrity is said to prohibit the taking of certain means to promote desirable outcomes, including the prevention of harm to that very individual. Hence the widely legislated duty to seek informed consent for invasive medical procedures. Yet constraints need not be absolute. Thus, an individual's right to physical integrity can be trumped by considerations of value in special circumstances, such as when the individual is a lethal threat to himself or others, and/ or is unable to control or otherwise exercise the relevant rights. Hence the widely legislated freedom to perform certain invasive procedures on patients whose lives are at risk and/or unable to consent. The presence of a constraint creates a special demand for ethical justification, yet not one that is obviously reducible to a matter of weighing values against each other on a scale of goods.[7]

Given the close association between the idea of a constraint and the idea of a right it is natural to think that the distinctive ethical significance of autonomy is partly to be explained in terms of the existence of constraints against the imposition of the will of some person(s) on that of another. In particular, it is natural to think that respect for agent autonomy imposes a substantial constraint that prohibits action to promote desirable outcomes where such action conflicts with the exercise of genuine self-governance. To think of agent autonomy in this way is to understand the constraints it generates as an important part of what we mean by saying that there is a special kind of respect that we owe to persons as self-governing rational agents, a respect we arguably fail to show if we are always prepared to put autonomy on a scale of goods along with other values. It is much less plausible to think of choice autonomy as a substantial constraint in this sense, except where it functions as a necessary condition of respecting agent autonomy. Absence of coercion as such may be a genuinely desirable thing in itself, but considered in isolation from the content of the options at stake, the effects of its exercise on the interests of those affected, or its embedding in a psychological profile of a being that exhibits a set of features that we can see as meriting a distinctive form of respect, the appeal to choice autonomy itself is arguably too thin a basis on which to ground the kinds of constraints we normally associate with the rights and duties

----

[7] The presence of a constraint can be thought to involve a lexical ordering (where no amount of some particular value can ever trump a certain constraint) or the imposition of some significant threshold (where no amount of a particular value is taken to weigh against a constraint up to a certain point of seriousness). For further discussion, see Scheffler (1988).

that are thought to characterize the more sophisticated ethical relationships we value as holding between paradigmatically moral persons (cf. O'Neill 2002).

Given my remarks in the previous section, however, the significance of this point should not be exaggerated. Its connection with agent autonomy is not the only thing that could explain the imposition of constraints against the infringement of choice autonomy. Having their autonomy of choice frustrated can have seriously negative effects on someone's well-being and thereby frustrate interests that are sufficiently important to justify the imposition of duties on others to protect them. Thus understood, a constraint to respect choice autonomy would be associated with a species of individual rights that do not presuppose that the subject of those rights can also be a duty holder and thereby capable of genuine self-governance (cf. Raz 1986). If so, there can be constraints against the infringement of choice autonomy even where agent autonomy is absent, such as in the case of patients with various kinds of mental illness and incapacity. Thus, it could be detrimental to the well-being of a severely demented patient to frustrate their preferences among a wide range of options, including some options between treatments or available medical procedures. According to the conception of choice autonomy just outlined, this would then count against pursuing a course of action running contrary to those preferences, even where that course of action is favoured by a previous, and agent autonomous, advance directive. To what extent, if ever, considerations of choice autonomy should trump considerations of agent autonomy would then come down to a question about the conflict between two different kinds of right, namely those that derive from our nature as self-governing agents on the one hand, and those that derive from our nature as agents with distinctive and ethically significant perspective on the world on the other. Given the aforementioned asymmetry in justification between agent autonomy and choice autonomy it may be tempting to think that any rights derived from the former source will necessarily trump rights derived from the latter. As it happens, I think this view is too simple. I shall not, however, argue for this claim here (cf. Dresser 1995; Shiffrin 2004).

Autonomy can be coherently thought of as an instrumental value, an intrinsic value, and also as a constraint on the promotion of value. On each model, agent autonomy is an uncontroversial source of ethical significance. Choice autonomy is ethically significant in the first two ways. And although its intrinsic ethical significance may not suffice to generate substantial constraints on promotion of value considered on its own, it is also possible to think that there can be genuine constraints on infringing choice autonomy, some of which are grounded independently of the fact that choice autonomy is a necessary condition for agent autonomy. We should therefore not think that choice autonomy is in principle unsuited to justify genuine constraints on ethically permissible action wherever agent autonomy is absent, as in the case of some persons who suffer from serious mental disorder or incapacity.

9.4 **Concluding remarks**

I have shown how considerations of autonomy normally play different roles in ethical thought from a first-person as opposed to an other-person perspective on practical reasoning. I have also shown that considerations of autonomy can be usefully distinguished into some that focus on a person's capacity for substantially self-governing agency and others that focus on an intellectually less demanding notion of voluntary choice or action. Finally, I have distinguished between three different ways of thinking about autonomy as a value, namely as a means to the promotion of desirable outcomes, as a desirable outcome in itself, and as a constraint on the promotion of desirable outcomes. I have argued that when these different aspects of claims about autonomy are kept distinct there is conceptual space for a view according to which we can reasonably consider ourselves to be under a duty to respect the autonomy of a person who does not have the capacities we normally associate with substantial, or genuine, self-governance.

Acknowledgements

I am grateful to Lubomira Radoilska and the participants in her Cambridge seminars on autonomy and mental health, as well as to the audience of the January 2010 CRASSH conference on the same topic, for observations that have aided me during the writing of this paper. I am also grateful to Ben Colburn and Gemma Mitchell for many informative discussions in the context of their own work on the nature and value of autonomy.

References

Alzheimer's Society. (2010). Factsheet on Advance Directives. [Online] http://www.alzheimers.org.uk/factsheet/463 (accessed 21 August 2010).

Arpaly, N. (2003). *Unprincipled Virtue*. Oxford: Oxford University Press.

Beauchamp, T.L. (2005). Who deserves autonomy, and whose autonomy deserves respect? In J. Stacey Taylor (ed.) *Personal Autonomy: New Essays on Personal Autonomy and Its Role in Contemporary Moral Philosophy*. Cambridge: Cambridge University Press, pp. 310–25.

Christman, J. (1988). Constructing the inner citadel: Recent work on autonomy. *Ethics* 99: 109–24.

Darwall, S. (2006). *The Second Person Standpoint: Morality, Respect & Accountability*. Cambridge, MA: Harvard University Press.

Dresser, R. (1995). Dworkin on dementia. *Hastings Center Report* 25: 32–38.

Dworkin, G. (1988). *The Theory and Practice of Autonomy*. Cambridge: Cambridge University Press.

Dworkin, R. (1994). *Life's Dominion*. New York: Vintage.

Elster, J. (1984). *Ulysses and the Sirens*. Cambridge: Cambridge University Press.

Foucault, M. (1989). *Madness and Civilization*. London: Routledge.

Frankfurt, H. (1987). *The Importance of What We Care About*. Cambridge: Cambridge University Press.

Keown, J. (2002). *Euthanasia, Ethics and Public Policy*. Cambridge: Cambridge University Press.

Kittay, E. (2005). At the margins of moral personhood. *Ethics* 116: 100–31.

Korsgaard, C. (2009). *Self-Constitution*. Oxford: Oxford University Press.

McMahan, J. (1996). Cognitive disability, misfortune and justice. *Philosophy and Public Affairs* 25: 3–35.

Nozick, R. (1974). *Anarchy, State and Utopia*. Oxford: Basil Blackwell.

Nozick, R. (1997). *Socratic Puzzles*. Cambridge, MA: Harvard University Press.

Nussbaum, M. (2009). The capabilities of people with cognitive disabilities. *Metaphilosophy* 40: 331–51.

Olsaretti, S. (2004). *Liberty, Desert and the Market*. Cambridge: Cambridge University Press.

O'Neill, O. (2000). *Bounds of Justice*. Cambridge: Cambridge University Press.

O'Neill, O. (2002). *Autonomy and Trust in Bioethics*. Cambridge: Cambridge University Press.

Rawls, J. (1970). *A Theory of Justice*. Cambridge, MA: Harvard University Press.

Raz, J. (1986). *The Morality of Freedom*. Oxford: Oxford University Press.

Scanlon, T.M. (1998). *What We Owe to Each Other*. Cambridge, MA: Harvard University Press.

Scheffler, S. (ed.) (1988). *Consequentialism and Its Critics*. Oxford: Oxford University Press.

Scoccia, D. (1990). Paternalism and respect for autonomy. *Ethics* 100: 318–34.

Shiffrin, S.V. (2004). Autonomy, beneficience, and the permanently demented. In J. Burley (ed.) *Dworkin and His Critics*. Oxford: Blackwell, pp. 195–217.

Singer, P. (2009). Speciesism and moral status. *Metaphilosophy* 40: 567–81.

Waldron, J. (ed.) (1984). *Theories of Rights*. Oxford: Oxford University Press.

Wikler, D. (1979). Paternalism and the mildly retarded. *Philosophy and Public Affairs* 8: 377–92.

Williams, B. (2006). The human prejudice. In A.W. Moore (ed.) *Philosophy as a Humanistic Discipline*. Princeton, NJ: Princeton University Press, pp. 135–52.

Part IV

Emerging alternatives

Chapter 10

Autonomy, dialogue, and practical rationality

Guy A.M. Widdershoven and
Tineke A. Abma

10.1 Introduction

In healthcare ethics, autonomy is often conceptualized as self-determination. A person is autonomous if he can make his own decisions regarding treatment and care. Autonomy can be limited because of external or internal factors. A crucial external factor is the attitude of healthcare providers. If a provider takes over the decision (acts paternalistically), autonomy is compromised (this may be for good reasons, but nevertheless). An internal factor hindering autonomy may be a lack of decision-making capacity in the patient. If the patient is unable to express a decision (either directly or, for instance, through an advance directive), there is no room for self-determination. If the patient is unable to base the decision on adequate information and reasoning, self-determination is problematic, since decisions are not well founded. If a patient would decide between treatment options through throwing a dice, this would not be regarded as an autonomous decision, unless the options would be in all aspects equivalent, and leaving it up to chance would therefore be a reasonable way to come to a conclusion.

In this chapter, we will propose an alternative approach to autonomy, focusing not on self-determination, but on moral development as dialogical and practical learning. From this perspective, a person is autonomous if he knows the right thing to do in his situation. We will argue that this does not require freedom from external interference, but support from others who may help the person to find out what is right for him through dialogue and deliberation. If a healthcare provider questions the views of the patient, this does not necessarily imply that autonomy is compromised. By urging the patient to reflect on his values, a healthcare provider may help the patient to develop a new and better understanding of his situation and a more adequate way of dealing with it. This alternative view on autonomy entails a different conceptualization of capacity. The focus is not on the ability of making individual decisions, but on the ability of finding ways of practically dealing with one's situation. A person who is unable to express a decision may be able to know what is good in a practical way; on the other hand, a person who is able to express what he wants to be done, does not necessarily know how to handle his situation. If capacity is regarded as being able to manage one's situation, the emphasis is not on understanding information and being able to reason, but on insight, or practical rationality (phronesis). A person does not have to be able to reason about options in a logically coherent way, but should be able to know the right way to live in the specific situation and to realize this in practice.

We will elucidate the importance of dialogue and practical rationality with an example from forensic psychiatry. In this setting, patients are not free to refuse treatment. Yet, they do have some choices. How can professionals respect patient autonomy in this situation? From the perspective of autonomy as self-determination, one should leave decisions to the person himself, unless this would lead to danger for the person or for others involved. From the perspective of autonomy as moral development, one should support the person in giving meaning to his life and handling his situation. This implies that one does not take the wishes and decisions of the person for granted as expressions of autonomy, but sees them as a starting point for a joint process of deliberation and practical experimentation, aimed at developing autonomy in daily life.

Case

David (pseudonym) is a man in his early fifties. After a sex offence 10 years ago, he was sentenced to treatment in forensic psychiatry. This included cognitive behavioural therapy, which made him realize that he is obsessed with sex. He wanted to get rid of the obsession, in order to have room for other concerns, such as friendship and work. In concert with his therapist, he agreed to testosterone-lowering medication.

This allowed him to leave the forensic clinic after a few years and to live a normal life, with a house, a job, and friends. He remains under outpatient supervision. Every month he has to come back to the clinic for an injection. At the place where he works, a contact person, who knows his history, keeps an eye on him and reports to the clinic. Since he is on medication, he is no longer constantly preoccupied with sex and can relax and, for instance, read a book. With women he is able to show his softer side.

David is positive about using the medication. He is now able to control himself and lead a normal life. Without the medication he would still be trapped in his obsession. Yet he also expresses negative experiences. The medication has significant side effects. He gained 20 pounds in 6 months. He can no longer take pride in his bodily appearance. The treatment resulted in breast growth, therefore his mammary glands were surgically removed. His genitals have shrunk. When he looks in the mirror, he no longer recognizes himself. A sexual relationship is no longer possible, he says. He feels he cannot present himself to a woman in his present condition. Moreover, the medication resulted in reduction of his muscles and brings a risk of osteoporosis. He thinks in the end he will become ill. 'I have a time bomb in my body', he says.

Did David decide for the treatment himself? This question is not easy for him to answer. He knows he needs the medication to control himself. He does not want to become obsessed with sex again, and therefore embraces the medication. The choice is in this sense clearly his own. At the same time he experiences a lot of pressure from the environment. He says, 'When you have to choose between medication and life imprisonment, who would go for the latter?'. He also experiences changes in society. When he was admitted to the forensic clinic, leave was still relatively easy to get; nowadays it is becoming increasingly difficult. It seems that medication has become a precondition for leave, even when it is not medically indicated, because testosterone levels are normal.

10.2 Two approaches to autonomy

In ethics, autonomy is often identified with self-ownership and self-determination. Somebody is autonomous when he or she can decide for himself what happens. Following John Stuart Mill (1859), autonomy as self-ownership describes the freedom of the individual to shape his own life unhindered by others. His renowned principle of liberty holds that an individual is sovereign in directing his own life, as long as his actions do not hurt others. Notable authors in the field of healthcare ethics have emphasized that respect for autonomy means that the healthcare professional should avoid meddling in the decision-making of the patient (Beauchamp and Childress 2008). When a patient makes an unwise decision, one should not intervene unless his safety or that of others is in jeopardy.

Non-intervention is stressed in this view of autonomy. The individual is to rule about his own life without interference from others. This implies a notion of negative freedom, meaning that the person is free from external influence or pressure. Negative freedom can be distinguished from positive freedom (Berlin 1969). The concept of positive freedom refers to a person's ability to be the source of his own decisions and to lead his life in accordance with his own value-commitments, goals, and plans. In the notion of positive freedom, the content of choices is taken into account. From this perspective, one does not have to respect every choice. A choice that is in accordance with the life-plan of the individual has greater importance than a choice based on a random impulse (Dworkin 1988). The ethical value of the continuation of one's life path and personal history can also be found in the work of Ricoeur (1992). People become incredible, untrustworthy, and irresponsible when they step outside their life history, and cannot keep up the promises they made to others and to themselves. When someone makes a choice he otherwise would regret, the choice is not an expression of what the person truly values in his or her life. Preventing the person to act according to this choice is not an obstruction of autonomy, but can be seen as helping the person to (re)gain autonomy.

Care ethicists hold on to the notion of autonomy as positive freedom (Verkerk 2001). They stress that autonomy is not the same as deciding without interference. Autonomy can only be developed in relationships with others, so in states of dependence. Hence care ethicists speak of relational autonomy (MacKenzie and Stoljar 2000). From a care perspective, people require support to gain insight into what is important in their lives and how to arrange their lives accordingly (Oeseburg and Abma 2006). Care professionals should help patients (or refer them to others who can help) to discover better ways to take part in society and live a meaningful life. This implies an active search for pursuits that fit with personal wishes and abilities and foster participation. Care professionals should help patients not to enter situations which may tempt them to do things they will regret later. They may arrange support and supervision to help patients to remain on track. Care professionals can check whether clients have kept their promises, and if not, why not, and try to improve the situation accordingly. In this way care professionals help to empower patients.

According to Agich (1993), individuals are never fully formed but they are part of a dynamic process of development, in interaction with their environment. Only for a person who lacks identity, freedom equals absolute independence. Dependency does not impair a person's freedom as long as that person can develop and mature. The same holds true for the mutual influence that care professionals and patients have on each other. According to Agich, it is more important to help patients to live with their vulnerabilities and to accept their limitations than to offer them freedom of choice (Agich 1993). This implies that it is more important to guard people against temptations, then to let them do whatever they want.

These two approaches to autonomy can be seen in the story of David. Placement in forensic psychiatry is experienced by David as an obstacle to his freedom. He is forced to undergo therapy. His autonomy as negative freedom is curtailed. This has a good reason: he is dangerous to others and should not be allowed to walk loose and be a risk to women. Although the forensic placement sets limits to his freedom to do what he likes, it also helps him to develop a new view of what is important in life. He learns to see that his behaviour was self-centred and lacked concern for other people. He becomes aware that sexual gratification is not the only relevant thing in life. He learns to see that he has obligations towards others and towards himself. This can be interpreted as a growth of positive freedom. Rather than being driven by impulses, David develops a life-plan in which he aims to realize values such as friendship and work. David says he has changed in a positive way, and had become more considerate and responsible.

Interestingly, therapy makes him realize that autonomy as negative freedom is one-sided. His former life was entirely dedicated to being independent and doing what he liked. He went after women only for his own gratification. Sexual pleasure was all that mattered to him. Paradoxically, his problems began when he was abandoned by his wife because he had an affair with another woman. Instead of feeling free, he felt frustrated because he could not see his child anymore.

This frustration made him angry towards other women, which ultimately led to the sexual offence for which he was sentenced. Through behavioural therapy and active help of others, he realizes that he must learn to control his sexuality so that he will not commit acts for which he is ashamed later. He realizes that there are other goals in life than immediate gratification. Thus, he comes to see the relevance of positive freedom, of living one's life according to the values which one endorses.

One might object that David's decision to agree with the proposal of the psychiatrist to try medication is, in the end, an instance of negative freedom. He has the choice between a possible discharge from the forensic clinic with medication, and staying in the clinic without it. In the first case, he will be free, but he will have to endure the side effects of treatment; in the second case he will not regain freedom to live in society, but his body will be free from the side effects. Since David is allowed to make this choice, the forensic situation is different from the situation in countries without any rights for people who have committed crimes. Although this is certainly relevant from a sociopolitical point of view, David does not seem to experience this as a free choice. The second alternative is so grave that he feels forced to choose for the first one. More significantly, David does not choose because, after considering the consequences of both options, he has concluded that he prefers one of them. He is aware that he needs the medication to become the person he wants to be, even if this comes at great costs. Thus, his choice is motivated in a positive way by his value-commitments.

Another objection would be that David is not really free, because he has taken over and internalized the view of the good life presented to him by the psychiatrist (acting as representative of society). The notion of positive freedom is problematic because people are induced to behave according to given sociopolitical ideas. We actually need the notion of negative freedom to protect us against instances of unfreedom resulting from the ideal of positive freedom. This is actually the way in which the distinction between the two concepts of freedom is elaborated by Berlin. He warns against the idea of positive freedom, because it can easily be misused to force people to accept views of others. Is this objection relevant in the case of David? The therapeutic alliance certainly aims to make him reconsider his views. The idea is to confront him with the consequences of his behaviour and make him aware of other, better options. These confronting conversations do have an element of interference. David is urged to reflect and to come to a new view of himself. Yet, he does not simply take over the views of the therapist or those of society at large. He investigates both his own views and those of others, and comes to a new position through a process of reflection and gaining insight. From a hermeneutic perspective, one may say that he develops his own views by entering into a dialogue with other views. This process is not totally under one's own control, since the other views are challenging and disturbing. Yet, taking over other views through reflection implies a critical appraisal. According to Gadamer, the antithesis between reason (making up one's own mind) and tradition (taking over given views and ideas) is wrong. Gadamer explains this as follows: 'Even the most genuine tradition does not persist because of the inertia of what once existed. It needs to be affirmed, embraced, cultivated (. . .) Preservation is an act of reason, though an inconspicuous one' (Gadamer 1960, p. 265). David affirms social values such as consideration and responsibility, not because he is induced to do so, but because he deems them relevant for his own life after critical examination. He considers himself freer than before, because he is able to manage his life and relate to others.

We conclude that David gained autonomy during the therapeutic process in the forensic clinic. He has developed a view on who he wants to be and what he owes to others, taking into account his limitations and sociopolitical restrictions. This process is the result of external influences and even pressure. Yet, David embraces the new view, identifies with it, and regards it as part of his own identity. Although David affirms his new role and responsibilities, he is ambivalent about the resulting changes in his body and appearance. He seems not to be able to adjust his life to the felt loss of male identity. His autonomy as a moral agent is not matched by autonomy as an embodied person. He misses views of male identity which can serve as a vehicle for learning, and seems to remain captured in the tradition of male sexuality which was part of his former life. The psychiatric treatment addressed his moral identity and responsibility, but not his bodily identity. A further step in becoming autonomous seems to require a process of reflection on and investigation of new views on embodiment and sexuality.

10.3 **Autonomy and dialogue**

In an interesting paper, Emanuel and Emanuel (1992) distinguish four models of the physician–patient relationship. The first is the paternalistic model. The doctor decides, acting in the best interest of the patient. In this model the doctor is the guardian of the patient. The second model is the informative, or consumer model. It is based upon autonomous choice of the patient, after being informed by the doctor. The values of the patient are considered to be given. In this model the doctor is the technical expert. The third model is the interpretive model. It aims at interpreting the patient's values and implementing the patient's selected intervention. The values of the patient are seen as inchoate and conflicting, and in need of interpretation. In this model the doctor is a counsellor or adviser. The fourth model is the deliberative model. It is based upon the presupposition that the patient's values are not only in need of interpretation, but also of discussion and deliberation. The doctor is regarded as a friend or teacher.

Emanuel and Emanuel show that the four models entail distinct views on patient autonomy. In the first model, patient autonomy is not an issue. The patient does not play a role in deciding what to do. A sensible patient agrees with and follows the physician's decisions. This entails neither negative nor positive freedom, since the patient is not regarded as a person who acts and decides for himself. In the second model, autonomy is seen as self-determination. This model focuses on negative freedom. In the third model, the emphasis is on finding out the true values of the patient. This means that the patient is supported in determining what he wants. This implies aspects of positive freedom. The physician does not simply follow the patient's wishes, but helps the patient to find out what he wishes and choose what is important for him. The fourth model regards patient autonomy as self-development: 'The conception of patient autonomy is moral self-development; the patient is empowered not simply to follow unexamined preferences or examined values, but to consider, through dialogue, alternative health-related values, their worthiness and their implications for treatment' (Emanuel and Emanuel 1992 p. 2222).

The role of dialogue in autonomy can be elaborated further with the help of the hermeneutic philosophy of Gadamer (1960). According to Gadamer, dialogue is a reciprocal relationship of mutual understanding. In a dialogue, two people listen to one another and learn to see better what is at stake by opening up to the horizon of the other. This means that one does not think to know best, but is open to the possibility that the other knows better. Yet, one does not simply take over the view of the other, but investigates it critically in order to understand its relevance for one's own situation. The paternalistic model is not dialogical, because it assumes that the physician knows best, and does not need to take into account the patient's point of view. The informative model is the opposite: it takes the values of the patient as leading, without attention for the physician's point of view. This is not dialogical either. The interpretive model is more open, in that it gives the physician a role in examining the patient's perspective. In the end, however, this perspective is considered as given. Neither the physician nor the patient learns to see the situation differently. In the deliberative model, the patient is challenged to broaden his perspective. This implies a dialogical view on patient self-development. Gadamer explains this as follows:

> When two people understand one another, this does not mean that one 'understands' the other in such a way that he sees the other from above, and thus oversees him ('Überschaut'). Likewise, to 'hear someone and respond to him' ('auf jemanden hören') does not mean to execute blindly what the other wants. A person who acts in such a way is called slavish ('hörig'). Openness towards the other entails the recognition that I myself will have to accept things that are against me, even if no one else pushes me to do so. (Gadamer 1960, p. 343)

Gadamer's hermeneutics shows that a dialogical approach to autonomy means that the patient learns to see what matters in life and changes his view in interaction with the physician. This is neatly expressed in the Emanuels' concept of autonomy as moral self-development. Gadamer's hermeneutics goes further than the deliberative model, in that it states explicitly that learning and development are mutually shared processes. Not only does the patient learn from the physician, but the physician also learns from the patient. The physician has to be open to the possibility that the patient perspective may be better. Sometimes, the patient is open to the physician's point of view, while the physician is not prepared to change. This is not reciprocal learning (Widdershoven and Abma 2007).

The importance of dialogue and deliberation can be seen in the case of David. He develops a new view on what is important in life through his contact with the behavioural therapist. This makes him realize that sexual gratification is not the only thing that counts. He wants to get rid of his obsession with sex, so that he can develop relationships in a more responsible way. With his psychiatrist, he discusses the effects of hormone-reducing medication. He agrees to use the medication, because it helps him to realize his new values. The dialogue with the psychiatrist is for David a vehicle of moral learning and moral development. While David learns a new way of looking at himself and his life, the psychiatrist does not seem to show much consideration for David's concerns about his body and his identity as a man. By focusing on the advantages of the medication for controlling sexual behaviour, the disadvantages get little attention. The possibility of reducing the dose is not discussed. David is not stimulated in reconsidering his bodily identity. The option of presenting oneself to a woman in a tender way is not addressed. The behavioural therapy seems to focus on fostering responsibility towards others, not on learning to live with a changing body. A truly dialogical approach would entail deliberation on the dose of the medication and support of David in reflecting on his body and his relationships with women (Slatman and Widdershoven, 2010). From a dialogical perspective, the interaction between David and his psychiatrist should be reciprocal, so that David's problems are addressed in a better way.

One may wonder whether the relationship between physician and patient can actually be reciprocal. Is not the relationship by definition asymmetrical? There is indeed an asymmetry here, since the focus is on the patient's problems. Unlike that of the patient, the personal life of

the physician is not relevant. Yet, although the issue under consideration is the patient's situation, the perspectives of both the physician
and the patient on this issue are equally relevant. The patient and the
physician both have knowledge; the physician has medical knowledge,
the patient has experiential knowledge. They both have a normative
perspective on what is important in the situation. The aim of the deliberation between physician and patient is to discuss facts and values, and
come to an agreement. On the factual level, the effects and side effects
of treatment are issues to be discussed. The physician has some authority, since he has general knowledge of and experience with the medication. Yet, this authority does not mean that he always knows best.
The patient will have to acknowledge the relevance of the physician's
knowledge, and come to understand his situation in the light of this
knowledge. In this process, the patient can raise questions which may
require further investigation by the physician. The patient's experience
can provide the physician with extra information about how to use the
medication in the concrete situation. Physician and patient have to
tune their knowledge in order to find the best dose. On the normative
level, the patient's responsibilities as well as his identity should be inves-
tigated. In regard to these issues, the symmetry between physician and
patient is clearer than in the cognitive domain. Both have a view on
what counts as a good life, including managing one's sexual impulses
and building relationships with other people.

In the case, David and the psychiatrist evidently have discussed
factual and normative aspects related to the use of medication. David
has learned a lot about the effects and side effects of treatment, and has
gained insight in how to behave towards other people. His perspective
is broadened through the interaction, both in the cognitive and in the
normative domain. As to the facts, he knows the effect of the medication on his impulses and on his body; in the normative area he has
come to understand the importance of friendship and trustworthiness
towards others. Whereas David has proven to be open to the cognitive
and normative aspects of the perspective of the psychiatrist, one may
wonder whether the psychiatrist was equally open towards David. The
psychiatrist did explain side effects, but did not address the possibility

of experimenting with the dose. As to the bodily changes, some solutions were tried (the removal of breast tissue), but according to David this did not really help him to live with his new appearance. The psychiatrist was not prepared to investigate with David how to build up a physical relationship with women given his decline of lust and bodily strength. From this we may conclude that reciprocity was compromised, not because David was unable to understand the perspective of the psychiatrist, but because the psychiatrist was not prepared to open up sufficiently to David's point of view. The idea that the relationship between physician and patient is asymmetrical because the physician knows and understands more appears not to be true; actually the patient is more open and understanding. Reciprocity is missing because the physician does not learn enough from the patient and thus does not optimally contribute to the process of investigation. The lack of reciprocity is not given a priori, but can be corrected, if the physician is prepared to listen to the patient's story and help him to find a solution which does justice to his problems and experiences.

10.4 **Autonomy as practical rationality**

The outcome of dialogical interaction and learning is a better understanding of what matters in life and what is to be done in the concrete situation. This is not primarily a matter of theoretical learning, but of practical understanding. According to Aristotle, moral knowledge is practical. It implies knowing what to do and how to act. Unlike for example mathematics, ethics does not require detached insight into eternal truth, but practical understanding of concrete and changing situations. Moral knowledge presupposes experience in life, and is developed by practicing. Autonomy is a matter of practical knowledge about what is important in everyday life and how to act accordingly.

From a dialogical perspective, autonomy is fostered by interaction with others. If autonomy is practical, this interaction also should be of a practical nature. This implies again an addition to the deliberative model of the Emanuels. Their view of dialogue is not just one-sided in that it focuses on patient learning only; it also has a bias towards theory. It tends to regard the examination of values as a matter of discussion and argumentation. The situation they seem to have in mind is that of the physician and the patient discussing various options of treatment with specific risks and benefits, for example, in oncology. The physician then invites the patient to investigate what is really important: living longer or having a smaller risk of serious side effects? In medical practice, choices are not always clear-cut. Moreover, values are not just theoretical issues, they are related to emotions and practical considerations. Interestingly, the interpretive model has more awareness of patients' emotions than the deliberative model, which seems to assume that patients are able to discuss their situation in a detached way.

How can the physician foster practical understanding of the patient and shared practical learning? This requires a dialogue on practical issues, taking into account practical experiences and considerations. The focus should be on concrete interests and concerns, not on abstract principles. Such a dialogue is not a theoretical exchange of viewpoints, but a practical process of negotiation about concrete actions. The physician can invite the patient to see his situation differently by offering concrete alternatives and urging the patient to consider them. At the same time, he has to be open to the patient's reaction and prepared to reconsider his proposal, in response to the patient's reaction.

An example of a dialogical approach focusing on practical interaction can be found in the work of Moody (1992). According to him, care does not merely consist of offering information and waiting for consent, but reaching a joint understanding through negotiation. By being involved with the patient, the physician should encourage the patient to handle the situation in a sensible and responsible way. This means that he should enter negotiations with the patient by actively discussing options and offering concrete alternatives. Moody mentions several practical actions which can be used in the process of negotiation. He discerns four types of intervention. The first is advocacy, or representation of interest. The physician acts as an advocate for the interests of the patient and tries to defend these. For this these interests must be understood. If necessary the care situation should be adjusted, for example when a patient does not want to be helped by a certain professional, but is open to another. The second form of intervention is stimulation. Here, the objective is to encourage the patient to look at himself differently. For example, invite the patient to regard himself as a person with responsibilities towards others. The third intervention is persuasion. The professional tries to persuade the client to be cooperative by offering convincing reasons. These must be tailored to the client's circumstances. The fourth and final intervention is deciding for the other. In this situation the physician takes over. According to Moody, however, communication and negotiation remain important, for example in explaining to the patient why and how one intervenes, and in staying in touch with other parties involved, such as family, or other professionals.

Let us again turn to the example of David. The approach of the psychiatrist offering him medication focused on fostering practical rationality. David was stimulated to regard his behaviour in a different way. He was invited to consider what he needs to live on his own and work. The interventions required are proposed with some pressure. The psychiatrist made clear that David would not be able to live in society without supervision. David agreed that he needed some external control to make sure that he would behave in a responsible way. Thus, David was persuaded to take medicine and accept supervision. In a similar way, the psychiatrist might address issues concerning David's experience with his body. Can David be stimulated to experiment with dating, can he be persuaded to see himself as a person who might be attractive to women in a different way than he used to be? Again, some pressure will be needed to get David to try and find out in practice whether he can combine being friendly and developing deeper feelings towards a woman. Like developing moral responsibility, presenting one's identity as a man is not a matter of theoretical considerations, but of practical experience and understanding.

10.5 Conclusion

Commonly, care professionals tend not to interfere in the lives and privacy of patients referring to the value of autonomy. Respect for autonomy, however, can be explicated in a number of ways. From the viewpoint of negative freedom one should give people the space and opportunity to make their own decisions and not interfere. The contents of their choices are irrelevant. People are seen as individuals who, ideally, live their lives independently of each other. From the perspective of positive freedom, people are free when they are allowed to develop and learn to handle the situation they are in. This requires an intersubjective context of care and support. Giving direction to one's life does not mean that a person can do whatever he wants without hindrance or impediment. Rather, it means that a person is able to structure and build his own life supported by the attention and involvement of others and that he learns how to handle his disabilities and cope with his limitations, finding new ways of expressing himself and relating to others.

In the context of forensic psychiatry, patients are only marginally free to determine whether or not to comply with treatment options. Of course they can refuse to cooperate, but this will result in being locked up longer. This situation is not experienced as one of freedom. Yet, paradoxically, the pressure put on patients in this situation can motivate them to change their views of themselves and learn to behave in a more responsible way. The minimalization of negative freedom can go along with the possibility to develop autonomy as positive freedom. This development requires openness on the side of the patient, who has to be prepared to broaden his perspective. It also requires openness on the side of the psychiatrist, who has to respond to the patient's concerns and help him to find new ways of dealing with vulnerability. If both parties are prepared to listen to one another and to learn from each other, a situation is created in which patient autonomy as moral self-development can be fostered.

References

Agich, G.J. (1993). *Autonomy and long-term care*. Oxford: Oxford University Press.

Beauchamp, T.L. and Childress, J.F. (2008). *Principles of biomedical ethics* (6th edn.). Oxford: Oxford University Press.

Berlin, I. (1969). *Four essays on liberty*. Oxford: Oxford University Press.

Dworkin, G. (1998). *The theory and practice of autonomy*. New York: Cambridge University Press.

Emanuel, E.J. and Emanuel, L.L. (1992). Four models of the physician-patient relationship. *Journal of the American medical Association* 267: 2221–26.

Gadamer, H.-G. (1960). *Wahrheit und Methode* (1st edn.). Tübingen: J.C.B. Mohr.

Mackenzie, C. and Stoljar, N. (eds.) (2000). *Relational Autonomy*. Oxford: Oxford University Press.

Mill, J.S. (1859). *On liberty*. Harmondsworth: Penguin.

Moody, H.R. (1992). *Ethics in an aging society*. Baltimore, MD: Johns Hopkins University Press.

Oeseburg, B. and Abma, T.A. (2006). Care as a mutual endeavour. *Medicine, Health Care and Philosophy* 9: 349–57.

Ricoeur, P. (1992). *Oneself as Another* (Trans. K. Blamey; original title: Soi-même, comme un autre). Chicago/London: The University of Chicago Press.

Slatman, J. and Widdershoven, G. (2010). Hand transplants and bodily integrity. *Body & Society,* 16(3): 69–92.

Verkerk, M.A. (2001). The care perspective and autonomy. *Medicine, Health Care and Philosophy* 4: 289–94.

Widdershoven, G.A.M. and Abma, T.A. (2007). Hermeneutic ethics between practice and theory. In R.E. Ashcroft, A. Dawson, H. Draper and J.R. McMillan (eds.) *Principles of Health Care Ethics* (2nd edn.). Chichester: John Wiley & Sons Ltd., pp. 215–21.

Chapter 11

How do I learn to be me again? Autonomy, life skills, and identity

Grant Gillett

11.1 Introduction

Autonomy is a key concept in contemporary ethics and particularly the ethics of mental healthcare. But what is it? When we ask about the term we are faced with related concepts like 'the will', 'volition', 'self rule', 'reason', and 'competence'.

Under this last guise, autonomy as an ethical value can function as the legitimation of what is effectively a search and disable policy aimed at those who are differently oriented in the human life-world. This policy can affect both the elderly and mental health survivors both of whom may be considered to suffer from a defect of volition due to mental incompetence. For many, experiences of marginalization have caused a re-evaluation of the values around which their lives are organized and that distances them from an all-in conception of reason-governed action in terms of the choices regarded by most as normal rather than pathological.

Autonomy, as many note, means self-rule and is often taken to imply that autonomous decisions are made according to consciously endorsed reasons or principles. But many reasons that are well within the range of 'normal' (in developed societies) can be so seriously distorted in favour of self-interest and individual economy that a psychopath can look normal and rational despite his obvious social dysfunction.

The idea of self-determination, wherever it leads, and whatever value or preference structure is in play, is a widely accepted norm in our understanding of autonomy despite the fact that none of us is an island and that some life plans are inadequate in terms of the realities of human well-being and our relational needs involving support, recognition, dependence, and so on. In fact, being 'held' in life can be the key to living well for many human beings (Nelson 2002). The mean and lean view of autonomy as self-determination falters, for instance, in the (sometimes skeletally thin) face of anorexia where a steely will drives an apparently rational person to die from starvation. The common take on responsibility and agency, based on an individualist ethos, has it that a person owns his or her own actions so that s/he is responsible for them, in the sense of having opted for them as a conscious expression of self and identity. A more inclusive or relational view relates *responsibility* and *responsivity* or right awareness and sensitivity to the life situation in which one finds oneself.

The individualist model has a further defect in that it often fails to distinguish between means-end reasoning where a person endorses pathological ends (reflecting desires and other inner states no matter how dysfunctional they are), and the autonomy of a strong-willed human being who exhibits self-governance such that s/he constructs a life that is sustainable. A sustainable life, richly aware of and appropriately in tune with others, is plausibly a healthy mode of being-in-the-world-with-others in which responsiveness to reason or argument informs projects and interactions (Nussbaum 1990). One might, for instance, think of the kinds of reason exhibited in anorexia (Giordano 2005) or psychopathy (Gillett 2009), as not showing this feature in very different ways. However, the difficulty with constructing an "ought" for autonomy that goes beyond plain matters of truth and ventures into prescriptions for a good life is that health and well-being are intrinsically evaluative concepts and, given the variations in human ways of being, permit a wide range of choices (Nussbaum 1994).

I will therefore discuss the notion of autonomy by trying to determine what constitutes a life that is genuinely meaningful and worthy of a human being and ask what is the proper role of reason in such a life. Phillipa Foot has described such a life as requiring a person to enlist in a collective of 'volunteers banded together to fight for liberty and justice and against inhumanity and oppression' (Foot 1978, p. 167), so that certain guiding values come into play.

The question of argument and the will allows me to examine the concept of the will within a neo-Aristotelian framework that grounds a discussion of Foucault's *cura sui* (care of the self). An interpretation of autonomy and *cura sui*, compatible with a journey metaphor, can then be developed such that autonomy, in mental health particularly but also on a wider stage, emerges as a collaborative project of acquiring the skills to translate the results of formative conversations (or 'argument', broadly construed) into effective action so that one makes sustainable and realistic decisions and, in the process, learns to participate in and take strength from the lives of others.

11.2 **Instrumental rationality and low animal cunning**

Kant in discussing freedom distinguishes between *arbitrium brutum* and *arbitrium liberum*. The former is a function of what moves a person as a result of their animal nature and the latter is a uniquely human kind of freedom in which the intellect plays a central part. I will argue that the variety of reason in question embeds a shared and interpersonal human sensibility that draws on sources of motivation and skills of living well developed by living with others. An alienated person has trouble with these negotiable motivations and the skills required to construct a sustainable life story. Too often the damaging effects of alienation are neglected in the ethical discussions of autonomy but they are essential to an understanding of mental health and recovery from mental disorder (Gillett 2009).

Aristotle, Kant, and Foucault, in diverse ways, noticed that a person can become alienated from the world in which they must act by various cognitive failures and as a result suffer from defects of volition that reveal a contrast between mere cleverness (the cunning required to obtain whatever ends one is inclined to aim for) and a genuine ability to reason about the values that ought to guide one's life.

A concept of autonomy and self-governance in the light of the truth drawing on *cura sui* enables a person to grasp the truths and skills needed for a sustainable life by linking the subject and the truth of his or her situation as a being-in-the-world-with-others. The techniques involved empower people to do things and make decisions about their lives (Foucault 1994). Aristotle notes that a person only learns techniques and life skills by enacting them and so a person trying to recover a sense of him or herself and the possibility of meaningful autonomy needs practical help in becoming capable of living as somebody again, perhaps starting with what seem very small steps.

An account that is both neo-Aristotelian and neo-Kantian begins with Kant's analysis of training in judgement whereby a fledgling thinker, in learning to apply concepts, is taught to judge rightly about things (and their properties) encountered in varying conditions and thus learns to ground his/her experience in the truths that make one capable of right thinking.

At B172 of the *Critique of Pure Reason*, Kant describes the faculty of judgment as 'the faculty of subsuming under rules' (1789/1929). The skill of subsuming a presentation (e.g. the presence of a frog in front of me) under a rule-governed concept (<frog>) is not merely discursive or propositional knowledge but is an ability possessed by human beings—'a special talent . . . that must be practiced'. In learning to exercise such a cognitive skill a human being builds on 'natural' human capacities and develops cognitive techniques that map how things are in the world onto a mirror of the world—a structure of thought. Well-grounded assessments of life situations make use of this mirror to organize experience and action in the light of human ways of thinking.

In his appeal to examples and the role of training, Kant gives an important role to other thinkers—those who are already adept at using the relevant concepts and can do the training. These cognitive masters engage with a thinker and introduce him or her into the world that is 'not only impersonal and also intersubjective in itself, but results in the constitution of an intersubjective world' (Jaspers 1957, p. 34). This is the real shared world, not a private or Cartesian domain in which somebody can become lost in their own thoughts and fantasies; it is a world in which things happen to us and we react, interact, and act in the presence of one another.

The mastery of concepts has a formative effect on my mind and my ability to think and act rightly, a process laid out clearly by Wittgenstein who discusses our rule governed ways of thinking about the world around us.

> But if a person has not yet got the concepts, I shall teach him to use the words by means of examples and by practice . . .
>
> I do it he does it after me; and I influence him by expressions of agreement, rejection, expectation, encouragement. I let him go his way, or hold him back; and so on.
>
> From a child up I learnt to judge like this. This is judging.
>
> A pupil and a teacher. The pupil will not let anything be explained to him, for he continually interrupts with doubts, for instance as to the existence of things, the meaning of words, etc. The teacher says, 'Stop interrupting me and do as I tell you. So far your doubts don't make any sense at all'.
>
> The child, I should like to say, learns to react in such and such a way; and in so reacting it doesn't so far know anything. Knowing only begins at a later level. (Wittgenstein 1953, *Philosophical investigations* p. 208; 1972 *On certainty* pp. 128, 310, 538)

His account is grounded in human ethology—the rules are not individual creations or dispositions in an internal information processor but essentially shared and connect our lives and minds. That connectedness is the basis of a distinctively human experience whereby one makes judgments about what is out there and how it is with others according to a shared symbolic order that shapes one's own moments of recognition, intentional activity, and knowledge of self and world. Thereby we become attuned (Neisser 1976) or adapted to the human life-world, our autonomy resting on an understanding of how to do meaningful things within a shared context of being. That context affords opportunities for action and satisfaction and a fulfilled life.

11.3 Freedom and strength of will

I have argued that skills of cognitive-emotive attunement and adaptation are taught and learnt through training, correction, and shaping by those who 'know what to do and how to do it'. These mentors or instructors do not compel, they teach and advise and help the neophyte to master their techniques and share their powers. Tasks are given and interactions in the context of those tasks create learning linked to the many 'oughts' that surround our abilities (as in 'You ought to do it like this!' or 'Think of it this way and you will see what is going on!'). Whether one does what is suggested or required is not merely a mechanistic outworking of natural processes (even though it may depend on such processes) but an engagement of intellect and interest. The learner must be engaged with and encouraged to develop his or her powers so as to learn that one *ought* to respond thus and so because doing so enhances one's ability to act effectively 'around here'. Catching on to these techniques of living makes autonomy a meaningful concept because the person learns that things in their world are ready to hand for various purposes (as Heidegger would have it (1953/1996)). One can only intend to act thus and so if one knows (to a sufficient degree) how and sets about it in a way that has a hope of success in appropriate conditions. For instance, intending to ski involves first learning to ski and one cannot intend presently to ski without first learning to put skis on, learning to stand upright on snow on skis, learning to move on skis without falling over, and so on. So in life more generally, learning to do the things one used to do after the mind has been disrupted or disconnected from the conversations, transactions and achievements that make up living a human life, takes step by step forming of abilities which can then in-form (re)new(ed) life skills.

Discursive abilities, the building blocks of a human life story, are developed not only in conventional teaching-learning settings (and the neurocognitive structures they help to shape) but also in the many informal and interpersonal situations that are part of the fabric of everyday human life. The ability to act or enact one's own story reflects one's participation in diverse relationships (doctor–patient; coach–athlete; parent–child; teacher–learner). For that reason, recovery is holistic, nothing is incidental, and everything contributes to everything else, even something as minimal as becoming competent at walking the neighbour's dog.

Therefore the discursive skills that create autonomy are techniques of self-empowerment acquired 'with a little help from one's friends' and their mastery allows one to translate into practice the results of conversations (or argument, broadly construed (Nussbaum 1994)) whereby reason-responsiveness and reflective abilities come into being. These skills empower by enabling a person to engage with, adapt to, and be effective in diverse situations and thereby learning to live again, in the real world. Imagine, for instance, that you feel trapped within four walls and then notice the outline of a door and something that might be a handle to open it. This perception links the visual array in front of you to a way of acting that can release you—a simple example of a cognitive technique but also a metaphor for the confinement that is often part of a discontent of the mind. The door is an *affordance*—it affords an opportunity for life affirming or enhancing action. Life is full of such but most social affordances are more subtle, requiring both cognitive and emotional attunement, to the world and others, to pick them up. A chance to get to know somebody better, a cue that you are welcome to participate in some activity, a suggestion that you make yourself known in some context or other where others may create social affordances for you, these things can be missed or not seen for what they are if a person has become alienated from others in certain ways. If the world is not in focus for you in the familiar way it is for others (as in psychosis) or if you are so obsessed with some aspect of your being-in-the-world that you try out ways of being that disrupt your present hierarchy of values (as in anorexia), you may not be able to determine the way your life goes with any degree of freedom whatsoever (Giordano 2005 esp. chapter 5; Gillett 2009 esp. chapter 11).

Discursive skills create autonomy and empower a person through shared adaptive techniques that attune the person to the human life-world and translate the results of conversation into action. Therefore autonomy is related to the ability to use the results of conversation to structure one's activity. That is genuine self-rule in the light of reason (or argument—reason responsive adjustment of attitudes) and it depends on (conscious and unconscious) brain function that is sufficiently in tune with the life world shared by others. A person is autonomous, therefore, to some extent in proportion to his or her ability to engage in ordinary human intercourse and insanity involves, as Kant puts it, 'loss of a sense for ideas that are common to all' (Kant 1798/1978). When we have mastered the requisite skills, life situations do not evoke poorly apprehended motives and patterns of response (perhaps manifesting unconscious mechanisms) but rather allow us to exercise of techniques whereby we affect things and exploit the opportunities they present. Kant also argues that agency[1] and potential autonomy cannot be easily linked to explanations on terms of underlying brain processes even though, from the point of view of a scientific understanding, our behaviour must be causally produced in ways that conform to the dictates of brain science. Nietzsche objects, noting that science embeds a kind of 'prevailing mechanistic stupidity' and therefore must get itself tangled up in inconclusive debates around freedom and unfreedom and mechanistic functions that make us behave in certain ways. Nietzsche, in place of this metaphysical to and fro about determinism, poses a question of strong and weak wills (Nietzsche 1886/1975, esp. #21). The will is strong, he argues, if a person can develop the life skills needed to enact the conclusions of his/her engagement in conversation, interaction, argument, and contestation, and so overcome ignorance, and weakness of will.

Notice that this line of argument undercuts the mechanistic or causal theory of action (supported by a suspect neurophilosophy of acts of will (Gillett 2008a, esp. chapter 6) and a reductive metaphysics of the mind) and adopts a much more promising account of volition for clinical and psychiatric ethics—and it also opens up the possibility of therapy for the soul. We could summarize the argument as follows.

11.4 The will to power argument

WP1. Empowering oneself by using shared techniques to modify one's life context makes a person effective in engaging with the world.

WP2. Taking control over one's environment in light of the contingencies it produces undercuts the idea of behaviour being determined by antecedent causes.

WP3. Reflective techniques and skills that allow a person to modify his or her own responses result in self-control.

WP4. Self-control and effectiveness in operating on the world are the basis one of effective agency. Therefore,

---

[1] By 'spontaneous', Kant means that can only be explained in terms of the reason an agent gives for initiating some cascade of events in the world even though the event concerned may also have a physical description.

WP5. Agency and self-formation (perhaps with help from others) depend on the mastery of life skills and result in genuine autonomy.

Nietzsche concedes that human beings in general (not just those suffering 'mental disorders') are torn his way and that by inner forces and urges of which they are often barely cognisant. These psychological influences are always obscured by the human need for self-validation. That is why human beings are vulnerable to coercion and persuasion by desires and inclinations that most would not endorse in the light of argument and critical interrogation. When a person can act in ways that are open to self-understanding and self-control, s/he can be said to have a strong will. If the resulting acts can be endorsed even after examination by arguments about what is admirable, then a strong will is a candidate for what we could call a good or virtuous will. Kant links the good will or virtue to intentions formed that way but his emphasis on the pure will and being governed by reason alone leaves him open to a charge of being other-worldly in his moral philosophy. In fact, 'between the motion and the act falls the shadow' and the shadow may be a mixed motive or disruptive contingencies—'I did it mainly to honour her but, of course it also earned me a certain recognition that may have affected my thinking'; 'I know I promised but my wife was distraught so what could I do?'. Aristotle and Nietzsche both regard an act as the outcome of practical reason (or the exercise of the will) and recognize the many and varied ways in which an agent's intention to act thus and so might fail. Thus, even though, through our thoughts and intentions, we can and do effect change in our own lives and the lives of others, we vary in our ability to do so. That ability is, however, the key to autonomy, and it can be deficient in a number of ways.

11.5 How shall I fail me, let me count some ways

One way in which autonomy can fail is a loss of what some call *ipseity*—the very familiar and practical knowledge of self as an acting subject (Stanghellini 2004; Sass and Parnas 2007). Agency is a matter of using well-practised techniques embedding an intuitive grasp of one's place in the world as the bedrock of everyday life. Doing things in ways that are second nature for a person lies at the heart of all knowing because knowledge is based on our dealings with things. It is in action space, therefore, that the body instinctively shapes the mind and a person's conception of who s/he is (Gallagher 2005). This is the domain of the self, where a person has an intuitive sense of belonging and knows how to go on in a diverse range of situations.

When the context of self is fractured in some way, the deployment of life skills takes place without a sure foundation—a place to stand and people among whom one belongs. That alienation is disconcerting and disempowering. It is produced by any of a number of disruptions in the three-way relationship between the subject, the world, and the meanings that make sense of the world and through which the world can be acted on. Autonomy and meaningful individuality is therefore subjectivity in context, an interwoven and complex structure of familiar and practised techniques that enable a person to do things and be somebody in the ways that constitute him or her as a self.

Mental illness can severely disrupt that essentially dynamic and interactive pattern of being. For instance, one might face an impasse: the world ahead is presided over by a demand and an expectation to meet it in some very limited way. The demand might be, for instance, to be a woman faced by a range of stereotyping choices dictated by others—to be thin and 'spiritual', in control, to be fecund, to be attractive to the opposite sex, to fulfil the expectations of parents, and so on. Such an impasse can be so profound as to be fatal and a young woman facing it can be desperate for indicators that she does not have to go there, that she can be her own self, the person she has always been, not becoming this or that at the behest of others (Giordano 2005).

Or a person might find he is out of touch, bombarded by stimulations which do not resolve into familiar patterns and people who no longer seem to be saying anything comprehensible or straightforward. The world may seem overly crammed with promise or meaning and with clamours for attention and resolution that are elusive. Even voices that are usually just in the background—part of one's own thinking, mere hints and under control—may seem to have taken on a life of their own with urgent and desperately important messages to convey (May, 2000).

Or the world, from the earliest memories you have, may seem an unforgiving and unwelcoming place, likely to be hostile with people all doing their own thing and serving their own agendae such that you have a stark choice between being the abuser or the abused. When the world conducts itself in those terms it is difficult to feel at home in it, or to know what a word like 'trust' might mean. Softness, welcome may seem no more than appearances that beguile the naïve and the soon-to-be-victims (among whom you are determined not to count yourself) (Gillett 2010).

In each of these cases something has gone terribly wrong and it may or may not be amenable to correction by conversation and restoration of right relationships between self and others. The loss of autonomy in each case is different but in each there is a break between the techniques deployed by the self and the context in which the self must live and construct a sustainable way of being.

This argument underpins both recovery ethics and the attainment of as-good-as-it-gets autonomy: self-government in the light of the truth or the ability to take control of your own actions and desires in the light of the realities of your life. Nietzsche's claim that psychology is the developmental theory of the will to power (Nietzsche 1886/1975) is therefore central in the current account of self-understanding and autonomy in that developing some efficacy or power in your life situation and the challenges it presents is a matter of learning techniques that empower oneself to act in real-life situations and discern the many truths that are implicit within them.

11.6 **Existential rationality**

Becoming me again after the me that I used to be has been broken or twisted out of shape is a journey that interweaves action and identity. The journey is gestured at by Jean Paul Sartre when he remarks that the free project is my being (Sartre 1958). It is a theme taken up in the narrative theory of identity, the view that we weave stories around our being-in-the-world-with-others (Schechtman 1996; Lindemann-Nelson 2001; McKenzie and Atkins 2008). The theory has it that human beings construct their existence around a question—'Who am I?'.

The question is other-directed and depends on the ways that others mirror our dealings with them and include us in their intercourse with each other. From this milieu of relationships and discourses each of us takes the ingredients out of which "my story" is made. Lacan notes that our very desires are themselves constructions out of surreal ingredients provided by this mirror world (Lacan 1977)—a world of reflections (or even smoke and mirrors). Each of us is mirrored in the glances, remarks, and relationships of others. What we see in these multifaceted mirrors are ourselves—the selves we take ourselves to be—and these selves come clothed with evaluations. Others not only register our presence but react to it with attitudes that situate us in their midst and give rise to significations held in place by a fragment of language, the currency of our conversations and cognitive-emotive dealings with each other.

> And I have known the eyes already, known them all—
> The eyes that fix you in a formulated phrase,
> And when I am formulated, sprawling on a pin,
> When I am pinned and wriggling on the wall,
> Then how should I begin
> To spit out all the butt-ends of my days and ways?
> And how should I presume?
>
> (T.S. Eliot *The love song of J. Alfred Prufrock*)

Such conversations empower and/or paralyse depending on the way that I figure in them. Autonomy is the ability to direct my own journey in such a context, where certain things are possible, permitted, or valorized and others are unacceptable. If I am in the process of re-emerging from a debility, I may ask myself: 'How should I presume to take my place in this context?'. Or, 'What is it ok to do around here for someone like me?'. Yet, these questions are universal, they apply to each of us in an unfamiliar domain or in a context from which we have become alienated. Relationships give rise to reasons, spoken and unspoken, that I may or may not be in a position or prepared to consciously endorse. This structure of reasons is a resource needed to get by in shared human life and to articulate human worth. As an agent, I can be disordered in a way not reflected in any defect of means-end reasoning (which could be both ingenious and manipulative, e.g. for an anorexic or bulimic woman, or a psychopath) but reflected in the direction or ethos of that reasoning. I can, particularly when suffering a discontent of the mind, enact (unreasonable) values that rule my life in ways that we may feel hesitant about calling autonomous.

The problem lies with a principled distinction between autonomous decisions and things that one finds oneself doing, perhaps consciously and voluntarily but which a part of oneself feels quite unhappy with. Where do we draw the lines between reason and unreason, given that:

1 Different people accept different constellations of values as reflecting a reasonable view of life, and

2 Our values, attitudes, and commitments seem to arise from within us partly as 'reasons of which reason knows not?'(Church 2005).

The present approach, arising from the work of Nietzsche and Foucault, relates autonomy, as self-rule in accordance with truth or an informed understanding of the world, to reasoned and sustainable self-efficacy—the ability to achieve what you judge, in the light of conversations with those you value, to be admirable or worth aiming at. This ability depends on a workable set of techniques of being-in-the-world-with-others given the actual situation in which you live and what it takes to sustain well-being in that setting. Human well-being is inescapably relational and therefore has moral content. It therefore embraces a concept of reason as that which relates us rightly to both truth (duly noting Pilate's question, 'What is truth?') and goodness where something like Foot's 'natural goodness' or sustainable well-being is in play (Foot 2001). Both over-arching values are cashed in terms of life-affirming social inter-course between human beings with different ways of being-in-the world. For the mental health survivor, participation in that discourse may have been disordered for a time and the techniques required to adapt to a context of being in a world of others have to be restored through inclusion and recognition as one who belongs to that world.

11.7 *Cura sui* or care of the self

Philosophers who follow Hume or Mill (as do many contemporary bioethicists) often focus on autonomy as unhampered individual choice based on means-end reasoning, so that the individual' s legitimate attitudes and values are formulated without any constraint (apart from the harm principle). But Kant's emphasis on self-rule in the light of reason seems to invoke what we might call 'all-in reason' an objectively reasonable set of beliefs and attitudes given the truth of our community of being with others (as members of a kingdom of ends). It is tempting to think that he develops this idea from Aristotle's *Nicomachean Ethics* VI.12, where we find a mere cleverness (which is instrumental and focuses on the most efficient means of achieving that which is its mark) distinguished from practical wisdom (in which the mark at which one aims is itself up for debate in the light of what it means to be a good human being).

Aristotle notes that sufficient cleverness allows a person to achieve what s/he sets out to do but that one can mistake cleverness for properly reason-governed action or practical wisdom. Aristotelian conceptions of reason concern what we should value and, if the current argument is correct, imply that we should be mindful of the ends (or guiding principles and purposes) worth subscribing to as part of our shared journey through the human life-world. It is hard, absent a divine revelation properly interpreted, to see any other way apart from engaging in the kind of reasoned argument and respect for others that is proper to Kant's 'kingdom of ends' to discern that more final end (or telos).

The thought that argument is therapy for the soul, also classical in its provenance, is further developed in Foucault's later writing on ethics where he endorses a certain kind of truth that which empowers and equips a person by imparting to them techniques of the self (Gillett 2008b). Such an approach yields a robust view of autonomy that finesses doubts about the reality of self-rule and displaces the idea that actions can be autonomous only in the sense of being caused by a person's own inner states of belief and desire, whatever they may be. The thought that autonomy requires sustainable self-efficacy (again in the human life-world) implicates co-creation in well-being whereby a person is nurtured by others, values their companionship, and, in a very real way, becomes banded together with them in the common cause of a good life (as Foot has it). The shared nature of sustainable real-world autonomy reinforces the claim that the journey through and out of mental illness is not one that is best taken alone.

11.8 **A journey in company out of a place of trial**

> The care of the self is ethical in itself; but it implies complex relationships with others insofar as this ethos of freedom is also a way of caring for others. . . Ethos also implies a relationship with others, insofar as the care of the self enables one to occupy his rightful position in the city, the community, or interpersonal relationships . . . proper care of the self requires listening to the lessons of a master. One needs a guide, a counsellor or a friend, someone who will be truthful with you. Thus the problem of relationships with others is present throughout the development of the care of the self. (Foucault 1994, *Ethics* p. 287)

Persons in conversation are subjective nodes in a life-world crisscrossed with significance in that the signs that we use in our discourse reveal or un-conceal the meanings that surround us, unlocking possibilities, prohibitions, and affordances (Harre and Gillett 1994). People act on, interact with, and are acted on by things around them as become somebody in the world. In doing so, they articulate aspects of themselves, as, for instance, when a rugby player finds the ability to shed tears as he tells of his descent into depression and the frustration and helplessness he felt at being engulfed by something he could neither overcome nor even name. Our decision-making as autonomous human beings draws on meanings that pick out points of significance in the world around us. These emerge as we are introduced to aspects of a situation as it is experienced by others. The intersubjective responses of those others can include or marginalize a person in ways that affirm or deny things that subjectively loom large or inspire that person. Either way, denial and silencing that renders a person inarticulate about what matters also makes him or her ineffective. When that happens, impaired, restricted, or less inclusive possibilities for the person to be themselves in the life world they inhabit are the result. It follows that restoring autonomy is not just switching on an inner circuit linked to voluntary action, though that may help, but creating significance and affordance in circumstances where significant things may have been obscured or lost.

Person-centred explanations pick out human beings as subjective, psychophysical beings and draw on the diverse patterns of human adaptation and shared attunement to an environment that people need to find meaningful ways of being in the world, whatever neurological functions underpin them. The actions or decisions available to somebody reflect or are informed by understandings of their world and the thoughts and attitudes concerned arise in human discourse. The relevant conversations embed what I have called argument and provide scaffolding for deliberation (Vygotsky 1978). Through conversations, others engage with a person's narrative and the moral and personal challenges inherent in their shared context of being. Many things affect a person's ability to engage in such contexts in ways that adequately manifest who they are, including the neurological capacities, cognitive abilities, and discursive skills required to perceive, make judgments, and order their thoughts. Only when these are in order and given the opportunity to be exercised can a person enact his or her own story rather than merely being an 'object' who is 'dealt with' by others. Being rightly connected to the truth, one could say, frees one from being merely a moral patient in any given life context and allows one to become a moral agent—to enact an identity that embodies certain values and that underpins being somebody around here.

11.9 Autonomy as equipping oneself to exercise power in the world

The growth of thinking, experiencing, meaning-making beings occurs through interactions that shape the brain so that the person concerned develops hexeis (or habits of being) incorporating life skills that link actions and decisions to his/her contexts, knowledge, and life projects. These modes of attunement to what is going down are the result of directed attention in touch with what others are noticing, learning to use appropriate terms in responsive and nuanced ways. They enable a person to take on an identity as somebody, an acquaintance and companion who acts in virtuous ways that others can endorse, who uses appropriate life skills to create and maintain satisfying relationships. In mental health recovery and the land of *Clinicum*, the supportive role must often be taken on by healthcare professionals, as has been recognized from the time of Hippocrates (Lloyd 1978):

> Although it were no easy thing for common people to discover for themselves the nature of their own diseases and the causes why they get worse or better, yet it is easy for them to follow when another makes the discoveries and explains the events to them.

When you are ill, you need a guide, an informant, someone who knows about your disease and its trajectory, who forms a partnership with you and who empowers you to play your part in co-creating a good regimen of care. Here again, participation is enhanced by 'argument'—reasoned, respectful discussion aimed at clarifying a situation in the light of the truth. That enables people to assume and enact identities and to live out life stories each with its unique value, rather than being helpless puppets of 'the slings and arrows of outrageous fortune' perhaps distorted by a malfunctioning biological information processing systems, or emotive reactions that interfere with relationships and shared achievements.

Attunement to the world, especially the world of the clinic and its workings, may require scaffolding (or cognitive support) by those with the skills required to negotiate it (Vygotsky 1978). That need casts the healthcare professional or any other companion in the recovery journey in the role of educator and counsellor, caring for the person and playing a part in equipping them to take a participant role in their mental healthcare. As a result, the decision-making becomes dynamic and interactive as are all the neurocognitive skills that equip us for an unfolding set of circumstances in identity affirming ways (Clark 1997). The reality of co-creation between the patient, whose story frames the clinical encounter, and healthcare professionals or others, who try and help the patient through the illness journey, means that the idea of autonomy as an individual property (dependent on inner mental, or neural, states and events) is seriously flawed. Autonomy is other-involving, it influences and reflects the context of action and those who help to form it and, when it is developed and empowered, it shapes a story that a person can feel good about as an expression of an identity that is worth something because it gives rise to a good-enough sense of well-being.

Reasoned decision-making, and the exercise of autonomy in general, is interactive; intelligent beings draw on a world of meaning and understanding and, in the light of the truth as they see it, participate in determining what happens in and around them as beings-in-the-world-with-others. That is the real-world meaning of autonomy, a radically relational property of a person who may, for a time, have strayed into the domain of *Clinicum* (Gillett 2004) (or into the margins of society) but who needs help to develop the skills to participate rather than merely having things done to them. Neuroscience may tell us important things about the vehicle of that dynamic identity—the brain and its neurocognitive operations—and brain dysfunction may derail autonomy and adaptation to the human life-world. But, whatever the role of the brain, autonomy based on the ability to affect the world in ways that begin in conversations, is not merely an illusion subscribed to by ethicists but an emergent property in the tryadic relation between human beings, meanings, and contexts of life. That autonomy effectively inscribes our brains with the life skills we need to enact our stories, even in the midst of illness journeys.

References

Church, J. (2005). Reasons of which reason knows not. *Philosophy, Psychiatry & Psychology* 12: 31–42.

Clark, A. (1997). *Being there: putting brain body and world together again*. Cambridge, MA: MIT Press.

Foot, P. (1978). *Virtues and vices*. Oxford: Blackwell.

Foot, P. (2001). *Natural Goodness*. Oxford: Oxford University Press.

Foucault, M. (1994). *Ethics: subjectivity and truth* (Ed. P. Rabinow). London: Penguin.

Gallagher, S. (2005). *How the body shapes the mind*. Oxford: Clarendon.

Gillett, G. (2004). *Bioethics and the clinic: Hippocratic reflections*. Baltimore, MD: Johns Hopkins University Press.

Gillett, G. (2008a). *Subjectivity and Being somebody: human identity and neuroethics* (St Andrews series on philosophy and Public Affairs). Exeter: Imprint Academic.

Gillett, G. (2008b) Autonomy and selfishness. *Lancet* 372: 1214–15.

Gillett, G. (2009). *The mind and its discontents* (2nd edn.). Oxford: University Press.

Gillett, G. (2010). Intentional action, moral responsibility and psychopaths. In L. Malatesti and J. McMillan (eds.) *Responsibility and Psychopathy: Interfacing Law, Psychiatry and Philosophy*. Oxford: Oxford University Press, pp. 283–98.

Giordano, S. (2005). *Understanding eating disorders*. Oxford: Oxford University Press.

Harre, H.R. and Gillett, G. (1994). *The Discursive Mind*. Thousand Oaks, CA: Sage.

Heidegger, M. (1953/1996). *Being and Time* (Trans. J. Stambaugh). New York: SUNY Press.

Jaspers, K. (1957). *Kant*. New York: Harcourt.

Kant, I. (1789/1929). *The Critique of pure reason* (Trans. N. Kemp Smith). St Martin's Press, New York.

Kant, I. (1798/1978). *Anthropology from a pragmatic point of view* (Trans. V.L. Dowdell). Carbondale, IL: Southern Illinois University Press.

Lacan, J. (1977). *Ecrits.* New York: Norton and Co.

Lindemann-Nelson, H. (2001). *Damaged Identities, Narrative Repair.* Ithaca, NY: Cornell University Press.

Lindemann-Nelson, H. (2002). What child is this? *Hastings Center Report* 32(6): 29–38.

Lloyd, G. (ed.) (1978). Tradition in medicine. In *Hippocratic Writings.* London: Penguin, pp. 70–86.

May, R. (2000). Routes to recovery from psychosis: The roots of a clinical psychologist. *Clinical Psychology Forum* 146: 6–10.

McKenzie, C. and Atkins, K. (eds.) (2008). *Practical Identity and Narrative Agency.* New York: Routledge.

Neisser, U. (1976). *Cognition and reality.* San Francisco, CA: Freedman and Sons.

Nietzsche, F. (1886/1975). *Beyond good and evil* (Trans. R.J. Hollingdale) London: Penguin.

Nussbaum, M. (1990). *Love's Knowledge.* New York: Oxford University Press.

Nussbaum, M. (1994). *The therapy of desire.* Princeton, NJ: University Press.

Sartre, J.P. (1958). *Being and Nothingness* (Trans. H Barnes). London: Methuen & Co.

Sass, L. and Parnas, J. (2007). Explaining schizophrenia: the relevance of phenomenology. In M.C. Chung, K.W.M. Fulford, and G. Graham (eds.) *Reconceiving Schizophrenia.* Oxford: Oxford University Press, pp. 63–96.

Schechtman, M. (1996). *The Constitution of Selves.* Ithaca, NY: Cornell University Press.

Stanghellini, G. (2004). *Disembodied spirits and deanimated bodies.* Oxford: University Press.

Vygotsky, L.S. (1978). *Mind in Society.* Cambridge, MA: Harvard University Press.

Wittgenstein, L. (1953). *Philosophical investigations* (Trans. G.E.M. Anscombe). Oxford: Blackwell.

Wittgenstein, L. (1972). *On certainty* (Eds. G.E.M. Anscombe and G. H. von Wright, Trans. D. Paul and G.E.M. Anscombe). New York: Harper & Row.

Chapter 12

Autonomy and Ulysses arrangements

Lubomira Radoilska

12.1 Introduction

In this chapter, I sketch the structure of a general concept of autonomy and then reply to possible objections with reference to Ulysses arrangements in psychiatry. In so doing, I commit to the claim that autonomy is best understood as a de facto contested concept rather than either an essentially contested one or an umbrella term covering a loose set of separate target concepts.[1]

The argument proceeds as follows. At the start of the inquiry, I explore three main strategies to conceiving autonomy in the current debate: value-neutral, value-laden, and relational. The objective is to bring into relief their distinctive rationales and draw attention to ensuing points of disagreement. Next, I identify two paradigm cases of autonomy by considering everyday instances of pre-commitment,[2] and then offer a first sketch of the concept of autonomy as opposed to the closely related

---

[1] Both the distinction between concepts and conceptions, and the notion of an essentially contested concept as employed in this chapter draw on Gallie (1956). On the thesis that autonomy is merely an umbrella term covering a loose set of separate target concepts, see Arpaly (2003, chapter 4). The differences between the two rejected models of understanding autonomy—an essentially contested concept and an umbrella term—are of no bearing to the present inquiry, since both models have similarly sceptical implications with respect to the project of articulating a general concept of autonomy. By sketching such a concept, it becomes clear that neither of these models is persuasive. On the importance of locating competing autonomy accounts with respect to a possible general concept, see Chapter 1, this volume, by Jane Heal.

[2] Unless stated otherwise (see in particular Section 12.4), the terms 'pre-commitment' and 'Ulysses arrangement' will be used interchangingly throughout the chapter.

freedom of action and intentional agency. Finally, I explain away the autonomy paradox to which the previously identified pair of paradigm cases seems to give rise in the context of mental disorder. By resolving this paradox, we learn two valuable lessons. The first is about the relationships between the three conceptions of autonomy just mentioned. The second is about the relationships between autonomy and mental disorder.

12.2 **Three approaches to autonomy**

A plausible way to map out the broader lines of disagreement on autonomy is to compare three main alternatives that have emerged from the current debate. These alternatives are often referred to as value-neutral, value-laden, and relational strategies (Christman 2003; Taylor 2005; Buss 2008).[3] The present section will look into each of these strategies in turn.

The first, value-neutral approach focuses on identifying the formal features that distinguish autonomous from non-autonomous actions and choices. These features are meant to capture the special relationship a person has to a particular category of her actions and motives that could be seen as her own in a suitably robust sense. This point becomes clear, if we consider cases where the autonomy conferring relationship has broken down, such as instances of coercion and compulsion. A person subjected to coercion does not act by choice. On this occasion, her motives to act are not fully her own. Similarly, a person in the grips of compulsion does not act by choice. In this respect, her motives are not sufficiently up to her.[4]

These two cases illustrate the kinds of constraints that need to be eliminated in order for a choice to be considered as autonomous: external constraints endangering a person's ownership of the motives from which she acts and internal constraints belying her authorship over

---

[3] The terms 'value-neutral' and 'procedural' are sometimes used interchangeably with respect to autonomy conceptions. The same goes for 'value-laden' and 'substantive'.

[4] Compare Robert Nozick's analysis of coercion as a successful attempt to modify a person's intentions by means of credible threats (1969) and Lennart Nordenfelt's account of compulsion as subjective unavoidability (2007).

these motives.[5] Value-neutral accounts define the relationship to one's motives that is free from these and similar constraints in a variety of ways.[6] According to a classical approach, the underlying attitude is captured in terms of endorsement, identification or, more modestly, acceptance (Frankfurt 1971; 1998, chapter 12; 1999, chapter 11; 2002). An alternative approach points to the significance of a historical perspective onto the formation of both first-order motives and higher-order attitudes, such as endorsement (Christman 2007). This further criterion aims to address less apparent threats to autonomy that may not be recognized as such by the person affected. Examples include so-called adaptive preferences, where the desirability of different options is inappropriately influenced by their perceived (un)availability as in Aesop's fable 'The Fox and the Grapes' (Elster 1983; Colburn 2011).

These variations notwithstanding, both alternatives concur on a central idea, according to which the autonomy conferring relationship of a person to her motives can be fully defined with no reference to further principles or values. A major implication is that autonomy is presented as a separate source of normativity, on a par with moral and prudential considerations, such as beneficence and efficiency.[7] The underlying reasoning can be reconstructed as follows:

1 Autonomous choices deserve special consideration simply by virtue of being a person's own in a suitably robust sense, such as being free from undue influences, both external and internal.

---

[5] See Feinberg (1980, chapter 1 and 1986, chapter 18) and Moran (2001). See also Chapter 3, this volume, where K.W.M. Fulford and I discuss the Aristotelian notion of being 'up to the agent' which underlies considerations of both ownership and authorship with respect to motives and actions.

[6] In the following, I shall comment on two alternatives only, for the aim is to pick out the underlying strategy that value-neutral accounts share rather than detail possible points of disagreement within it.

[7] On the notion of sources of normativity, see Korsgaard (1996). The interpretation of value-neutral autonomy as one source of normativity among others that I propose departs from Korsgaard's thesis, according to which autonomy is the ultimate source of normativity, since it underwrites a person's ability to put herself under obligation and to perceive certain actions as worth undertaking. This point will be further developed in the subsequent discussion on value-laden accounts of autonomy.

2 The significance of autonomous choices as previously defined cannot be duly acknowledged unless there is a protected sphere of action, where these kinds of choices may be followed through without further justification.

3 Within this sphere of action, an autonomous choice should be treated as authoritative, although it may happen to be morally objectionable or unwise.

The intuitive appeal of this line of thought is reflected in the liberal idea of toleration as a prerequisite for personal freedom within society. The implicit links between autonomy and toleration become clear once we notice that respect for either comes to matter in similar circumstances: whenever a particular choice faces solid objections and these can be enforced over dissenters. As Joseph Raz points out, we cannot tolerate other people's virtue but only their limitations (1987, p. 320). Similarly, respect for autonomy would be superfluous with regard to choices that are generally considered as admirable. In this regard, autonomy and toleration offer two complementary ways to define one and the same cluster of choices as particularly exposed to interference and worth protecting. The first point stems from the fact that the choices at issue are deemed to be objectionable in some conspicuous way, such as being foolish, perverse, or wrong, to paraphrase John Stuart Mill (1859, p. 53). An intuitive reaction would be to try and undo these kinds of choices. The second point expresses a core insight of the value-neutral approach indicating that there must be a sphere of action where autonomous choices need not be backed up by further reasons. It requires that the initial reaction in favour of interference is curtailed, but does not remove the grounds for disapproval that motivated it in the first instance. This is why toleration may appear paradoxical at first sight. For it involves both a strong negative evaluation and a commitment not to act upon it (Scanlon 1996). The idea of autonomy as an independent source of normativity helps dissipate the impression that toleration is odd. The underlying intuition is clearly expressed in Mill's classical treatise *On Liberty*:

> If a person possesses any tolerable amount of common sense and experience, his own mode of laying out his existence is the best, not because it is the best in itself, but because it is his own mode. (1859, p. 114)

Turning to the second key approach to autonomy, we are in a position to notice an immediate contrast. For value-laden accounts intertwine autonomy and practical rationality and argue that responsiveness to reasons is the distinctive feature of autonomous choices (Watson 1975, 2004; Hill 1991; Korsgaard 1996). A direct implication is the idea that, ultimately, the source of normativity can only be one. It is supported by an intuitive line of reasoning that could be summed up as follows:

1 Autonomy could hardly be a plausible normative concept if its task were to uphold morally objectionable choices or prop up other forms of practical irrationality.

2 Instead, choices are worthy of special consideration only if they respond to reasons, the validity of which could also be appreciated from an impartial or ideal observer's viewpoint.

3 A choice is autonomous to the extent that it is responsive to reasons in the sense specified here rather than to mere incentives.[8]

The value-laden interpretation of autonomy as practical rationality and ultimate source of normativity could be grounded in a strong analogy between motivation and cognition. This analogy is well captured by the concept of 'orthonomy' or correct determination as applicable to desires (Pettit and Smith 1996). To bring out this point, let us consider, following Pettit and Smith, the nature and scope of freedom in theoretical settings. For instance, our intellectual freedom would be effectively undermined by a licence to brave the laws of logic, believe in patent falsehoods, and ignore evidence on hand. These examples suggest that, in the realm of belief, freedom presupposes rules and constraints that forestall hindrances to reliably getting things right, such as wishful thinking and hasty conclusions. In fact, following these rules and respecting these constraints are key expressions of our freedom of thought. Conversely, forming a belief without sufficient reason and refusing to revise an earlier opinion in the face of contrary evidence are paradigm cases of having one's freedom of

---

[8] The contrast between reasons and incentives here draws on Kant's distinction between motives and incentives (*Groundwork* 4: 427).

thought compromised. The core idea is that what holds a person back as a thinker boils down to an inadequate relationship between beliefs and supporting reasons. From this perspective a belief is unfree to the extent that it is unwarranted.

Drawing on this account of freedom with respect to beliefs, it is plausible to conclude that freedom with respect to desires would be equally undermined by a licence to satisfy any fancy, ignore reasonable demands, or abandon long-term commitments on a whim. For the kind of volitional arbitrariness these examples have in common structurally resembles the inadequate relationship between beliefs and supporting reasons that we have seen to erode freedom of thought. Following this line of reasoning, it is natural to stipulate that freedom of will should depend in a similar way on a fitting relationship between motives and reasons for action. This relationship would only obtain if motives are responsive to reasons as opposed to what we may call unexamined incentives.

The notion of orthonomy offers an insightful way of thinking about freedom with respect to desires. In particular, it enables us to identify anything that holds a person back from engaging in worthwhile pursuits as an obstacle to her freedom. On this view, a choice is unfree to the extent that it is idiosyncratic rather than responsive to reasons. The outcome leaves no room for a principled asymmetry between first- and other-person perspectives on individual choices. In doing so, it corroborates the underlying assumption of value-laden accounts of autonomy, which is to reject the possibility of alternative sources of normativity.

Orthonomy is not the only possible interpretation of responsiveness to reasons. This essential idea could be also presented in Kantian terms, such as universalizability of our motives for action or ability to recognize and fulfil unconditional requirements (Hill 1991; Korsgaard 1996). In each instance, however, the main ambition is relevantly similar, that is, to contrast autonomy with various forms of arbitrary, idiosyncratic, or otherwise indefensible expressions of the will, independently of whether they have been initiated by the agent herself or prompted by a third party.

The third major strategy to defining autonomy offers a critical stand-point to both the preceding value-laden approach and its value-neutral rivals. Its essential idea is that interpersonal relationships are constitutive of personal autonomy rather than contingent factors that may impede or facilitate it (Meyers 1989; Stoljar 2000). This leads to a distinctive claim, according to which personal autonomy is best presented in terms of a particular social-relational status. As Marina Oshana puts it:

> [T]o be autonomous is to stand in a certain position of authority over one's life with respect to others. (2006, p. 94).

In support of this claim, relational accounts argue that unless we take on an interpersonal perspective on autonomy, we are bound to overlook the effects of oppressive arrangements on an oppressed person's capacity for autonomy. As a result, we would end up with a flawed distinction between autonomous and non-autonomous choices that effectively condones the loss of personal autonomy incurred by members of dominated social groups.

A related worry is that socialization into a deferential role typically leads to earnest acceptance so that a person thus socialized naturally gives way to the preferences of powerful others and, moreover, does so without a trace of resentment. This is not to say that there is something inherently suspect in motivations that depart from self-interest. Nor is the idea to suggest that personal ambition is a prerequisite for personal autonomy. Instead, the point is to draw attention to a pervasive way in which imposed choices could be mistaken for autonomous from both first- and other-person perspectives.

This conclusion could be disputed. For both value-neutral and value-laden accounts seem in a position to address the psychological threats that oppressive socialization poses to autonomy. For instance, a value-neutral notion of adaptive preferences would be able to identify as non-autonomous individual choices traceable to a systematically abusive environment. A value-laden approach to autonomy could also spot that autonomy is being compromised in such instances because the choices at issue are clearly not responsive to reasons, but manipulated from outside.

Although persuasive, this line of reasoning does not tackle the main challenge raised by the relational strategy, which is to account for the social nature of autonomy rather than concentrate on psychological manifestations that may turn out to be secondary. The thought is that what goes wrong in circumstances of oppression has to do primarily with the social-relational status of the person oppressed rather than the way she relates to her motives or is able to track valid reasons for action. In other words, an oppressed person lacks autonomy by virtue of being oppressed, independently of how candid she is about her reasons for action and whether, counterfactually, she would have chosen to do the very same things that are now imposed on her. If this is correct, a focus on the psychology rather than politics of autonomy would obscure the real threats to autonomy. Moreover, it would make them appear as personal rather than social problems. This result is paradoxical in so far as it implies that an oppressed person should take it upon herself to become autonomous whilst being oppressed in the same way as before. The relational strategy to autonomy aims to resolve this paradox by adopting a social and interpersonal stance in opposition to both the intrapersonal and, in a sense, impersonal viewpoint championed respectively by the value-neutral and value-laden approaches.

12.3 **Ulysses arrangements as paradigm cases of self-determination**

Having set out these three approaches in general terms, let us consider their possible interactions in the context of a challenging case where competing concerns about autonomy appear to be equally plausible. This case relates to the use of Ulysses arrangements in psychiatry. But before fleshing out the autonomy paradox, to which this use seems to give rise, I shall look in some detail into paradigm cases of pre-commitment outside psychiatry. The idea is to establish whether there is something paradoxical in the very notion of pre-commitment, in advance of discussing its possible applications to contexts of mental disorder.

Drawing on Elster (1984, 2000) and Bratman (1999, 2007), it is persuasive to interpret pre-commitment broadly conceived as an essential aspect of intentional agency over time. This becomes clear as soon as we think of everyday planning, which requires routine decision-making about future and counterfactual situations just as much as immediate action. For instance, planning to go to the cinema next weekend requires not only that I book my ticket when I make up my mind, say, on Tuesday (immediate action), but also that a few days later I try to turn up for the screening I booked (commitment to a particular course of action in the future). A final element of my planning is to rule out foreseeable alternatives, such as staying at home or taking up last minute offers for a weekend break (commitment to stick to the plan). This latter commitment not only gives my plan to go to the cinema a better chance to succeed, but effectively distinguishes it as a plan of mine rather than a mere fall-back option that I create for myself, i.e. booking a cinema ticket for the weekend on Tuesday in case I have nothing better to do over the weekend. In contrast, booking a cinema ticket for the weekend on Tuesday amounts to planning in so far as I pre-commit to both try to attend the screening I booked and resist obvious alternatives, like staying at home. With respect to my planned cinema going, such alternatives count as 'distractions' or even 'temptations'. Opting for them equals failure for my cinema project.

In fact, it is in such circumstances—various failures or at least difficulties to stick to the plan—that the role of pre-commitment for intentional agency over time becomes salient. To return to the earlier example, my booking of a cinema ticket for a screening a few days later usually suffices to keep in check 'distractions', such as arbitrary changes of mind and sheer procrastination when it is time to get ready and go out. Moreover, my pre-commitment to resist such distractions and go to the cinema instead may not even come to attention as long as I go ahead with the plan wholeheartedly and am not the least attracted by alternative courses of action. Conversely, I may book my ticket in advance not because I am swayed by the idea of going to the pictures, but in order to make sure that, at the weekend, I will have good reason to go out rather than stay at home as usual. In this second scenario, pre-commitment comes to the forefront of my thinking because I wish to bring my plan to fruition, whilst being aware that my commitment to it is less than wholehearted. By booking a cinema ticket in advance, I give myself additional leverage against a temptation I foresee. As a result, I am able to realize a plan that I am otherwise unlikely to follow through. In this respect, pre-commitment broadens the scope of my freedom to act and opens up avenues that were previously closed or nearly closed for me.

This function of pre-commitment is well illustrated by Ulysses' encounter with the Sirens which, following Elster (1984), I propose to consider as a paradigm case. Drawing on the *Odyssey*, the options available to Ulysses without pre-commitment are two: either to sail away from the Isle of the Sirens and not hear their enchanting song, or to approach them and perish, for this song lures the sailors to their deaths. However, by implementing an ingenious form of pre-commitment (Ulysses orders his crew to tie him to the mast and plugs their ears up with beeswax), he is able to create a new option: to hear the song and not be lured to his death. Let us call this function of pre-commitment trailblazing.

There is a further function of pre-commitment relevant to the present inquiry that may slip under the radar if the focus stays with individual actions rather than agency over time. In this respect, the second cinema going scenario offers a better reference point than Ulysses and the Sirens. This is because it brings into relief a separate way in which resilience against what I see as temptation may increase my freedom. Here the benefit of pre-commitment is not so much that it expands the range of options from which to choose, but that it enables me to exert indirect influence over the kind of person I will be in the future. As the reluctant cinema going example indicates, this can be achieved by devising courses of action (booking my cinema ticket in advance) to counteract emerging trends in my behaviour, which I dislike (doing nothing over the weekends). In this case, pre-commitment is undertaken not as a one-off, but as a series of actions that I plan in advance in such a way as to make difficult to abandon for the sake of foreseeable and strong temptations. To return to the previous example, if I am worried about becoming inactive as soon as my working hours are over, booking a cinema ticket for the weekend on Tuesday is part of a bigger project, finding things to do over the weekends. If this kind of pre-commitment is successful, it will help to gradually change my routine to the point that no further pre-commitment will be necessary in order for me to engage in various exciting activities in my spare time. This is because, with respect to leisure, I would have become the kind of person I wanted to be when I began reshaping my weekend habits by ensuring that, albeit reluctantly, I would go to the cinema for the sake of a prepaid ticket.

This second function of pre-commitment is well accounted for by Aristotle's theory of moral development as character habituation outlined in *Nicomachean Ethics*, 2.[9] Drawing on this account, a person is able to develop virtuous character traits by engaging into praiseworthy activities in spite of the fact that at the beginning they have no immediate attraction to her. This is particularly salient if we think of acts of courage and temperance as they both require the suppression of strong intuitive responses, to avoid imminent danger in the former case and to forego instant gratification in the latter. The ability to do so may seem unsurprising once the virtues—courage and temperance—have been developed. For, a person of virtue considers virtuous actions not only as admirable but also as agreeable to perform. The question is how anyone could perform such actions without already being of virtuous character. Pre-commitment offers a plausible answer. Thus, although I am bound to perceive acting in accordance with virtue as onerous at the start of my ethical habituation, the fact that I live in a human society puts me in a good position to take control over my intuitive reactions to apparent danger and promised pleasures. In particular, the anticipated disapproval of others, especially significant ones, offers me—under the guise of a sense of shame—the required motivational leverage so that I make myself more resilient to distractions that could induce me to act in a cowardly or an intemperate manner. If my character habituation is successful, I grow out of my sense of shame and begin to act in accordance with virtue for virtue's sake. Disapproval avoidance

---

[9] I have developed the subsequent point in more detail elsewhere, see Radoilska (2007, pp. 233–290).

no longer figures among my reasons for doing the right thing. In fact, it is natural to expect that in so far as I am a person of virtue, I will do so even in the face of strong though misguided societal disapproval.

The preceding considerations point to a second paradigm case where the lead function of pre-commitment is no longer trailblazing but what I propose to call character-building. The focus here is on moulding the kind of person I am turning into over time rather than enabling the performance of a particular kind of action in the future. Clearly, trailblazing and character-building are not mutually exclusive. Quite the reverse, many instances of pre-commitment would combine both as in the case of booking a cinema ticket whereby I not only give myself an extra reason to go to the pictures this weekend (pre-commitment as trailblazing) but also start getting myself into a more proactive mind-set (pre-commitment as character-building).

Having identified and explored these two paradigm cases of pre-commitment, we are in a position to see that neither of them is likely to lead to an autonomy paradox in the sense specified at the start of the section, that is, to contribute to autonomy on one plausible conception, but be hostile to it on another, and beside the point on a third. This is because the two central cases of pre-commitment, trailblazing and character-building, are at the same time central cases of active self-determination. In both instances, a person steps in and takes charge of her situation instead of accepting it as a given. Thus, by means of trailblazing, I make possible the course of action I wish to undertake rather than go along with the range of pre-existing options. In so doing, I expand my domain of self-determination. Similarly, by means of character-building I work my way up to the kind of person I would like to be rather than settle for the character I inadvertently turn into, e.g. a 'couch potato', to return to the reluctant cinema going example. In so doing, I strengthen my capacity for self-determination.

Moreover, by considering these two central cases of pre-commitment, we are able to observe a particular feature that distinguishes active self-determination from two closely related categories, freedom of action and intentional agency. Both are consistent with taking up an option from a pre-set range about which one has no say, a mode of self-determination I propose to call passive. Furthermore, if the course of action I would like to undertake is within the range of options available to me and if I am happy with the kind of person I am becoming, there is no reason for me to engage in active self-determination as a separate project, in addition to what I already do. In fact, to the extent that they meet with success, the two discernible forms of active self-determination, trailblazing, and character-building, are also bound to slip back into the background of intentional agency. As suggested by the preceding discussion of pre-commitment, active self-determination becomes salient only when things risk getting out of hand.[10]

So there are at least three categories of self-determination to be distinguished: firstly, passive self-determination, which is consistent with freedom of action and intentional agency but not autonomy; secondly, inconspicuous active self-determination or trouble-free autonomy; and thirdly, active self-determination in the spotlight or autonomy as express pre-commitment, which takes the form of trailblazing, character-building, or both.

Given the centrality of express pre-commitment, it is plausible to consider aptitude to account for its two main forms as a test for eligible autonomy conceptions. More precisely, if a conception treats either of these forms as irrelevant or hostile to autonomy, this would count as a strong reason against this conception. Let us now turn to the three autonomy conceptions I presented in the previous section: value-neutral, value-laden, and relational, and see how each of them fares on this test.

Firstly, a value-neutral conception would have no difficulty accounting for either paradigm case since it already considers autonomy in terms of a dual relationship of ownership and authorship applicable to both actions and motives. As clarified in the previous section, this is to reflect that possible constraints to self-determination may be external, that is, ownership affecting or internal, that is, authorship affecting. Trailblazing and character-building enable a person to address both types of constraints, the first at the level of actions and the second at the

---

[10] For a related point, see Chapter 9, this volume, by Hallvard Lillehammer.

level of motives. For instance, trailblazing provides us with means to act only on motives that we endorse and to resist desires that we may find puzzling, disturbing, or repugnant. This type of pre-commitment is consistent with a Frankfurtian notion of identification as the hallmark of autonomous actions.[11] Similarly, character-building enables us to affect our underlying motivations rather than relate to them as 'passive bystanders' (Frankfurt 1971). By allowing us to remove various obstacles to becoming a well-integrated self, such as ambivalence, indifference, and other forms of self-alienation, this type of pre-commitment concurs with Frankfurt's analysis of 'wholeheartedness' as a distinctive feature of autonomous persons (1998, chapter 12).

Secondly, a value-laden conception would be able to accommodate the two paradigm forms of pre-commitment to the extent that they enable a person to respond to good reasons as opposed to mere incentives. For instance, trailblazing would amount to exercise of autonomy only if the option I aim to resist is bad or unworthy in some objective sense, over and above its being incompatible with a plan that matters to me.[12] To return to the cinema example, my advance booking of a ticket so that I do not stay at home over the weekend would be a plausible exercise of self-determination only if it is bad to spend one's weekends this way, not just something I happen to dislike. In a similar vein, character-building would count as autonomous only if the dispositions or traits I aim to develop are good, in addition to being aspirational.

Finally, a relational conception could take on board both trailblazing and character-building to the extent that each of them puts the spotlight on interpersonal dynamics as key aspect of self-determination. In this respect, the cinema example would not be considered of relevance to autonomy, at least not without providing further details about the social-relational standing of the person who engages

---

[11] See, in particular, Frankfurt (1998, chapter 5).

[12] Watson (2004, chapter 3) offers an example of this line of reasoning, since its central claim is that addiction is incompatible with autonomy not only because it typically jeopardizes projects that a person with addiction cares about, but mainly because it allows 'disordered appetites' and unworthy commitments to become the centre of her life.

in pre-commitment. However, both the original Ulysses arrangement (trailblazing) and the Aristotelian account of moral development I sketched earlier (character-building) could be adopted as central instances of relational autonomy, since they aptly point to the significance of warranted interpersonal trust. Thus, Ulysses would have been unable to safely hear the Sirens' song if his companions could not be trusted to both tie him to the mast as arranged and release him afterwards. Similarly, a person's moral development would be severely hampered if the community in which she grows up cannot be relied upon for ethical guidance. Both points are in line with the core insight of relational approaches to autonomy highlighting that oppressive social relationships make self-determination impossible, not merely difficult, whenever they prevent us from developing empowering kinds of reliance on others, like the original Ulysses arrangement and an Aristotelian character-building (cf. Stoljar 2000).

So, all three types of autonomy conceptions are consistent with the centrality of express pre-commitment and could therefore be considered as conceptions of the general concept I began to sketch in this section, that is, autonomy as active self-determination. This is a promising ground for both addressing apparent incongruities between different autonomy conceptions and distinguishing them from conceptions of neighbouring concepts, such as freedom of action and intentional agency.

However, to pursue this line of inquiry we should first resolve a difficulty raised by some discussions of pre-commitment in psychiatric contexts. The worry is that these discussions support the conclusion that express pre-commitment is an autonomy paradox in the sense ruled out by the preceding analysis. If correct, this conclusion would leave us with an uneasy choice: either to reject the general autonomy concept sketched earlier or to abandon some of the conceptions we just acknowledged. Either option would undermine the argument proposed here.

12.4 Ulysses arrangements as a possible paradox of self-determination

The challenge anticipated at the end of the previous section seems particularly to the point since the instances of pre-commitment in psychiatry that give rise to the putative autonomy paradox match the central cases of active self-determination, trailblazing and character-building, I described earlier.

The first instance relates to advance directives anticipating various situations that could arise in later stages of dementia when a person is no longer able to make or express competent decisions.[13] It is compelling to consider this kind of pre-commitment as an obvious case of trailblazing, for it extends this person's range of options to encompass choices which would otherwise be outside her control.

The second instance has to do with the use of Ulysses arrangements in order to anticipate various situations, in which a person loses insight into the effects of mental disorder on her thinking, but still fulfils the criteria for decisional capacity.[14] As a result, she is likely to make legally competent decisions which, however, she does not recognize as her own on recovery. Key Redfield Jamison's memoir of an expert on bipolar disorder who is also living with this condition offers a poignant testimony to this effect (1995). Drawing on her account, Ulysses arrangements offer a particularly efficient way to forestall related threats to self-determination, such as acting out of character during manic episodes. This is because these arrangements enable a person to appoint trusted others, including professionals and personal relations so that they may act as her guardians for the duration of such periods of confusion. The direct link with the second paradigm case of pre-commitment, character-building becomes apparent as soon as we take into consideration the tendency of this kind of Ulysses arrangements not merely to pre-empt the implementation of perplexing decisions (immediate objective), but also to remove the need for pre-emption (indirect objective). To return to the memoir above, having specified the conditions under which she could be given involuntary psychiatric treatment in a

---

[13] Consider, for instance, the situation of Mrs Day, a person with dementia who lacks decisional capacity and whose care has to be agreed by third parties, including healthcare professionals and relatives because she has not drafted advance directives whilst still having capacity (Chapter 8, this volume, by Elizabeth Fistein). On the notion of decisional capacity, see the Introduction to this volume.

[14] On the relationship between capacity and insight, see Chapter 7, this volume, by Jules Holroyd.

Ulysses arrangement, Jamison was able to spot the warning signs for herself so that it never had to be enforced in the following two decades. This is confirmed by recent research on the psychiatric treatment received by people with bipolar disorder who have previously signed similar kinds of Ulysses arrangements (Gremmen 2008): it reported a steady, statistically significant correlation with improved insight and almost exclusively voluntary treatment in contrast to people with the same condition who have not signed such an arrangement. Both Jamison's experience and this further evidence are consistent with the analysis of successful character-building I proposed in the previous section.

In light of these observations, it is safe to conclude that there is no relevant difference between, on the one hand, these two uses of pre-commitment in psychiatry and, on the other, the two paradigm cases of active self-determination in general. This is why the thought that these kinds of pre-commitment may lead to an autonomy paradox in psychiatry deserves careful consideration.

With respect to the first kind of pre-commitment, advance directives re later stages of dementia, this thought follows from a recent critique of the practice put forth by Agnieszka Jaworska (1999). According to Jaworska, the advance directives of people with dementia, who no longer have decisional capacity, should not be taken for an ultimate expression of their self-determination, but may be overridden by carers and family to protect the interests these people appear to have developed in their new situation. This central claim rests on a broader account of autonomous agency, which ties the latter in with a capacity to value or deeply care about things as opposed to a capacity to implement one's values. Drawing on empirical evidence, Jaworska suggests that, although people with dementia eventually lose the latter capacity, which she considers as inessential for autonomy, they still retain the former, which, on her account, is autonomy-conferring. So advance directives re later stages of dementia lead to an autonomy paradox on this view. This paradox is as follows: if this kind of pre-commitment is honoured, the people whose self-determination it means to uphold are denied self-determination. This is because, instead of being supported to implement the projects they have come to care about, people in the later stages of dementia are made to live by the decisions of their earlier, more articulate selves, with whom they no longer identify.

The interest of this challenge becomes apparent as soon as its implicit reliance on a relational approach to autonomy comes to attention. For the underlying intuitions that motivate Jaworska's critique seem to be the following. Firstly, whenever respect for a person's self-determination is confined to sticking to her earlier instructions as opposed to giving credence to her current preferences, she is unavoidably attributed lesser standing than that of a fully autonomous person who may revisit her prior commitments at any point.[15] Secondly, the assumption of lesser autonomy is self-fulfilling for it leads to closing down opportunities for self-determination that this person could have otherwise taken up.

With respect to the second kind of pre-commitment, Ulysses arrangements re manic episodes, the conclusion that they lead to an autonomy paradox is reached in a recent discussion by Theo van Willigenburg and Patrick Delaere (2005). Unlike the preceding critique, the underlying concern here is not so much that Ulysses arrangements are inimical to autonomy, but that they are beside the point. The supporting argument builds on the thesis that the kind of self-control that these arrangements promote does not amount to exercise of self-determination. This is because this kind of pre-commitment allows only for self-control in terms of self-enforcement, whereas self-determination requires a different category of self-control, that is, self-legislation. Although in both instances the goal is set by the person herself as opposed to an interfering third party, the authors reason, there is a significant difference between the ways, in which she goes about realizing this goal. In the case of self-legislation, she readily carries out her plan, whilst in the case of self-enforcement she merely goes along with it, since it has become impossible for her to pull out. Following this line of reasoning, Ulysses arrangements could be seen as paradoxical. For they turn out to

---

[15] For a compelling analysis of changing one's mind as an inherent aspect of self-determination, see Radden (2005).

be irrelevant to what the authors consider as autonomy in the strict sense (self-legislation) and at the same time preserving what they call autonomy as authenticity (self-enforcement).

The interest of this second challenge could be better appreciated if we bring into relief the value-laden approach to autonomy, on which it apparently rests. More precisely, Kant's distinction between acting from duty and acting in conformity with duty[16] seems to yield support to a stark contrast between self-legislation and self-enforcement. The point could be that, as a kind of self-enforcement, Ulysses arrangements are consistent only with acting in conformity with duty but not with acting from duty. Yet, only the latter mode of action is truly autonomous, for it responds directly to reasons as opposed to mere incentives. So the autonomy paradox, to which Ulysses arrangements give rise on van Willingeburg and Delaere's view, has to do with the supposition that self-enforcement does not leave room for responsiveness to reasons since it becomes relevant when only incentives, but no good reasons for action impress on an agent.

To recap, the conjunction of these two critiques of pre-commitment in psychiatry leaves us with the following paradox: instead of being central, the cases of active self-determination where alternative approaches to autonomy converge—trailblazing (in the guise of advance directives re dementia) and character-building (in the guise of Ulysses arrangements re manic episodes)—look like essentially contested cases displaying how unbridgeable the gaps between alternatives effectively are. Arguably, the first is to be dismissed as compromising self-determination proper on relational grounds, whereas the second seems to be beside the point from a value-laden perspective. It looks as though only if a value-neutral view is adopted, both cases remain steadily associated with self-determination.[17]

---

[16] *Groundwork* 4: 398–9. See also Timmermann (2009).

[17] See, for instance, Ronald Dworkin's defence of advance directives and the underlying 'integrity view of autonomy', according to which the right to autonomy is meant to protect 'the ability to act out of genuine preference or character or conviction or a sense of self' (1993, p. 225). I have not expanded on this or alternative value-neutral discussions of pre-commitment in psychiatry since they are fully consistent with my analysis of

My reply to this challenge will take two steps. The first will be to explain away the paradox above by identifying the mistake on which it rests. The second will be to expand on the valuable lessons about autonomy and its relationship to mental disorder that we learn from this mistake.

The mistake in question becomes apparent once we recall the distinction between two ways of exercising autonomy which emerged from the analysis of pre-commitment in the previous section: on the one hand, trouble-free autonomy, where the workings of pre-commitment remain inconspicuous, and, on the other, autonomy as express pre-commitment in view of considerable threats to the authorship or ownership of one's actions or motives. As argued earlier, although both ways of self-determination share the same structure, it is clearly visible only in express pre-commitment, but not in trouble free-autonomy where it fuses with freedom of action.

With the distinction between trouble-free autonomy and autonomy as express pre-commitment in mind, let us now return to the disputed conclusion that pre-commitment in psychiatry is a paradoxical form of self-determination. Clearly, this conclusion hangs on the idea that something akin to trouble-free autonomy is the genuine item, with respect to which express pre-commitment falls short. This is because, in order to make sense of the concern that pre-commitment in psychiatry may promote some lesser kind of self-determination at the expense of what is perceived as self-determination proper, a concern expressed by both Jaworska (1999) and van Willigenburg and Delaere (2005), we need to conceptualize express pre-commitment as an imperfect and potentially misleading replica of trouble-free autonomy.

However, there is good reason to reject this conceptualization, namely that it effectively misplaces the locus of autonomy from active self-determination to effortlessness. The upshot is unavoidable once trouble-free autonomy is set out as a standard. Express pre-commitment is bound to fail this standard since it is a trouble-shooting exercise

---

pre-commitment as paradigm case of self-determination and, therefore, are not conducive to the paradox under consideration.

of autonomy. The problem is not that, following this conceptualization, we end up with a view of autonomy that is unduly restrictive but that this view is simply mistaken. By focusing on effortlessness, which distinguishes trouble-free autonomy from autonomy as express pre-commitment, we not only begin to lose sight of the underlying feature they share, namely, that they are both instances of active self-determination. Moreover, the distinction between trouble-free autonomy and passive self-determination becomes blurred, for effortlessness is also typical of the latter, yet it is not compatible with autonomy. In fact, building on the point I made earlier about passive self-determination, we could say that its effortlessness boils down to making no effort toward self-determination. In contrast, the effortlessness of trouble-free autonomy is the outcome of successful self-determination. The apparent absence of obstacles to self-determination in this latter case can be traced back to a series of effective pre-commitments whereby a person has managed to influence the range of options open to her (trailblazing) as well as develop stable dispositions she approves of (character-building).[18] By looking in isolation at instances where no obstacles to self-determination seem to be present, it is easy to take the effortlessness of active self-determination that has become trouble-free, that is, the effortlessness of an achievement for the effortlessness of passive self-determination, that is, the effortlessness of not giving it a go.

The upshot of shifting attention away from active self-determination toward effortlessness can be observed in two related moves that critics of pre-commitment in psychiatry frequently make. The first is to argue that advance directives are inimical to autonomy since they fail to put on a par a person's past and future selves. The second is to locate the

---

[18] Aristotle's account of eudaimonia or an accomplished life of virtue offers a good illustration of trouble-free autonomy. See, in particular, *Nicomachean Ethics* 9.4 which expands on virtue as a state of friendship with oneself. A distinctive feature of this state is that there is nothing a person wishes either to change in herself or to have done otherwise. The notion of externality introduced by Frankfurt (1999, chapter 5) provides a helpful contrast to trouble-free exercise of autonomy with respect to internal obstacles. See, in particular, the case of a person who struggles with unexpected jealousy at the news of a friend's success.

significance of choice in the availability of options to choose from rather than the choice itself. Let us briefly consider each of them in turn.

The first move is key to critiques of pre-commitment, such as Jaworska's which, by denying that temporal asymmetry has a crucial role to play in self-determination, are able to present pre-commitment as enforcing the will of a forceful 'then-self' upon a vulnerable 'now-self' (Dresser 1995). Following this line of thought, it seems plausible to consider pre-commitment as hostile to the autonomy of this 'now-self' which may have developed new interests and values, neither shared, nor anticipated by the 'then-self'. Yet, if applied to self-determination in general rather than specific psychiatric contexts, this thought becomes extremely implausible. For it would open any plan to paternalistic interventions on grounds that one's future self may no longer stand for the same kind of thing as one's current self and the potentially different interests of the former have to be protected by society from the latter. In fact, a recent defence of hard paternalism draws on a similar line of reasoning in order to reach the conclusion that decisions of competent adults may be routinely ignored for their own good, whenever the prospective intrusion will only violate their abstract right to self-determination but no specific and substantive rights, such as freedom of religion or association (Scoccia 2008, pp. 371–379). This argument is instructive as it makes explicit the link between the claim that earlier 'selves' are not any weightier than later 'selves' (temporal neutrality) and the reduction of self-determination to a somewhat redundant confirmation of specific rights. As soon as we adopt the temporal neutrality thesis, self-determination loses both its object and purpose, for there is no longer a self to determine but only specific actions to undertake or abstain from. As a result, self-determination is reduced to mere freedom of action.

The second move is also related to the temporal neutrality thesis since its focus is the potentially irreversible character of pre-commitment in psychiatry. At the heart of this kind of critique lays the idea that, with respect to autonomy, pre-commitment is ambivalent an achievement to the extent that it forecloses options rather expands a person's range of choices. This intuition underlies van Willigenburg and Delaere's account of self-enforcement as incompatible with autonomy proper. For this account implies that autonomy proper or self-legislation can only take place if there is no lapse of time to speak of between decision and action. More precisely, only if the decision to act is either made or confirmed at the time of action, can self-legislation be contrasted with self-enforcement as proposed by van Willigenburg and Delaere. This becomes apparent if we consider the demarcation point between the two: whether reasons for action are immediately present to the agent or in need of enforcement. By confining instances of self-legislation to contemporaneous actions, van Willigenburg and Delaere are able to interpret temporal asymmetry as a flaw of self-determination, typical of self-enforcement. Yet, the apparent contrast between the two boils down to focusing on one and the same phenomenon, choice, from different viewpoints in time. This is because irreversibility, for which self-enforcement is critiqued, is in fact a feature of successful agency over time. Implicitly, every plan that we bring to fruition in the present becomes a piece of self-enforcement in relation to future actions. Moreover, the fact that options get foreclosed is the flipside of self-determination having taken place. To complain about pre-commitment for enabling courses of action that I may later regret is to fail to appreciate the significance of choice as key exercise of autonomy.

Aristotle's account of *proairesis* helps bring out this point.[19] Drawing on this account, we are able to observe that choice is an immediate cause of action which works by blocking alternatives. This is not to say that the chosen action gets carried out instantly, but that once an agent has made up her mind, there is no logical space for further deliberation either about other possible actions or the advantages of the action she already opted for.[20] So if a chosen course of action is not carried out, this can only mean that the agent has been prevented from following through by one kind of obstacle or another. Irreversibility and

---

[19] *Nicomachean Ethics* 3.1–5. See also Radoilska (2007, pp. 211–232).

[20] If there is still room for deliberation, this only tells us that the agent has not yet made a choice. See Raz (1975) whose conception of exclusionary reasons expands on this line of reasoning.

foreclosure of options turn out to be the signs of success at determining one's actions as opposed to having one's choices overturned. Moreover, the scenario, in which one's reasons for action are no longer apparent at the moment of action, looks like the standard case of acting for a reason rather than a paradoxical feature indicating a lesser kind of self-determination, as suggested by van Willigenburg and Delaere. Following this line of thought, self-legislation is at variance with pre-commitment only in so far it presents an aspiring kind of self-determination or self-determination which has not yet taken place. As soon as it achieves its objective, it becomes indistinguishable from self-enforcement.

Having dispelled the air of a paradox surrounding pre-commitment in psychiatry, we are able to draw two valuable lessons about autonomy and mental disorder. The first is as follows: not only are the three approaches to autonomy as set out at the start of the chapter conceptions of the same concept, there is an underlying hierarchy between them emerging from the discussion. More precisely, by considering key problems for critiques of pre-commitment in psychiatry, we are able to establish that a value-neutral conception of autonomy in terms of authorship and ownership of one's motives and actions is central. In contrast, questions about reasons-responsiveness and social-relational status, which are defining respectively for a value-laden and a relational conception, become significant when either side of self-determination, authorship or ownership, no longer holds firm. For instance, by trying to elicit the reasons for a particular choice that looks unlikely to be autonomous, we get clearer about its authorship, that is, the extent to which it is up to a person rather than being the upshot of internal or internalized obstacles to her self-determination. To decide one way or the other, a spotlight has to be put on the putative reasonableness or choiceworthiness of the option taken. This is because, if this option can be asserted as something choiceworthy, over and above this person's professed preference for it, her authorship is clearly confirmed, despite the initial appearances.[21] Thus understood, choiceworthiness

---

[21] See, however, Chapter 5, this volume, by Bortollotti et al. for an alternative account of the links between authorship and the ability to conceive one's choices as responsive to reasons.

offers an additional guarantee that a putative choice is indeed a choice. This line of reasoning is well illustrated by the presumption of non-voluntariness Joel Feinberg proposes to take as a starting point when considering cases of self-harm (1986, chapter 20). The thought is not that self-harm can never be chosen voluntarily, but that there is need for further scrutiny. In a similar vein, we could say that responsiveness to reasons should come to the fore whenever the presence of internal obstacles to self-determination makes the assumption of non-autonomy more likely than not. The same argument applies, mutatis mutandis, to considerations of social-relational status in instances where the ownership of a choice requires closer examination. The idea is to ascertain whether the external obstacles present are so pervasive as to undermine active self-determination. In this respect, an assumption of non-autonomy could be thought of by analogy with the impact coercive offers may have on a recipient's circumstance of choice.

The second lesson that we learn from looking into the paradox, to which pre-commitment in psychiatry seemed to give to rise, is that there is a strong, though implicit assumption of non-autonomy that attaches to mental disorder. This would explain both the salience of value-laden and relational concerns in the critiques of advance directives and Ulysses arrangements I examined earlier and the intuitive appeal of these critiques. Moreover, since pre-commitment is a clear-cut, paradigm case of autonomy, the assumption at issue can plausibly target only the context of mental disorder in which pre-commitment takes place, not pre-commitment itself. How cogent is this assumption? To the extent that it is treated as defeasible, in continuity with the preceding reflection on cases, such as self-harm and coercive offers, the assumption of non-autonomy could be a good starting point in some instances of mental disorder, where outcomes of self-determination are not easily distinguished from obstacles to self-determination. However, drawing on the account of pre-commitment developed earlier, it is implausible to consider these instances as different in kind from standard cases of active self-determination. In this respect, we should be wary of a broad assumption of non-autonomy that attaches to mental disorder as such. More precisely, the worry is that by focusing on the gravity of obstacles to self-determination or the experiential unmanageability of mental disorder, we may be employing an unduly demanding but also misleading success criterion for autonomy, such as effortlessness.[22] As argued in this chapter, absence of obstacles is not a prerequisite for autonomy, nor is effortlessness an essential feature of its exercise. Failing to realize this, we shall run into a similar paradox to that faced by critics of pre-commitment in psychiatry who end up removing, instead of obstacles to self-determination linked to mental disorder, a vital means to get on top of them.

12.5 **Summary and conclusions**

The structure of the concept of autonomy that emerged from the preceding discussion is as follows. Unlike the related freedom of action and intentional agency, autonomy is, firstly, incompatible with passive self-determination and, secondly, dependent upon a temporal asymmetry privileging prior over later commitments. More specifically, it takes the form of active self-determination with respect to one's actions, on the one hand, and, one's motives, on the other. There are two ways to exercise active self-determination: trouble-free autonomy and express pre-commitment. The effortlessness that distinguishes the former from the latter makes it difficult to perceive their shared form, which is pre-commitment. In contrast, this comes to light when active self-determination takes place against identifiable threats affecting either a person's authorship (internal obstacles) or ownership (external obstacles) over her actions and motives. The two paradigm kinds of express pre-commitment—trailblazing and character-building—articulate the underlying form, the first with respect to actions, the second with respect to motives.

In light of this analysis, it is plausible to consider a value-neutral conception of autonomy as an independent source of normativity as more fundamental than value-laden and relational alternatives. This is

---

[22] On the notion of mental disorder as unmanageable distress, see Chapter 4, this volume, by Derek Bolton and Natalie Banner. See also Chapter 3 where K.W.M. Fulford and I reflect on the role of different success criteria in alternative accounts of mental disorder.

because such a conception is focused on the complex relationship of authorship and ownership over one's actions and motives, which is at the heart of active self-determination. In contrast, considerations about responsiveness to reasons as opposed to mere incentives, which underpin value-laden conceptions, gain salience only when the presence of significant internal obstacles makes an assumption of non-autonomy plausible. Similarly, concerns about social and interpersonal standing central to relational conceptions legitimately come to the fore when the external obstacles present are so overwhelming as to clearly back an assumption of non-autonomy. The latter two conceptions are therefore best understood as offering each an additional test for distinguishing unobvious outcomes of active self-determination from apparent obstacles to it rather than rival theories of autonomy.

By making explicit the structure of the concept of autonomy, we are able to explain away the paradox to which express pre-commitment seems to give rise in the context of mental disorder. This paradox turns out to be the outcome of a flawed conceptualization which takes effortlessness to be the form of autonomy, not active self-determination. As a result, express pre-commitment is downgraded to a secondary kind of autonomy. Moreover, irreversibility and the foreclosure of alternatives, key aspects of successful self-determination, are misconceived as undermining autonomy. By dispelling this misconception, it becomes clear that the obstacles to autonomy associated with mental disorder are not different in kind from the obstacles addressed by standard instances of pre-commitment. Consequently, there is no special case to be made for an assumption of non-autonomy attaching to mental disorder.

References

Aristotle. (1984). Nicomachean Ethics (Trans. W.D. Ross). In J. Barnes (ed.) *The Complete Works of Aristotle*. Princeton, NJ: Princeton University Press.

Arpaly, N. (2003). *Unprincipled Virtue: An Inquiry into Moral Agency*. New York: Oxford University Press.

Bratman, M. (1999). *Faces of Intention: Selected Essays on Intention and Agency*. Cambridge: Cambridge University Press.

Bratman, M. (2007). *Structures of Agency*. Oxford: Oxford University Press.

Buss, S. (2008). Personal autonomy. In E.N. Zalta (ed.) *The Stanford Encyclopedia of Philosophy* (Winter 2008 Edition). [Online] http://plato.stanford.edu/entries/personal-autonomy/

Christman, J. (2003). Autonomy in moral and political philosophy. In E.N. Zalta (ed.) *The Stanford Encyclopedia of Philosophy* (Winter 2008 Edition) [Online] http://plato.stanford.edu/entries/autonomy-moral/

Christman, J. (2007). Autonomy, history, and the subject of justice. *Social Theory and Practice* 33(1): 1–26.

Colburn, B. (2011). Autonomy and adaptive preferences. *Utilitas* 23(1): 52–71.

Dresser, R. (1995). Dworkin on dementia: Elegant theory, questionable policy. *Hastings Center Report* 25(6): 32–38.

Dworkin, R. (1993). *Life's Dominion: an Argument about Abortion and Euthanasia.* London: Harper Collins.

Elster, J. (1983). *Sour Grapes: Studies in the Subversion of Rationality.* Cambridge: Cambridge University Press; Paris: Editions de la Maison des Sciences de l'Homme.

Elster, J. (1984). *Ulysses and the Sirens: Studies in Rationality and Irrationality.* Cambridge: Cambridge University Press.

Elster, J. (2000). *Ulysses Unbound: Studies in Rationality, Precommitment, and Constraints.* Cambridge: Cambridge University Press.

Feinberg, J. (1980). *Rights, Justice and the Bounds of Liberty: Essays in Social Philosophy.* Princeton, NJ: Princeton University Press.

Feinberg, J. (1986). *The Moral Limits of the Criminal Law: Vol. 3 Harm to Self.* New York: Oxford University Press.

Frankfurt, H. (1971). Freedom of the will and the concept of a person. *Journal of Philosophy* 68(1): 5–20.

Frankfurt, H. (1998).*The Importance of What We Care About: Philosophical Essays.* Cambridge: Cambridge University Press.

Frankfurt, H. (1999). *Necessity, Volition, and Love.* Cambridge: Cambridge University Press.

Frankfurt, H. (2002). Reply to Gary Watson. In S. Buss and L. Overton (eds.) *Contours of Agency: Essays on Themes from Harry Frankfurt.* Cambridge, MA: MIT Press, pp. 160–64.

Gallie, W.B. (1956). Essentially contested concepts. *Proceedings of the Aristotelian Society* 56: 167–98.

Gremmen, I. (2008). Ulysses arrangements in psychiatry: from normative ethics to empirical research and back. In G. Widdershoven, J. McMillan, T. Hope, and L. van der Scheer (eds.) *Empirical Ethics in Psychiatry.* Oxford: Oxford University Press, pp. 171–85.

Hill, T. E. (1991). *Autonomy and Self-Respect.* Cambridge: Cambridge University Press.

Jamison, K.J. (1995). *An Unquiet Mind: a Memoir of Moods and Madness.* London: Picador.

Jaworska, A. (1999). Respecting the margins of agency: Alzheimer's patients and the capacity to value. *Philosophy and Public Affairs* 28(2): 105–38.

Kant, I. (1785). Groundwork of the metaphysics of morals. In I. Kant *Practical Philosophy* (Ed. and trans. M.J. Gregor, 1996). Cambridge: Cambridge University Press.

Korsgaard, C. M. (1996). *Sources of Normativity*. Cambridge: Cambridge University Press.

Mill, J.S. (1859). *On Liberty*. Indianapolis, IN: Bobbs Merrill [1959].

Moran, R. (2001). *Authority and Estrangement: an Essay on Self-Knowledge*. Princeton, NJ: Princeton University Press.

Nordenfelt, L. (2007). *Rationality and Compulsion: Applying Action Theory to Psychiatry*. Oxford: Oxford University Press.

Nozick, R. (1969). Coercion. In S. Morgenbesser, P. Suppes, and M. White (eds.) *Philosophy, Science, and Method: Essays in Honour of Ernest Nagel*. New York: St. Martin's Press, pp. 440–72.

Oshana, M. (2006). *Personal Autonomy in Society*. Aldershot: Ashgate.

Pettit, P. and Smith, M. (1996). Freedom in belief and desire. *Journal of Philosophy* 93(9): 429–49.

Radden, J. (2005). Second thoughts: revoking decisions over one's future. *Philosophy and Phenomenological Research* 54(4): 787–801.

Radoilska, L. (2007). *L'Actualité d'Aristote en morale*. Paris: Presses Universitaires de France.

Raz, J. (1975). Reasons for action, decisions and norms. *Mind* 84(336): 481–99.

Raz, J. (1987). Autonomy, toleration, and the harm principle. In R. Gavison (ed.) *Issues in Contemporary Legal Philosophy: The Influence of H.L.A. Hart*. Oxford: Clarendon Press, pp. 313–33.

Scoccia, D. (2008). In defense of hard paternalism. *Law and Philosophy* 27: 351–81.

Scanlon, T. (1996). The Difficulty of tolerance. In D. Heyd (ed.) *Toleration: An Elusive Virtue*. Princeton, NJ: Princeton University press, pp. 226–39.

Stoljar, N. (2000). Autonomy and the feminist intuition. In C. Mackenzie, and N. Stoljar (eds.) *Relational Autonomy: Feminist Perspectives on Autonomy, Agency and the Social Self*. New York: Oxford University Press, pp. 94–111.

Taylor, J.S. (2005). Introduction. In J.S. Taylor (ed.) *Personal Autonomy: New Essays on Personal Autonomy and Its Role in Contemporary Moral Philosophy*. Cambridge: Cambridge University Press, pp. 1–29.

Timmermann, J. (2009). Acting from duty: inclination, reason and moral worth. In J. Timmermann (ed.) *Kant's Groundwork of the Metaphysics of Morals: A Critical Guide*. Cambridge: Cambridge University Press, pp. 45–62.

van Willigenburg, T. and Delaere, P.J.J. (2005). Protecting autonomy as authenticity using Ulysses contracts. *Journal of Medicine and Philosophy* 30(4): 395–409.

Watson, G. (1975). Free agency. *Journal of Philosophy* 72(8): 205–20.

Watson, G. (2004). *Agency and Answerability*. New York: Oxford University Press.

Index

Frankfurt, H. xiv, xviii, xxiv*fn*, 44, 90, 163,
197, 254, 265, 272*fn*
freedom
of action 26–7, 81, 263–4
in beliefs 256–7
from interference x, xvii, 81, 185–6, 220
negative *vs.* positive 52, 220–3
free will 31–8
arbitrium brutum and *arbitrium
liberum* 235
illusion of 27–8, 31–2
lay judgements 33, 35–8
substance dualism 32–4
uncaused will 35
Friedman, M. 90, 164
Fulford, K.W.M. 45, 50, 56, 58, 59, 62, 66*fn*,
67, 71, 152, 153, 154*fn*

Gadamer, H.-G. 223, 225
Gazzaniga, M. 110, 112
Gerrans, P. 103, 112–13
good, conceptions of 175–6, 179–80; *see also*
value

Hacking, I. 7
Haggard, P. 30
happiness 182–3, 184
harm 89, 124, 197
legal violation of confidentiality 134–5
see also self-harm
Harm principle xii–xiii, xxviii
Havens, L. 130
health
evaluative content of health
assessments 152–6
norms of 94–5, 152–6, 158
Hill, T. 44, 256, 257
Hope, T. 50, 157

identity
identity formation of confabulation 115–16
narrative theory 243–4
incompatibilism 26–7
indeterministic causation 27
indifference 39–40
insanity 45, 239; *see also* mental disorder
insanity defence 48–9
insight 46–8, 87, 150, 151–2, 267
instrumental rationality 235–7
intention 101, 107, 108, 241
conscious intentions 29–30
intentional agency 44–5, 263–4
breakdown of 45, 53, 65–6, 68–70
International Classification of Diseases
(ICD) 63, 78
intersubjective world 236
involuntary treatment 49–50
ipseity 241

irrational decisions xiv–xvi, xvii–xix, xxiii
irrationality xv, xvii, xviii, 118, 198, 256

Jamison, K.R. 65, 267–8
Jaworska, A. x*fn*, 5, 13, 17–20, 173, 268, 271
Jehovah's Witnesses xx–xxi, 161–2, 163

Kant, I. ix*fn*, 8–9, 92, 235, 236, 239, 240, 241,
246, 256*fn*, 270
Kapur, S. 112–13
Kennett, J. 90, 113–14
Korsgaard, C., 197, 254*fn*, 256, 257
Kvaran, T. 35–6

Lacan, J. 244
learning 221, 225–6, 236, 238
liberalism ix, 81, 92
Libet, B. 27–31, 32*fn*, 38–9
life stories 13
loss of insight 46–8, 267

Mackenzie, C. 7, 12, 44, 91, 93, 220
McNaughton, D. (McNaughton Rules) 48–9
Martin, A. xx, xxi, 159, 161, 162–3, 164
Matthews, S. 113–14
Mele, A. 26, 27*fn*, 28, 30, 32, 33, 38, 39, 40,
41, 68*fn*
Mental Capacity Act (2005)
best interests 170–91
conditions for capacity 146–7, 172–3
evaluative components 148–56
paternalism 178
reasonableness xvi–xvii, xx
value-laden conditions for capacity 160,
167
value-neutrality xvi–xvii
mental disorder 77–99
agential success 66–9
autonomy and 79, 80, 88–95
breakdown of intentional agency 45, 53,
65–6, 68–70
decisional capacity 127–8, 129, 267
definitions of 78
full legal excuse 49
loss of insight 46–8, 267
naturalism *vs.* social construction 77–8
privacy and 130–4
psychotic 46
religious experience xxi*fn*, 64
unmanageable distress 78–9, 81–8
value and 3–25
Mental Health Act (2007) 146
Mill, J. S. xiii, 219, 255
Montague, P.R. 32
Moody, H.R. 229
moral autonomy 7, 12, 81, 218, 223–4,
225, 256
moral knowledge 228